2ND EDITION

NANDA, NOC, *and* NIC
Linkages

NURSING DIAGNOSES, OUTCOMES, & INTERVENTIONS

Editors

Marion Johnson, RN, PhD
Gloria Bulechek, RN, PhD, FAAN
Howard Butcher, RN, PhD, APRN, BC
Joanne McCloskey Dochterman, RN, PhD, FAAN
Meridean Maas, RN, PhD, FAAN
Sue Moorhead, RN, PhD
Elizabeth Swanson, RN, PhD

Center for Nursing Classification & Clinical Effectiveness
Sharon Sweeney, Center Coordinator
University of Iowa
College of Nursing

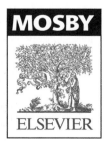

MOSBY

ELSEVIER

MOSBY
ELSEVIER

11830 Westline Industrial Drive
St. Louis, Missouri 63146

NANDA, NOC, and NIC Linkages:
Nursing Diagnoses, Outcomes, & Interventions, ed 2

ISBN-13 978-0-323-03194-3
ISBN-10 0-323-03194-3

NOTICE

Knowledge and best practice in this field are constantly changing. As new research and experience broaden our knowledge, changes in practice, treatment and drug therapy may become necessary or appropriate. Readers are advised to check the most current information provided (i) on procedures featured or (ii) by the manufacturer of each product to be administered, to verify the recommended dose or formula, the method and duration of administration, and contraindications. It is the responsibility of the practitioner, relying on their own experience and knowledge of the patient, to make diagnoses, to determine dosages and the best treatment for each individual patient, and to take all appropriate safety precautions. To the fullest extent of the law, neither the Publisher nor the Editors assume any liability for any injury and/or damage to persons or property arising out or related to any use of the material contained in this book.

Previous edition copyrighted 2001.

ISBN-13 978-0-323-03194-3
ISBN-10 0-323-03194-3

Executive Publisher: Barbara Nelson Cullen
Senior Developmental Editor: Victoria Bruno
Publishing Services Manager: Deborah L. Vogel
Senior Project Manager: Ann E. Rogers
Book Design Manager: Mark Oberkrom
Marketing Manager: Andrew Eilers

Printed in United States of America
Last digit is the print number: 9 8 7 6 5 4 3 2 1

Preface

This second edition of the linkage book has a title change to better reflect the focus of the book. The emphasis is now on the linkage work, *NANDA, NOC, and NIC Linkages: Nursing Diagnoses, Outcomes, & Interventions.* The standardized languages used in the book are the diagnoses developed by the North American Nursing Diagnosis Association, now NANDA International (NANDA), the outcomes of the Nursing Outcomes Classification (NOC), and the interventions of the Nursing Interventions Classification (NIC). Showing how these three languages can be used together to describe the content of nursing—the diagnoses, outcomes, and interventions that nurses use—will facilitate the use of each of the languages and make it easier for clinicians and educators to use the languages in practice. They also make it easier to develop clinical information systems using standardized language. The links also provide excellent opportunities for nurse researchers to explore the associations among diagnoses, outcomes, and interventions in conjunction with patient and organizational characteristics that might influence outcome achievement.

The first part of the book has minor changes. It continues to provide an introduction to the NANDA, NOC, NIC links that are presented in Part II. A brief description of the three languages, including their development and current status, is provided in Chapter 1. This orients users who are unfamiliar with one or more of the languages to the structure of each of the languages and provides references for learning more about each of the languages. The method used to develop the linkages in the first and second editions is described, and issues relevant to the development and use of the linkage work are identified. As with the first edition, the links were developed at the University of Iowa by the researchers who developed the NIC and NOC classifications with the assistance of graduate students and clinicians. The links are based primarily on expert opinion and therefore are not prescriptive. Testing in the clinical setting is an important step to gather information to support or modify the links presented here. Research studies are also needed to evaluate and test the linkages. The last chapter in Part I describes the use of the links in care planning, electronic information systems, nursing education, and nursing research. **This chapter is important for the user because it illustrates how to use the linkage book in clinical practice and education and suggests other helpful resources.** A number of case studies are provided to illustrate the use of the links.

The major portion of the book continues to be devoted to the links among the three languages. Entry to the links is through the NANDA diagnoses. The diagnoses are listed alphabetically with two exceptions: (1) all of the risk diagnoses appear in one section at the end of the linkages; and (2) the major concept, for example *thermoregulation,* has been used in the alphabetical listing rather than the modifier *ineffective.* Suggested NOC outcomes are linked to each of the diagnoses, and NIC interventions are linked to each of the NOC outcomes. Definitions are provided for each of the NANDA diagnoses and NOC outcomes in the linkage tables, and definitions for the NOC outcomes and the NIC interventions are found in the appendixes.

This linkage work does not attempt to link the taxonomic structures of each of the languages. However, the links will provide language developers and users the opportunity to evaluate the similarities and dissimilarities among the languages, to suggest modifications in the links, and to evaluate the work put forth in this book. The authors appreciate all feedback from users concerning missing elements or links that are not used in the practice situation.

Marion Johnson

Contents

PART I Languages and Applications, 1

Chapter 1 The Languages, 3
Chapter 2 Development of the Linkages, 13
Chapter 3 Linkage Applications, 21

PART II NANDA, NOC, and NIC Linkages, 49

Introduction, 51
Diagnoses Linked to NOC and NIC, 53
"Risk for" Diagnoses Linked to NOC and NIC, 511

PART III Appendixes, 619

A NOC Outcome Labels and Definitions, 621
B NIC Interventions Labels and Definitions, 639

LANGUAGES
AND
APPLICATIONS

The Languages

The need for uniform or standardized nursing language (SNL) has been discussed in nursing literature for more than 30 years (Dochterman & Jones, 2003; Jones, 1997; Keenan & Aquilino, 1998; Maas, 1985; McCloskey & Bulechek, 1994; McCormick, 1991; and Zielstorff, 1994). A uniform nursing language serves several purposes, including the following:

- Provides a language for nurses to communicate what they do among themselves, with other health care professionals, and with the public
- Allows the collection and analysis of information documenting nursing's contribution to patient care
- Facilitates the evaluation and improvement of nursing care
- Fosters the development of nursing knowledge
- Allows for the development of electronic clinical information systems and the electronic patient record
- Provides information for the formulation of organizational and public policy concerning health care and nursing care
- Facilitates teaching of clinical decision making to nursing students

The contribution of standardized languages to the practice and development of nursing has been described in detail in the articles cited previously as well as in the books describing the Nursing Interventions Classification (McCloskey & Bulechek, 1992, 1996, 2000; Dochterman & Bulechek, 2004) and the Nursing Outcomes Classification (Johnson & Maas, 1997; Johnson, Maas, & Moorhead, 2000; Moorhead, Johnson, & Maas, 2004).

This book illustrates linkages between three of the standardized languages recognized by the American Nurses Association (ANA): the diagnoses developed by NANDA (North American Nursing Diagnosis Association) International, the interventions of the Nursing Interventions Classification (NIC), and the outcomes of the Nursing Outcomes Classification (NOC). The provision of links between these classifications is a major step forward in facilitating the use of these languages in practice, education, and research. For those unfamiliar with the languages, a brief overview of each classification follows.

NANDA INTERNATIONAL

The use of standardized nursing language began in the 1970s with the development of NANDA's diagnostic classification. A nursing diagnosis is "a clinical judgment about individual, family, or community responses to actual or potential health problems/life processes. A nursing diagnosis provides the basis for selection of nursing interventions to achieve outcomes for which the nurse is accountable" (NANDA International, 2005, p. 277). Nursing diagnoses are both actual and potential (at risk for development). The elements of an actual NANDA diagnosis are the label, the definition of the diagnosis, the defining characteristics (signs and symptoms), and the related factors (causative or associated), as illustrated in Table 1-1. The elements of a potential diagnosis as defined by NANDA are the label, the definition, and the associated risk factors.

NANDA was formed in 1973 when a group of nurses met in St. Louis, Missouri, and organized the first National Conference Group for the Classification of Nursing Diagnoses (North American Nursing Diagnosis Association, 1999). In 2002 the name of the organization was changed to NANDA International to better reflect the membership from multiple countries. NANDA International is a membership organization directed by an elected President and Board. A Diagnosis Review Committee reviews new and refined diagnoses submitted by members and a Taxonomy Committee adds diagnoses to the taxonomic structure and refines the taxonomy. In 2005, the NANDA classification included 172 diagnoses and Taxonomy II with 13 domains and 47 classes (NANDA International, 2005). NANDA representatives, along with representatives from NIC and NOC, participated in the development of the Taxonomy of Nursing Practice, a unifying structure for the placement of diagnoses, interventions, and outcomes, published in 2003 (Dochterman & Jones, 2003). NANDA terminology has been translated into many languages and is used in more than 20 countries throughout the world. The NANDA organization publishes a classification book every other year and sponsors *The Journal of Nursing Language and Classification.* More information about the organization and the classification can be found at www.NANDA.org.

NIC

Research to develop a vocabulary and classification of nursing interventions began in 1987 with the formation of a research team led by Joanne McCloskey (now Joanne Dochterman) and Gloria Bulechek at The University of Iowa. The team developed the Nursing Interventions Classification (NIC), a comprehensive, standardized classification of interventions that nurses perform, first published in 1992. Unlike a nursing diagnosis or patient outcome, for which the focus of concern is the patient, the focus of concern with nursing interventions is nurse behavior; those things that nurses do to assist the patient to move toward a desired outcome.

An intervention is defined as "Any treatment, based upon clinical judgment and knowledge, that a nurse performs to enhance patient/client outcomes. Nursing interventions include both direct and indirect care; those aimed at individuals, families, and the community; and those for nurse-initiated, physician-initiated, and other provider-initiated treatments" (Dochterman & Bulechek, 2004, p. *xxiii*). Each NIC intervention

Table **1-1**   **One Example of a NANDA Diagnosis**

Anxiety

Definition: Vague uneasy feeling of discomfort or dread accompanied by an autonomic response (the source often nonspecific or unknown to the individual); a feeling of apprehension caused by anticipation of danger. It is an altering signal that warns of impending danger and enables the individual to take measures to deal with threat.

Defining Characteristics

Behavioral	Diminished productivity; scanning and vigilance; poor eye contact; restlessness; glancing about; extraneous movement (e.g., foot shuffling, hand/arm movements); expressed concerns due to change in life events; insomnia; fidgeting
Affective	Regretful; irritability; anguish; scared; jittery; overexcited; painful and persistent increased helplessness; rattled; uncertainty; increased wariness; focus on self; feelings of inadequacy; fearful; distressed; apprehension; anxious
Physiological	Voice quivering; trembling/hand tremors; shakiness; increased respiration (sympathetic); urinary urgency (parasympathetic); increased pulse (sympathetic); pupil dilation (sympathetic); increased reflexes (sympathetic); abdominal pain (parasympathetic); sleep disturbance (parasympathetic); tingling in extremities (parasympathetic); cardiovascular excitation (sympathetic); increased perspiration; facial tension; anorexia (sympathetic); heart pounding (sympathetic); diarrhea (parasympathetic); urinary hesitancy (parasympathetic); fatigue (parasympathetic); dry mouth (sympathetic); weakness (sympathetic); decreased pulse (parasympathetic); facial flushing (sympathetic); superficial vasoconstriction (sympathetic); twitching (sympathetic); decreased blood pressure (parasympathetic); nausea (parasympathetic); urinary frequency (parasympathetic); faintness (parasympathetic); respiratory difficulties (sympathetic); increased blood pressure (sympathetic)
Cognitive	Blocking of thought; confusion; preoccupation; forgetfulness; rumination; impaired attention; decreased perceptual field; fear of unspecific consequences; tendency to blame others; difficulty concentrating; diminished ability to problem solve, learn; awareness of physiological symptoms

Related Factors

Exposure to toxins; unconscious conflict about essential goals/values of life; familial association/heredity; unmet needs; interpersonal transmission/contagion; situational/maturational crises; threat of death; threat to self concept; stress; substance abuse; threat to or change in role status, health status, interaction patterns, role function, environment, economic status

From NANDA International. (2005). Nursing diagnoses: Definitions & classification 2005-2006, Philadelphia: Author.

consists of a label name, a definition, a set of activities that indicate the actions and thinking that go into the delivery of the intervention, and a short list of background readings as illustrated in Table 1-2. The intervention label name and the definition are the content of the intervention that is standardized and should not be changed when NIC is used to document care. Care can be individualized, however, through the choice of activities. From a list of approximately 10 to 30 activities per intervention, the nurse selects the activities most appropriate for the specific individual or family. The nurse can add new activities if needed; however, all modifications and additions should be congruent with the definition of the intervention. The classification is continually updated

Table **1-2**   **One Example of a NIC Intervention**

Anxiety Reduction

Definition: Minimizing apprehension, dread, foreboding, or uneasiness related to an unidentified source of anticipated danger

Activities

Use a calm, reassuring approach
Clearly state expectations for patient's behavior
Explain all procedures, including sensations likely to be experienced during the procedure
Seek to understand the patient's perspective of a stressful situation
Provide factual information concerning diagnosis, treatment, and prognosis
Stay with patient to promote safety and reduce fear
Encourage family to stay with patient, as appropriate
Provide objects that symbolize safeness
Administer back rub/neck rub, as appropriate
Encourage noncompetitive activities, as appropriate
Keep treatment equipment out of sight
Listen attentively
Reinforce behavior, as appropriate
Create an atmosphere to facilitate trust
Encourage verbalization of feelings, perceptions, and fears
Identify when level of anxiety changes
Provide diversional activities geared toward the reduction of tension
Help patient identify situations that precipitate anxiety
Control stimuli, as appropriate, for patient needs
Support the use of appropriate defense mechanisms
Assist patient to articulate a realistic description of an upcoming event
Determine patient's decision-making ability
Instruct patient in use of relaxation techniques
Administer medications to reduce anxiety, as appropriate
Observe for verbal and nonverbal signs of anxiety

From Dochterman, J. M., & Bulechek, G. M. (Eds.). (2004). *Nursing interventions classification (NIC)* (4th ed.). St. Louis: Mosby.

and has been published in four editions; the 2004 edition contains 514 interventions grouped into 30 classes and 7 domains for ease of use. NIC can be used in all settings (from acute care intensive care units to home care, hospice care, and primary care settings) and in all specialties (from pediatrics and obstetrics to cardiology and gerontology). Although the entire classification describes the domain of nursing, some of the interventions can be provided by other disciplines. Health care providers other than nurses are welcome to use NIC to describe their treatments.

The classification book as well as multiple other publications cited therein document the years of research undertaken to develop and test the classification and its taxonomic structure. NIC interventions have been linked with NANDA diagnoses, to Omaha System problems, to the Resident Assessment Instrument used in nursing homes, to OASIS (Outcome and Assessment Information Set) assessment categories for home health care, and to NOC outcomes. The NIC classification has been translated into nine languages. The classification is continually updated through an ongoing process of feedback and review. Work that is done between editions of the NIC book and other relevant publications that enhance the use of the classification are available from the Center for Nursing Classification and Clinical Effectiveness at The University of Iowa, College of Nursing, Iowa City, IA 52242. Current information is available at www.nursing.uiowa.edu/cnc.

NOC

In 1991 a research team led by Marion Johnson and Meridean Maas was formed at The University of Iowa to develop a classification of patient outcomes correlated with nursing care. The work of the research team resulted in the Nursing Outcomes Classification (NOC), a comprehensive, standardized classification of patient outcomes that can be used to evaluate the results of nursing interventions, first published in 1997.

Patient outcomes serve as the criteria against which to judge the success of a nursing intervention. An outcome is defined as "An individual, family, or community state, behavior, or perception that is measured along a continuum in response to a nursing intervention(s)" (Moorhead, Johnson, & Maas, 2004, p. xix). It is recognized that a number of variables, in addition to the intervention, influence patient outcomes. These variables range from the process used in providing the care, including the actions of other health care providers, to organizational and environmental variables that influence how interventions are selected and provided to patient characteristics, including the patient's physical and emotional health, as well as the life circumstances being experienced by the patient. Because the outcomes describe the status of the patient, other disciplines may find them useful for the evaluation of their interventions.

Each NOC outcome has a label name, a definition, a list of indicators to evaluate patient status in relation to the outcome, a five-point Likert scale to measure patient status, and a short list of references used in the development of the outcome, as illustrated in Table 1-3. The scales allow measurement of the outcome status at any point on a continuum from most negative to most positive, as well as identification of changes in patient status at different points in time. In contrast to the information provided by a goal statement, that is, whether a goal is met or not met, NOC outcomes can be used to

Table **1-3**   **One Example of a NOC Outcome**

Anxiety Self-Control

Definition: Personal actions to eliminate or reduce feelings of apprehension, tension, or uneasiness from an unidentifiable source

Outcome Target Rating: Maintain at ____   Increase to ____

Anxiety Self-Control	Never Demonstrated (1)	Rarely Demonstrated (2)	Sometimes Demonstrated (3)	Often Demonstrated (4)	Consistently Demonstrated (5)
Monitors intensity of anxiety	1	2	3	4	5
Eliminates precursors of anxiety	1	2	3	4	5
Decreases environmental stimuli when anxious	1	2	3	4	5
Seeks information to reduce anxiety	1	2	3	4	5
Plans coping strategies for stressful situations	1	2	3	4	5
Uses effective coping strategies	1	2	3	4	5
Uses relaxation techniques to reduce anxiety	1	2	3	4	5
Monitors duration of episodes	1	2	3	4	5
Monitors length of time between episodes	1	2	3	4	5
Maintains role performance	1	2	3	4	5
Maintains social relationships	1	2	3	4	5

Table **1-3**   **One Example of a NOC Outcome—cont'd**

Anxiety Self-Control	Never Demonstrated (1)	Rarely Demonstrated (2)	Sometimes Demonstrated (3)	Often Demonstrated (4)	Consistently Demonstrated (5)
Maintains concentration	1	2	3	4	5
Monitors sensory perceptual distortions	1	2	3	4	5
Monitors adequate sleep	1	2	3	4	5
Monitors physical manifestations of anxiety	1	2	3	4	5
Controls anxiety response	1	2	3	4	5

From Moorhead, S., Johnson, M., & Maas, M. (Eds.). (2004). *Nursing outcomes classification (NOC)* (3rd ed.). St. Louis: Mosby.

monitor progress, or lack of progress, throughout an episode of care and across different care settings. The outcomes have been developed to be used in all settings, all special-ties, and across the care continuum. The third edition of the classification published in 2004 contains 330 outcomes grouped into 31 classes and 7 domains for ease of use. The classification is continually updated to include new outcomes and to revise older out-comes based on new research or user feedback.

The NOC classification books and numerous other publications document the exten-sive research undertaken to develop and validate NOC. The outcomes have been linked to NANDA diagnoses, to Omaha System problems, to Gordon's functional patterns, to the Long-Term Care Minimum Data Set, to the Resident Assessment Instrument used in nursing homes, to the International Classification of Functioning (ICF), and to NIC interventions. The NOC classification has been translated into eight languages and is experiencing growing use across the United States and in other countries. Current infor-mation about NOC is available on the Center for Nursing Classification and Clinical Effectiveness web page: www.nursing.uiowa.edu/cnc.

CONCLUSION

NANDA, NIC, and NOC can be used together or separately. Together they represent the domain of nursing in all settings and specialties. They have been recognized by the ANA, included in the National Library of Medicine's Metathesaurus for a Unified Medical Language System (UMLS), included in the Cumulative Index to Nursing Literature (CINAHL), recognized by HL7 (Health Level 7, the electronic messaging standards organization in the United States), and included in SNOMED (Systematized Nomenclature of Medicine). Representatives from the three developing groups created the Taxonomy of Nursing Practice published by the ANA in 2003 (Dochterman & Jones, 2003). This common organizing structure should facilitate the use of all three languages. Multiple clinical agencies and educational settings across the United States and in many other countries are using one or more of these nursing languages for the documentation of patient care and for the education of nursing students. In this book, we provide linkages between NOC outcomes and NIC interventions for NANDA diagnoses. Linking the three languages provides assistance to clinicians and students in selecting the outcomes and interventions most appropriate for their clients, related to the nursing diagnoses. The next chapters describe the process of determining the linkages and how to use the linkages.

References

Dochterman, J. M., & Bulechek, G. M. (Eds.). (2004). *Nursing interventions classification (NIC)* (4th ed.). St. Louis: Mosby.

Dochterman, J. M., & Jones, D. A. (Eds.). (2003). *Unifying nursing languages: The harmonization of NANDA, NIC, and NOC*. Washington, D.C.: American Nurses Association.

Johnson, M., & Maas, M. (Eds.). (1997). *Nursing outcomes classification (NOC)*. St. Louis: Mosby.

Johnson, M., Maas, M., & Moorhead, S. (Eds.). (2000). *Nursing outcomes classification (NOC)* (2nd ed.). St. Louis: Mosby.

Jones, D. L. (1997). Building the information infrastructure required for managed care. *Image: Journal of Nursing Scholarship*, 29(4), 377-382.

Keenan, G., & Aquilino, M. L. (1998). Standardized nomenclatures: Keys to continuity of care, nursing accountability, and nursing effectiveness. *Outcomes Management for Nursing Practice,* 2(2), 81-85.

Maas, M. L. (1985). Nursing diagnosis: A leadership strategy for nursing administrators. *Journal of Nursing Administration*, 1(6), 39-42.

McCloskey, J. C., & Bulechek, G. M. (Eds.). (1992). *Nursing interventions classification (NIC)*. St. Louis: Mosby.

McCloskey, J. C., & Bulechek, G. M. (1994). Standardizing the language for nursing treatments: An overview of the issues. *Nursing Outlook,* 42(2), 56-63.

McCloskey, J. C., & Bulechek, G. M. (Eds.). (1996). *Nursing interventions classification (NIC)* (2nd ed.). St. Louis: Mosby.

McCloskey, J. C., & Bulechek, G. M. (Eds.). (2000). *Nursing interventions classification (NIC)* (3rd ed.). St. Louis: Mosby.

McCormick, K. A. (1991). Future data needs for quality of care monitoring, DRG considerations, reimbursement, and outcome measurement. *Image: Journal of Nursing Scholarship*, 23(1), 29-32.

Moorhead, S., Johnson, M., & Maas, M. (Eds.). (2004). *Nursing outcomes classification (NOC)* (3rd ed.). St. Louis: Mosby.

NANDA International. (2005). *Nursing diagnoses: Definitions & classification 2005-2006*. Philadelphia: Author.

North American Nursing Diagnosis Association. (1999). *Nursing diagnoses: Definitions & classification 1999-2000*. Philadelphia: Author.

Zielstorff, R. D. (1994). National data bases: Nursing's challenge, classification of nursing diagnoses. In Carroll-Johnson, R. M., & Paquette, M. (Eds.), *Classification of nursing diagnoses: Proceedings of the Tenth Conference* (pp. 34-42). Philadelphia: J.B. Lippincott.

Chapter 2

Development of the Linkages

Part II of the book links NANDA diagnoses, NIC interventions, and NOC outcomes. The work represents the judgment of selected members of the NIC and NOC research teams, including academicians, clinicians, and students. Data collected during the evaluation of NOC outcomes in clinical sites were used when available. The data, as illustrated in Table 2-1, show aggregated links among NOC outcomes, NIC interventions, and NANDA diagnoses based on the clinician's selections for individual patients. The aggregated data provided information about the outcomes and interventions that clinicians select for nursing diagnoses, which served as a resource to compare clinical decisions and expert opinion for some of the diagnoses. *However, it is important to recognize that the linkages in this book are not meant to be prescriptive and do not replace the clinical judgment of the practitioner.* In addition to the linkages provided in this book, users may select other outcomes and interventions for a particular diagnosis for an individual patient. The linkages presented here illustrate how three distinct nursing languages can be connected and used together when planning care for an individual patient or a group of patients.

DESCRIPTION OF THE LINKAGES

The linkages in this book are the NANDA International diagnoses, the Nursing Interventions Classification (NIC) interventions, and the Nursing Outcomes Classification (NOC) outcomes. A linkage can be defined as that which directs the relationship or association of concepts. The links between the NANDA diagnoses and the NOC outcomes suggest the relationships between the patient's problem or current status and those aspects of the problem or status that are expected to be resolved or improved by one or more interventions. The links between the NANDA diagnoses and the NIC interventions suggest the relationship between the patient's problem and the nursing actions that will resolve or diminish the problem. The links between the NOC outcomes and the NIC interventions suggest a similar relationship: that between the resolution of a problem and the nursing actions directed at problem resolution, that is, the outcome that the intervention(s) is expected to influence.

The concept names and definitions used in the linkages are those in the 2005-2006 edition of *Nursing Diagnoses: Definitions & Classification* (NANDA International,

Table **2-1**   **Top Four NOCs and Top Four Associated NICs for NANDA Diagnosis Knowledge Deficit**

NANDA	N*	NOC	N*	NIC	N*
Knowledge Deficient	665	Knowledge: Medication	155	Teaching: Prescribed Medication	114
				Teaching: Disease Process	75
				Medication Management	66
				Teaching: Individual	65
		Knowledge: Disease Process	128	Teaching: Disease Process	101
				Teaching: Individual	69
				Teaching: Prescribed Medication	46
				Learning Facilitation	43
		Knowledge: Treatment Regimen	113	Teaching: Disease Process	63
				Teaching: Prescribed Medication	55
				Teaching: Individual	50
				Discharge Planning	49
		Knowledge: Health Resources	106	Discharge Planning	60
				Teaching: Individual	42
				Teaching: Prescribed Medication	41
				Teaching: Disease Process	38

*N refers to the number of patients for whom the diagnoses, outcomes, and intervention were used.

2005), the fourth edition of *Nursing Interventions Classification (NIC)* (Dochterman & Bulechek, 2004), and the third edition of *Nursing Outcomes Classification (NOC)* (Moorhead, Johnson, & Maas, 2004). The NANDA diagnosis is the entry point for the linkages. The diagnoses are listed in alphabetical order except for the risk diagnoses, which are listed alphabetically following the other diagnoses. However, the NANDA diagnostic name has been reordered when the beginning term does not specify the concept of concern in the diagnostic label; for example, *Ineffective Thermoregulation* is presented in these linkages as *Thermoregulation, Ineffective*. This reordering was done to facilitate the ease with which a diagnosis can be found by listing the diagnostic concept before the modifier. Each diagnosis contains the diagnostic name and the definition. Suggested NOC outcomes with associated NIC interventions are provided for each diagnosis. The definition for each of the selected outcomes is provided in the linkage table and in Appendix A. The interventions are identified as major, suggested, and optional interventions for achieving each of the suggested outcomes for a particular diagnosis. This is consistent with the way the NIC interventions have been presented for NANDA diagnoses (Dochterman & Bulechek, 2004). Definitions of the NIC interventions used in the linkages are provided in Appendix B.

The alphabetical ordering of the diagnoses does not reflect the taxonomic structure used by NANDA. Likewise, the taxonomic and coding structures of NIC and NOC are not reflected in these linkages. The current taxonomic structure for each of these languages can be found in the books describing each language. The current editions of the NIC and NOC classifications also include placement of the languages in the common organizing structure, the Taxonomy of Nursing Practice (Dochterman & Jones, 2003), as mentioned in Chapter 1.

DEVELOPMENT OF THE LINKAGES

Previous linkage work provided the starting point for developing the links in the first edition (Johnson, Bulechek, Dochterman, Maas, & Moorhead, 2001), and for revising and updating the links in this edition. Prior linkage work used for the first edition included the development of links between NANDA diagnoses and NIC interventions, NANDA diagnoses and NOC outcomes, and NIC interventions and NOC outcomes. Linkage work used for the current edition included the suggested outcomes for each NANDA diagnosis from the third edition of the *Nursing Outcomes Classification (NOC)* (Moorhead, Johnson, & Maas, 2004) and suggested interventions for each NANDA diagnosis in the fourth edition of the *Nursing Interventions Classification (NIC)* (Dochterman & Bulechek, 2004). In addition, linkages from the clinical evaluation of NOC were considered in the second edition. Table 2-1 illustrates the top four NOC outcomes selected for the NANDA diagnosis, Knowledge Deficient, and the top four associated NIC interventions selected for each of the NOC outcomes. The diagnosis was used with 665 patients, representing one of the most commonly used diagnoses across all clinical sites. It is interesting to note that the NIC intervention, Teaching: Individual, was a top intervention selected for each of the outcomes. All of the linkage work mentioned in the preceding text provides multiple links between each of the diagnoses, outcomes, and interventions. The methods used in the development of each of the links are described in the publications in which they appear. As with the preceding linkage work, the current work is based primarily on expert judgment and is not intended to be prescriptive.

The linkage work in the first edition (Johnson, Bulechek, Dochterman, Maas, & Moorhead, 2001) was used as the basis for the NANDA-NOC-NIC links in this book. Development of the links for the first edition will be described, and this description is followed by the method used to revise and update this book.

First Edition Development

Development of the NANDA-NOC-NIC links in the first edition proceeded in the following three phases:
1. Creating an initial list of linkages
2. Refining the first level of linkages
3. Refining the second level of linkages

Creating the initial list required that the format for presenting the links be determined. Diagnoses were selected as the entry point for the linkages because traditionally they are considered the second step in the nursing process, following assessment and preceding the selection of interventions and outcomes.

Suggested outcomes from the NANDA-NOC links (Johnson, Maas, & Moorhead, 2000) were linked to each diagnosis. The diagnosis can be thought of as a standardized term that represents the initial condition or present state of the patient and the outcome as the desired or end state that results from nursing interventions (Pesut & Herman, 1999). Therefore, the desired outcome is identified before selection of nursing interventions. Bulechek and McCloskey identify the desired patient outcome and the characteristics of the diagnosis as two of the factors to be considered when selecting a nursing intervention (Bulechek & McCloskey, 1999). After the suggested outcomes were linked to the diagnosis, a publication (Iowa Interventions Project, 1998) linking the NIC interventions to the first edition NOC outcomes (NOC-NIC) was used to link interventions to the outcomes selected for each diagnosis. The interventions were used as they appeared in the NOC-NIC linkage work, including the identification of an intervention as major, suggested, and optional for each outcome.

In summary, the initial links were derived by linking the suggested outcomes from the second edition of NOC with the NANDA diagnosis, and then linking the major, suggested, and optional interventions from the NOC-NIC linkage work with each of the outcomes. The outcomes and interventions were not linked to the defining characteristics (signs and symptoms) or the related factors (etiologies) of each diagnosis because this would generate multiple repetitive links for each diagnosis.

The work then moved into the second phase, the initial refinement of the linkage work. Throughout this phase, the defining characteristics and related factors of the diagnosis were considered as the links were further developed. For example, when the NANDA diagnosis is related to a specific etiologic factor, such as with functional or stress urinary incontinence, the suggested outcomes and interventions for that diagnosis are more specific for the etiology. When the NANDA diagnosis requires further specification, such as the type of altered tissue perfusion or sensory deficit, a diagnosis with associated outcomes and interventions was provided for each diagnostic type presented in NANDA. In all instances, the definition, characteristics, and related or risk factors were considered when refining the links. Refinement was done using the following steps.

1. The relevance of the interventions associated with each outcome for the specific diagnosis was evaluated, and interventions linked to and appropriate for the outcome but not appropriate for the diagnosis were eliminated. The decision to eliminate an intervention was based on the clinical judgment of the reviewer and comparison with the NANDA-NIC linkage work (McCloskey & Bulechek, 2000). For example, *Tissue Integrity: Skin & Mucous Membranes* is a suggested outcome for the diagnosis *Oral Mucous Membrane, Altered*. However, some of the interventions such as *Bathing*, *Foot Care*, and *Pressure Ulcer Prevention*, although appropriate interventions for the outcome *Tissue Integrity: Skin & Mucous Membranes*, are not appropriate for the diagnosis, *Oral Mucous Membrane, Altered*.

2. The interventions previously linked to the diagnosis (NANDA-NIC linkages) were compared with the interventions associated with each of the outcomes selected for the diagnosis. If an intervention in the NANDA-NIC linkage was not linked to the diagnosis via one of the outcomes, the relevance of the intervention for each of the outcomes was considered and the missing intervention was linked to one of the outcomes if appropriate.

3. As the interventions linked to the outcomes for a diagnosis (NOC-NIC) were compared with the interventions linked to the diagnosis (NANDA-NIC), some discrepancies among the linkages became evident. In some instances the interventions linked to the suggested outcomes were quite different from the interventions linked to the diagnosis. When this occurred, outcomes not associated with the interventions recommended for the diagnosis were reviewed to determine if the outcome should be retained or if other outcomes would be more appropriate for the diagnosis. As a result of the decisions made at this step, some of the outcomes selected for the NANDA diagnoses were not consistent with the suggested outcomes in the NANDA-NOC linkages in the second edition of *Nursing Outcomes Classification (NOC)* (Johnson, Maas, & Moorhead, 2000).

4. As the previous steps were being carried out, the placement of each intervention as major, suggested, and optional was evaluated for appropriateness for the particular diagnosis. In some cases the placement of the interventions remained the same as in the previous NOC-NIC linkages (Iowa Interventions Project, 1998), and at other times the interventions were moved to a different level of importance for the diagnosis. One of the factors used to determine the appropriate placement level of an intervention was the placement of the intervention when linked to the diagnosis. If appropriate for the outcome, the intervention level was retained as identified in the NANDA-NIC linkages (McCloskey & Bulechek, 2000).

The final phase in the development of the linkages was second level refinement. Because one person completed the initial links, it was important that others review the linkage work. Reviewers were the other authors of the book and, in some instances, clinicians and graduate students with clinical expertise. Suggested changes were made in the linkages if there was agreement among the reviewers. If reviewer agreement was not reached, the suggested changes were brought to the authors for discussion and for a final decision.

Second Edition Revision and Update

Linkages and methods developed for the first edition served as the basis for linkage revision in the second edition. The following steps were used to develop the current linkages.

1. Outcomes used in the first linkage book were compared with outcomes suggested for a diagnosis in the third edition of the NOC book (Moorhead, Johnson, & Maas, 2004). In many instances the outcomes in the first linkage book and the suggested outcomes in the current NOC book were the same. In other instances, additional outcomes had been added to the list of suggested outcomes in the NOC book and these were added to the diagnosis in the linkage book. In a few

instances, some of the outcomes in the first linkage book were no longer on the suggested list in the current NOC book. Before these outcomes were removed, they were reviewed by all of the authors; in some cases the decision was made to retain them in the linkage book. It was during this phase that outcomes and interventions selected by clinicians in the NOC evaluation study were compared with the proposed linkages.

2. Interventions selected for each outcome in the first linkage book were reviewed against the interventions selected for the diagnosis in the current NIC book (Dochterman & Bulechek, 2004). Again, removal or addition of interventions was based on author review and comparison with data, if available, from the NOC evaluation study. The general tendency is to retain interventions rather than eliminate them. This provides more realistic options for clinicians when selecting interventions for patients of various ages and with various medical diagnoses and related problems.

3. Formatting and technical changes were made in the linkages. Terminology for all three languages was updated to reflect changes in the editions used for each of the languages. Changes made in NANDA diagnoses included the addition of 24 new diagnoses, the revision of 15 diagnoses, and editorial changes in how a number of the diagnoses were labeled. A number of NOC outcomes had language revisions without changes in the concept. For example, 10 NOC outcomes had major changes in the label name and 38 outcomes had minor, editorial changes in the label name. Six NOC outcomes were retired (deleted) and do not appear in this edition of the linkage work. Only one NIC intervention had a label name change and one intervention was retired. A number of interventions had revisions in the definition. A change made in this edition was to include the definition of the outcome in the linkage table. This was done to assist the user when selecting interventions for a patient or a care plan. Definitions for the interventions appear in Appendix A, since the number of interventions precludes including the definition in the linkage table.

The revision of linkages for this book required scrutiny of previous and current linkage work. As a result, the linkages in this book, although similar to previous linkage work, are not identical to the linkages found in the first edition of *Nursing Diagnoses, Outcomes, & Interventions*; the fourth edition of the *Nursing Interventions Classification (NIC)*; or the third edition of the *Nursing Outcomes Classification (NOC)*. Discrepancies may occur because a particular link is not appropriate when the three components—diagnosis, outcome, and intervention—are linked; but are appropriate when considering only the relationship between the diagnosis and outcome or the diagnosis and the intervention. The judgment to include or eliminate a particular outcome for a diagnosis on the basis of the interventions recommended for the diagnosis is another source of differences. For example, there are a few times when an outcome used in the linkage book is not linked to the diagnosis in the NOC book. This occurred if the appropriateness of the outcome became apparent when considering the interventions recommended for the diagnosis. Although rare, another difference occurs when not all of the interventions selected for a specific diagnosis in the NIC book are found in the linkage table. This can occur because not all possible outcomes that might be selected for a diagnosis are included in the linkage table and some of the interventions would be more appropriate for the missing outcomes. Given the number of diagnostic, outcome, and intervention linkages in this edition, the number of times there are significant differences between these linkages and those in the NOC and NIC books is minimal.

Clinical evaluation and testing of the linkages found in this book is needed. Clinical sites that use the three languages can aggregate and analyze data collected at their site to determine the outcomes and interventions selected for both nursing and medical diagnoses. The data can also be analyzed to determine which diagnoses, outcomes, and interventions are selected for patient populations delineated by age, medical diagnosis, or other parameters of interest. The linkages can also be tested in research studies that focus on select patient populations or select practice sites. Feedback from clinicians and others using the work will assist the authors to refine the linkages for future editions.

References

Bulechek, G. M., & McCloskey, J. C. (Eds.). (1999). *Nursing interventions: Effective nursing treatments* (3rd ed.). Philadelphia: W.B. Saunders.

Dochterman, J. M., & Bulechek, G. M. (Eds.). (2004). *Nursing interventions classification (NIC)* (4th ed.). St. Louis: Mosby.

Dochterman, J. M., & Jones, D. A. (Eds.). (2003). *Unifying nursing languages: The harmonization of NANDA, NIC, and NOC.* Washington, D.C.: American Nurses Association.

Iowa Interventions Project. (1998). *NIC interventions linked to NOC outcomes.* Iowa City, IA: Center for Nursing Classification.

Johnson, M., Bulechek, G., Dochterman, J. M., Maas, M., & Moorhead, S. (2001). *Nursing diagnoses, outcomes, & interventions: NANDA, NOC, and NIC Linkages.* St. Louis: Mosby.

Johnson, M., Maas, M., & Moorhead, S. (Eds.). (1997). *Nursing outcomes classification (NOC).* St. Louis: Mosby.

Johnson, M., Maas, M., & Moorhead, S. (Eds.). (2000). *Nursing outcomes classification (NOC)* (2nd ed.). St. Louis: Mosby.

McCloskey, J. C., & Bulechek, G. M. (Eds.). (2000). *Nursing interventions classification (NIC)* (3rd ed.). St. Louis: Mosby.

Moorhead, S., Johnson, M., & Maas, M. (Eds.). (2004). *Nursing outcomes classification (NOC)* (3rd ed.). St. Louis: Mosby.

NANDA International. (2005). *Nursing diagnoses: Definitions & classification 2005-2006.* Philadelphia: Author.

North American Nursing Diagnosis Association. (1999). *Nursing diagnoses: Definitions & classification 1999-2000.* Philadelphia: Author.

Pesut, D. J., & Herman, J. (1999). *Clinical reasoning: The art & science of critical & creative thinking.* Boston: Delmar Publishers.

Chapter 3

Linkage Applications

The linkages provided in this book have a number of uses. They can be used for the development of care plans and critical paths for patient populations or for individual patients. They provide a standardized language that can be used in software development for electronic nursing information systems. The linkages can assist educators in developing curricula and teaching clinical decision-making, and they can be used by researchers for testing nursing interventions, evaluating the connections suggested in the linkages, and developing mid-range nursing theories.

CARE PLANNING

Nurses use a decision-making process to determine a nursing diagnosis, to project a desired outcome, and to select interventions to achieve the outcome. The linkages in this book can assist the nurse in making decisions about the outcome and interventions to be selected. It is important to keep in mind that the linkages are only guides; the nurse must continually evaluate the situation and adjust the diagnoses, outcomes, and interventions to fit the unique needs of each patient or patient population. The use of suggested links does not alter the skills that nurses need and use in making decisions about patient care. "The skills the nurse must have to use the nursing process are: intellectual, interpersonal, and technical. Intellectual skills entail problem solving, critical thinking, and making nursing judgments" (Yura & Walsh, 1973, p. 69). When using the linkages, these intellectual skills are directed toward evaluating and selecting or rejecting the outcomes and interventions provided for each nursing diagnosis.

The first judgment the nurse must make when using the linkages is to determine the nursing diagnosis. There is general agreement that prior to making a nursing diagnosis, an assessment of the patient status must be made. Rubenfeld and Scheffer (1999) state that assessment includes both data collection and data analysis or, as they describe it, "finding clues" and "making sense of the clues" (p. 130). They detail a number of steps used in assessment that enable the nurse to draw conclusions about the patient's strengths and health concerns, that is, to make a diagnosis. They further suggest categorizing health concerns as (1) problems for referral (issues addressed by other health providers), (2) interdisciplinary problems addressed collaboratively with other providers, and (3) nursing diagnoses for which the nurse has primary responsibility for treating the patient.

Pesut and Herman (1999) use terms other than assessment to describe the stage of data gathering. They indicate that the nurse listens to the client's story and then uses "cue logic" to discern the meaning of the story and "framing" to connect cues and discern between the central issue or problem and peripheral problems. This allows the nurse to develop a description of the initial condition of the patient (referred to as the present state) and select the desired outcome (referred to as the end state). The present state can then be compared to the end state following a nursing intervention to determine the effectiveness of that intervention in achieving the desired outcome. Both the present state and the end state can be defined by standardized terms, for example, a NANDA diagnosis and a NOC outcome. The present state may be specified with the diagnosis *Altered Thought Processes* and possible desired outcomes might be *Cognitive Ability, Distorted Thought Control, or Memory,* depending upon the etiology and type of thought alteration. Following the intervention(s), the end state can be compared with the projected, desired outcome to determine the effectiveness of the intervention in achieving the predicted outcome. The end state can also be compared with the beginning, present state to determine the change in patient status achieved by the interventions, another measure of effectiveness. A discussion of how to measure this type of change and aggregate findings is available in the literature (Johnson, Moorhead, Maas, & Reed, 2003) as is a description of how data from a computerized clinical documentation system using NANDA, NOC, and NIC were used to determine the effect of nursing interventions (Scherb, 2002).

Determining a nursing diagnosis is an essential first step for accessing the links in this book, since the diagnosis is used as the entry point for the linkages. This is true when planning the care for one patient (an individual care plan) or for a group of patients (a critical path). However, identification of the nursing diagnosis for a group of patients requires an additional step: the collection and analysis of data to determine the diagnoses that occur most frequently and are important to address for the entire population. Once a nursing diagnosis is determined, the nurse can locate the diagnosis in the linkage tables and determine if any of the suggested outcomes are appropriate for the individual patient or patient group. When selecting the outcome, the nurse should consider the following factors: (1) the defining characteristics of the diagnosis, (2) the related factors of the diagnosis, (3) the patient characteristics that can affect outcome achievement, (4) the outcomes generally associated with the diagnosis, and (5) the preferences of the patient. It is important to note that the outcomes presented in the linkage work reflect a desired end state outcome related to the patient state to be achieved. For example, the suggested outcomes for *Noncompliance* are *Adherence Behavior, Compliance Behavior,* and *Treatment Behavior: Illness or Injury.* However, intermediate outcomes that address the related factors (etiologies) in a NANDA diagnosis must often be met before the actual end state outcome is achieved. For example, if *Noncompliance* is related to inadequate knowledge of the disease process, the nurse might want to select the outcome *Knowledge: Disease Process* as well as the outcome *Compliance Behavior.* Examples of outcomes selected by clinicians for six NANDA diagnoses are reported in the literature with a discussion of some of the factors that might influence selection (Moorhead & Johnson, 2004).

After the outcome is selected, the nurse can use the interventions suggested in the linkage work to assist in the selection of an intervention(s) for the individual or group.

The major interventions are the most closely related to both the diagnosis and outcome and should be considered first. If the major intervention is not selected, consideration should be given to the suggested interventions and the optional interventions. Bulechek and McCloskey (1999) identify six factors to consider when selecting a nursing intervention. They are (1) the desired patient outcome, (2) the characteristics of the nursing diagnosis, (3) the research base associated with the intervention, (4) the feasibility of implementing the intervention, (5) the acceptability of the intervention to the patient, and (6) the capability of the nurse. In addition to the capability of the nurse, the clinician will find information about estimates of time and education necessary to perform the interventions helpful when selecting interventions (Center for Nursing Classification & Clinical Effectiveness, 2001; Dochterman & Bulechek, 2004). All of these factors should be considered when using the linkage work; the linkages can assist the nurse by suggesting interventions associated with both the outcome and the diagnosis, but cannot replace the nurse's judgment when selecting an intervention.

The use of the NANDA-NOC-NIC linkages in the development of individualized care plans is illustrated in the case studies at the end of this chapter following the references. Each case study illustrates one way in which the linkages can be used in preparing an individualized care plan. Although each case study could have a number of NANDA diagnoses, only one or two diagnoses have been selected. One or more NOC outcomes and NIC interventions have been selected for each diagnosis. Indicators considered helpful or important in evaluating outcome achievement and pertinent intervention activities have been provided. In some cases the scale that would be used with the NOC outcome is presented.

Each case is preceded by a brief description of the patient and includes some discussion of the reason the diagnoses, outcomes, or interventions were selected, and in some cases suggest other diagnoses, outcomes, or interventions that might be considered. Each case presents a slightly different format for preparing the plan of care.

ELECTRONIC INFORMATION SYSTEMS

Computerized clinical information systems are more prevalent in health care organizations, as the need to capture clinical data that are useful for evaluation has increased. Health care purchasers and managed care entities rely on statistical information derived from these systems to determine how health care dollars will be spent. As one author so aptly noted, "if nurses do not develop and adopt the tools needed to participate in this information-driven environment, opportunities to provide nursing services may significantly diminish in the future" (Jones, 1997, p. 377). Although the development of nursing information systems was identified as a high priority as early as 1988 (National Center for Nursing Research, 1988), the development of systems that use standardized data elements, while making progress, is still in the early stages of development. As health care information systems expand, each discipline must identify the data elements required to evaluate the processes and outcomes of care.

Database development requires a common language and a standard way to organize data. A uniform data set establishes standard measurements, definitions, and classifications (Murnaghan, 1978) for use in electronic information systems. The NANDA-NOC-NIC linkages are a beginning step in the organization of nursing information and provide meaningful categories of data for analysis. In an effort to move nursing forward in preparation for the electronic patient record, the American Nurses Association (ANA) developed a set of standards for nursing data sets in information systems. Standards include those related to nomenclatures, clinical content linkages, the data repository, and general system requirements (American Nurses Association, 1997). The ANA recognizes the NANDA, NOC, and NIC vocabularies as approved nomenclatures. All three languages have been registered in HL7 (Health Level 7), the U.S. standards organization for health care. They are all licensed for inclusion in SNOMED (Systematized Nomenclature of Medicine), a comprehensive reference terminology that is poised to become the recognized terminology for the electronic record.

Nurses' documentation of the diagnoses they treat, the interventions used to treat the diagnoses, and the resulting outcome responses to interventions in computerized information systems is necessary for the development of large local, regional, national, and international nursing databases (Iowa Interventions Project, 1997; Keenan & Aquilino, 1998). Large clinical databases are needed to assess nursing effectiveness, generate hypotheses for testing with controlled research designs, and refine the linkages among diagnoses, interventions, and outcomes based on clinical and research evidence. These database uses are essential for nursing knowledge development, for research-based practice, and to influence health care policy. Busy clinicians, however, cannot afford the time to repeatedly sort through each standardized language in alphabetical form in a computerized system. Nurses also are reluctant to fully document their data if they must access a large number of computer screens for recording. The NANDA-NOC-NIC linkages presented in this book assist with the organization and structuring of nursing clinical information systems that are the most efficient for nurses' documentation of their practice. The taxonomies provide an organizing scheme for the arrangement of computer screens that ease clinicians' access for documentation. Likewise, the linkages offer greater efficiency by supplying groupings of diagnoses, interventions, and outcomes with a high probability of effective relationships for patient care.

Although not prescriptive, the linkages also offer some decision support. A review of the outcomes and interventions that experienced nurses selected for a diagnosis will help clinicians consider possible treatments and responses that might be overlooked in the context of hectic and demanding clinical decision-making. This decision support is sure to be even more helpful to novice nurses who also need clinical reasoning options available for review, but who often have difficulty identifying the critical and priority outcomes and interventions for a diagnosis.

TEACHING CLINICAL DECISION-MAKING

The linkages can be used in conjunction with the three languages (NANDA, NOC, and NIC) to assist students in developing the skills necessary for clinical decision-making. Case studies and computer simulations have been developed on the basis of the linkages in this book and instructions for access are included with the book. Faculty who teach clinical decision-making can use the linkages to develop their own case studies and simulations. Discussion of the cases can focus on the adequacy of the diagnosis selected to address the problem, the appropriateness of the outcomes and interventions selected and the rationale for their selection, and the identification of other outcomes or interventions that might be more appropriate in a given situation. A database with the linkages can be made available for students to use when planning care for a patient or a group of patients. Students can use the linkages to evaluate the relationship between the patient's signs and symptoms, the defining characteristics and related factors of the diagnosis, the outcome and its indicators, and the intervention and its activities. They can select the outcome indicators and intervention activities for a patient according to the patient's status and the elements of the nursing diagnosis. The linkages will facilitate the teaching of clinical decision-making through the application of teaching strategies such as the Outcome-Present State Test (OPT) model (Pesut & Herman, 1999).

The linkages also can be used in planning content for the curriculum. They can assist the faculty in selecting a body of content and distributing the content among the various courses. The linkages among diagnoses, outcomes, and interventions can be a starting point to identify a body of content related to the nursing diagnoses and where the content will be taught in the curriculum. For example, the faculty may choose to teach content related to the diagnosis *Anxiety* and the outcome *Anxiety Control*. Although these concepts may be covered in a number of courses, the interventions might be most appropriately distributed among courses. For example, *Active Listening*, *Calming Technique*, and *Exercise Promotion* might be taught early in the curriculum, whereas *Hypnosis, Simple Guided Imagery*, and *Therapeutic Touch* might be taught later in the curriculum or even in a graduate program. A publication describing the implementation of the three languages in an undergraduate curriculum (Finesilver & Metzler, 2002) is available through the Center for Nursing Classification and Clinical Effectiveness at The University of Iowa, College of Nursing.

There are a number of advantages to using NANDA-NOC-NIC vocabularies and linkages in a nursing curriculum. The vocabularies are comprehensive and can be used for patients across the continuum of care and in all settings in which care is provided. The terminology is useful for nurses in all nursing specialties and in various nursing roles. This makes the vocabularies and associated linkage work useful in both under-graduate and graduate curricula. As the electronic patient record becomes a reality, the use of standardized languages in the health care setting will become commonplace and a circumstance that nurses should be prepared for as students.

RESEARCH AND KNOWLEDGE DEVELOPMENT

The development of nursing knowledge requires evaluation of the effectiveness of various nursing interventions and the appropriateness of the decision-making process in selecting interventions to resolve a diagnosis or to achieve a particular outcome. The linkage work contained in this book provides numerous relationships that require testing and evaluation in a clinical setting. Questions about which of the suggested interventions achieve the best outcome for a particular diagnosis, which of the outcomes are most achievable for a particular patient population, and what diagnoses and interventions are associated with specific medical diagnoses are just a sample of the questions that can be addressed. Studies, such as the one by Peters (2000), which test the use of the outcomes and interventions with specific patient populations also add to the body of knowledge.

Empirical work, as just described, will build mid-range theories unique to nursing (Blegen & Tripp-Reimer, 1997a; 1997b). The labels as defined in the taxonomies provide the concepts; the linkages among the diagnoses, interventions, and outcomes provide the connections between the concepts. As this work unfolds, we will have a clear articulation between theory, practice, and research, and this will build the body of knowledge unique to the discipline.

As well as studying the relationships between interventions and outcomes, the relationships among the environment, the structure of the health care organization, the processes of care, and the patient outcomes need to be studied. Without this type of data, organizations have little information on which to adjust staff mix or determine the cost-effectiveness of structural or process changes in the nursing care delivery system. Issues related to the study of organizational factors that influence patient outcomes have gained increased emphasis in recent literature. The November 1997 supplement (Vol. 35, No. 11) of *Medical Care,* the Official Journal of the Medical Care Section of the American Public Health Association, is devoted to a discussion of these factors.

Identification of patient factors that influence outcome attainment, referred to as risk factors, is another area that needs to be studied to carry out effectiveness research related to nursing interventions. These factors need to be identified to reduce or remove the effects of confounding factors in studies where the cases are not randomly assigned to different treatments, as is typical in most effectiveness research (Iezzoni, 1997). Identification of the personal factors that influence outcome achievement for a particular diagnosis or the effectiveness of an intervention for patients with various personal characteristics and life circumstances will add to the body of nursing knowledge and allow nurses to provide the highest quality of care possible. As effectiveness research and evidence-based practice gains momentum in nursing, both organizational and personal factors that need to be considered in the analysis of data are being identified in the literature (Johnson, 2002; Titler, Dochterman, & Reed, 2004).

Professional practice languages and classification systems are the fundamental categories of thought that define a profession and its scope of practice. Although the nursing profession has made considerable progress in developing languages and classification systems, there is a need to use the languages to promote knowledge development. It is hoped that these linkages will suggest questions for study, including comparisons of the various languages currently used in nursing.

References

American Nurses Association. (1997). Nursing informatics & data set evaluation center (NIDSEC) standards and scoring guidelines. Washington, DC: Author.

Blegen, M.A., & Tripp-Reimer, T. (1997a). Implications of nursing taxonomies for middle-range theory development. *Advances in Nursing Science*, 19(3), 37-49.

Blegen, M. A., & Tripp-Reimer, T. (1997b). Nursing theory, nursing research, and nursing practice: Connected or separate? In McCloskey, J. C., & Grace, H. K. (Eds.). *Current issues in nursing* (5th ed.). (pp. 68-74). St. Louis: Mosby.

Bulechek, G. M., & McCloskey, J. C. (Eds.). (1999). *Nursing interventions: Essential nursing treatments* (3rd ed.). Philadelphia: W.B. Saunders.

Center for Nursing Classification & Clinical Effectiveness. (2001). *Estimated time and educational requirements to perform 486 nursing interventions.* Iowa City, IA: Center for Nursing Classification & Clinical Effectiveness, The University of Iowa College of Nursing.

Dochterman, J. M., & Bulechek, G. M. (2004). *Nursing interventions classification (NIC).* (4th ed.). St. Louis: Mosby.

Finesilver, C., & Metzler, D. (Eds.). (2002). *Curriculum guide for implementation of NANDA, NIC, and NOC into an undergraduate nursing curriculum.* Iowa City, IA: Center for Nursing Classification and Clinical Effectiveness, The University of Iowa College of Nursing.

Iezzoni, L. I. (1997). Dimensions of risk. In Iezzoni, L. I. (Ed.). *Risk adjustment for measuring healthcare outcomes.* (2nd ed.). (pp. 43-115). Chicago: Health Administration Press.

Iowa Interventions Project. (1997). Proposal to bring nursing into the information age. *Image: Journal of Nursing Scholarship*, 29(3), 275-281.

Johnson, M. (2002). Tools and systems for improved outcomes: Variables for outcomes analysis. *Outcomes Management* 6(3), 95-98.

Johnson, M., Moorhead, S., Maas, M., & Reed, D. (2003). Evaluation of the sensitivity and use of the nursing outcomes classification. *Journal of Nursing Measurement*, 11(2), 119-134.

Jones, D. L. (1997). Building the information infrastructure required for managed care. *Image: Journal of Nursing Scholarship*, 29(4), 377-382.

Keenan, G., & Aquilino, M.L. (1998). Standardized nomenclatures: Keys to continuity of care, nursing accountability and nursing effectiveness. *Outcomes Management for Nursing Practice*, 2(2), 81-85.

Moorhead, S., & Johnson, M. (2004). Diagnostic-specific outcomes and nursing effectiveness research. *International Journal of Nursing Terminologies and Classifications*, 15(2), 49-57.

Murnaghan, H. (1978). Uniform basic data sets for health statistical systems. *International Journal of Epidemiology*, 7, 263-269.

National Center for Nursing Research. (1988, January 27-29). Report on the national nursing research agenda for the participants in the conference on research priorities in nursing science. Washington, DC: National Center for Nursing Research.

Pesut, D. J., & Herman, J. (1999). *Clinical reasoning: The art & science of critical & creative thinking.* Boston: Delmar Publishers.

Peters, R. M. (2000). Using NOC outcome of risk control in prevention, early detection, and control of hypertension. *Outcomes Management for Nursing Practice*, 4(1), 39-45.

Rubenfeld, M. G., & Scheffer, B. K. (1999). *Critical thinking in nursing: An interactive approach* (2nd ed.). Philadelphia: Lippincott.

Scherb, C.A. (2002). Outcomes research: Making a difference. *Outcomes Management*, 6(1), 22-26.

Supplement. (1997). *Medical Care, the Official Journal of the Medical Care Section of the American Public Health Association,* 35:11.

Titler, M., Dochterman, J., & Reed, D. (2004). *Guideline for conducting effectiveness research in nursing & other health care services.* Iowa City, IA: Center for Nursing Classification & Effectiveness, The University of Iowa College of Nursing.

Yura, H., & Walsh, M. B. (1973). *The nursing process: Assessing, planning, implementing, evaluating* (2nd ed.). New York: Appleton-Century-Crofts.

CASE STUDY 3–1

Casey Schumacher, R.N., M.S.N., A.R.N.P., doctoral candidate

JC is an 82-year-old Caucasian male with a history of chronic obstructive pulmonary disease (COPD) and congestive heart failure (CHF). JC's 87-year-old wife prepares his meals and assists him with activities of daily living. JC is unable to attend to his personal care independently. JC's neurologic status is within normal limits. Vital signs are: blood pressure 144/88 mm Hg, afebrile, apical pulse 108 and regular, respirations of 38 per minute, slightly labored at rest. JC is wearing nasal oxygen at 2 liters per minute. Breath sounds are diminished in the bases with crackles noted in the right upper lobe (RUL), although the crackles cleared with cough. JC's wife stated he is taking his medication routinely, displaying the system she had organized to keep up with his QID schedule. JC's inhalers were not found with his scheduled medications. His wife explained that JC kept his inhalers by his recliner and only took them when he felt he could not breathe. JC's wife and JC shared their concerns regarding the expense of taking the inhalers as prescribed. JC has a history of four readmissions to the hospital in the last 3 months related to respiratory difficulties.

PLAN OF CARE FOR JC

Nursing Diagnosis	Nursing Outcomes	Nursing Interventions
Ineffective Health Maintenance	**Health Beliefs: Perceived Resources**	**Case Management**
Defining Characteristics: Reported lack of financial resources Lack of knowledge regarding health practice (e.g., importance of using inhaler as ordered) **Related Factors:** Lack of material resources	**Scale:** Very weak [1] to very strong [5] **Indicators:** Perceived adequacy of personal finances Perceived adequacy of health insurance Perceived access to prescribed medications	**Activities:** Explain role of the case manager to patient and family Develop relationships with patient, family, and other health care providers Use effective communication skills with patient, family, and other health care providers Treat patient and family with dignity and respect Maintain patient and family confidentiality and privacy Assess patient's physical health status, mental status, functional capability, formal and informal support systems, financial resources, and environmental conditions as needed Determine plan with input from patient and/or family

Case Study 3–1—cont'd

Nursing Diagnosis	Nursing Outcomes	Nursing Interventions
Ineffective Health Maintenance	Health Beliefs: Perceived Resources	**Case Management** **Activities:—cont'd** Discuss plan of care and intended outcomes with patient's primary provider Evaluate progress toward established goals on a continual basis Identify resources and/or services needed Coordinate provision of needed resources or services Coordinate care with other pertinent health care providers Encourage appropriate patient and/or family decision-making activities Monitor plan for quality, quantity, timeliness, and effectiveness of services Assist patient and/or family in accessing and navigating health care system Advocate for patient as necessary Promote efficient use of resources
	Knowledge: Medication **Scale:** None (1) to extensive (5) **Indicators:** Recognition of need to inform health care professional of all medications taken Description of actions of medication, especially inhaler Description of precautions for medications	**Teaching: Prescribed Medication** **Activities:** Instruct on the purpose and action of inhaler Review patient's knowledge of medication Inform of consequences of not taking medications Determine the patient's ability to obtain required medications Provide information on cost-saving programs Include family as appropriate

Continued

Case Study 3–1—cont'd

Nursing Diagnosis	Nursing Outcomes	Nursing Interventions
	Knowledge: Medication	Teaching: Prescribed Medication
	Indicators:—cont'd	
	Description of correct administration of medications	
	Description of how to obtain required medications	

Discussion of Case

The outcomes and interventions are aimed at the defining characteristics of the diagnosis: the lack of financial resources and lack of knowledge. The selection of the intervention is particularly appropriate, as the case manager can assess for other problems and plan to address them; this is especially important because of the inability of the patient to carry out functional activities and the age of his wife. Another diagnosis that might have been considered is Ineffective Therapeutic Management, with the defining characteristic being: Verbalizes difficulty with one or more prescribed regimens for the treatment of the illness. However, the problem does not appear to be with following the regimen except for the financial concern of purchasing medications, a defining characteristic of Ineffective Health Maintenance.

CASE STUDY 3–2

Casey Schumacher, R.N., M.S.N., A.R.N.P., doctoral candidate

Maria is a well-nourished, pregnant 29-year-old Hispanic woman, presenting to the free medical clinic for her first time at approximately 36 weeks of gestation. Maria speaks Spanish, requiring translator services. Maria's Hispanic husband works at the local meat packing plant on a seasonal basis; he speaks very limited English. Their 3-year-old son accompanied them. Both father and son appear to be well nourished, without obvious health issues. A Hispanic woman who had accompanied another patient provided translation. The usual translator, a matriarch in the community, was not present. The translator was able to communicate that Maria had only one prior pregnancy (G2P1ab0) delivered by cesarean section in Mexico. Records were requested, although the address provided from the patient via the translator was minimal. Maria was cooperative throughout the physical examination. No abnormal findings were noted. Vital signs were within normal limits (WNL). Measurements and an ultrasound evaluation were completed supporting the estimated delivery date. Laboratory work was collected and an appointment for the following week was scheduled. Instructions were provided through the translator regarding possible signs/symptoms for which Maria should call the physician immediately. Contact information was supplied. Maria was prescribed prenatal vitamins and instructed to keep them out of reach of children.

Maria kept her next appointment. On this visit, the matriarch was available for translation. Maria had a slight weight gain of 1.5 lbs., blood pressure was 128/86 mm Hg, no protein was noted in her urine, and nonpitting edema was noted in Maria's ankles. Maria stated she was experiencing a slight headache but did not want to take medication for the headache. Maria stated she had not been hungry today. She stated she was tired and would lie down when she finished fixing dinner for her family that evening. Routine prenatal examination and care was unremarkable. Marie was provided instructions should the headache persist; signs and symptoms of preeclampsia were reviewed with Maria. Contact information was again provided and an appointment was made for the following week.

Four days later Maria is admitted to the area hospital with elevated blood pressure of 172/108 mm Hg; 3+ pitting edema in her hand, forearms, and ankles; and a urine dipstick reveals protein spill. Maria arrives at the hospital with her husband and son and two other children. A translator from the hospital arrives and relays the fact that Maria has gone to bed in a dark room for the past three days except to fix her family meals. Maria has been unable to eat due to nausea and vomiting but refused to call in spite of concerns from her husband.

The following plan of care presents two diagnoses and related outcomes and interventions that might be appropriate for Maria.

Continued

CASE STUDY 3–2—cont'd

PLAN OF CARE FOR MARIA

Nursing Diagnosis	Nursing Outcomes	Nursing Intervention
Noncompliance: Prenatal	**Maternal Status: Antepartum**	**Prenatal Care**
Defining Characteristics: Behavior indicative of failure to adhere	**Scale:** Severe deviation from normal range (1) to no deviation from normal range (5)	**Activities:** Monitor blood pressure Monitor urine glucose and protein levels
Evidence of development of complications as noted below:	**Indicators:** Weight change Cognitive orientation Neurologic reflexes	Monitor ankles, hands, and face for edema Monitor deep tendon reflexes Monitor fetal heart rate
History of persistent headache, nausea, vomiting for several days	Blood pressure Apical pulse rate Urine protein	
Activity limited to lying down in darkened room for past two days	**Scale:** Severe (1) to none (5)	
Blood pressure 172/108 mm Hg; 3+ pitting edema in hands, forearms, and ankles	**Indicators:** Edema Headache Seizure activity	
Urine dipstick reveals protein spill	Nausea Vomiting	

CASE STUDY 3–2—cont'd

Nursing Diagnosis	Nursing Outcomes	Nursing Interventions
Noncompliance Prenatal	Maternal Status: Intrapartum	Intrapartal Care: High-Risk Delivery
Related Factors:	**Scale:**	**Nursing Activities:**
Knowledge related to prenatal care may be inadequate due to communication and cultural factors	Severe deviation from normal range (1) to no deviation from normal range (5)	Inform patient and support person of extra procedures and personnel to anticipate during birthing process
Gravidity 2, parity 1 Pregnancy previous cesarean delivery	**Indicators:** Blood pressure Apical heart rate	Communicate changes in maternal or fetal status to primary practitioner, as appropriate
Cultural barrier to communication	Urine output Cognitive orientation Neurologic reflexes	Prepare appropriate equipment Notify extra assistants to attend birth
	Scale: Severe (1) to none (5)	Provide assistance for gowning and gloving obstetrical team
	Indicators: Seizure activity	Use universal precautions Assist with administration of
	Headache Nausea	maternal anesthetic, as needed (e.g., intubation)
	Vomiting	Record time of birth
		Assist with neonatal resuscitation, as needed
		Document procedures
		Explain newborn characteristics related to high-risk birth
		Assist mother to recover from anesthetic
		Observe mother for postpartum complications

Continued

Case Study 3–2—cont'd

Nursing Diagnosis	Nursing Outcomes	Nursing Interventions
Impaired Verbal Communication	Client Satisfaction: Cultural Needs Fulfillment	Culture Brokerage
Defining Characteristics: Inability to speak dominant language	**Scale:** Not at all satisfied (1) to completely satisfied (5)	**Nursing Activities:** Facilitate use of a translator, accurate nonverbal communication
Related Factors: Cultural differences	**Indicators:** Use of creative methods to establish communication due to language differences	Provide information to other health care providers about the patient's language differences
	Respect for cultural health behaviors	Assist other health care providers to understand and accept patient's reasons for non-adherence
	Respect for personal values	Modify typical interventions (e.g., patient teaching) in culturally competent ways
	Incorporation of cultural beliefs health teaching	Appear relaxed and unhurried in interactions with the patient and family
	Care consistent with cultural beliefs	
	Respect for family members' participation in care	

Discussion of Case

Maria will most likely have a cesarean section soon after admission because of her symptoms and previous history of cesarean section. The medical diagnosis in this situation is likely to be preeclampsia, a diagnosis that requires immediate attention for the relief of symptoms. Noncompliance is one nursing diagnosis that can be selected based on the fact that her physical condition has deteriorated and complications have occurred. Although the development of symptoms was likely not related to Maria's behavior, her failure to follow directions to get medical attention for symptoms as she was instructed makes this an appropriate diagnosis for the patient. The outcomes and interventions selected are those related to immediate pre-delivery and delivery care, since the pregnancy is the condition for which she is receiving care.

Meridean Maas, R.N., Ph.D., F.A.A.N.

Mr. Lehman is an 80-year-old man, widowed for 10 years, who is residing in his own home. Mr. Lehman had a cholecystectomy when he was 65 and a transurethral resection of the prostate for benign hypertrophy when he was 70. He has been treated for congestive heart failure for the last 5 years, and during the last 3 months he has been taking 80 mg of Lasix each morning. Mr. Lehman has had reduced activity because of his cardiac decompensation and has experienced loss of strength and mobility for self-care activities. He has particular difficulty with small motor tasks, including putting on and removing his clothing. He often does not remove his clothing at night and resists changing his clothing more than once or twice a week. Frequently, the home health nurse or aide finds his underwear and trousers wet with urine. His voidings are usually in large amounts. He is a heavy coffee drinker and does not like decaffeinated coffee. Urinalysis revealed that the urine was clear of bacteria and fungi. Mr. Lehman reports that he knows when he has to urinate, but that emptying often comes before he has time to reach the toilet. He states that he has reduced his fluid intake other than coffee in an effort to reduce the need to urinate. Following a comprehensive assessment, the nurse documents the following signs and symptoms (defining characteristics) and etiologies for three primary urinary incontinence diagnoses; Urge Incontinence, Iatrogenic Incontinence, and Functional Incontinence.

Urinary Incontinence Diagnoses	Critical Signs and Symptoms	Etiologies/Related Factors
Urge Incontinence	Aware of need to void	Bladder irritation from caffeine
	Voids in large amounts	Limited fluid intake
	Low volume fluid intake	
	Large amount of coffee intake	
	Underclothing frequently wet	
Iatrogenic Incontinence	Taking diuretic (Lasix)	Effects of diuretic medication
Functional Incontinence	Difficulty removing clothing	Impaired mobility
	Loss of strength/mobility	
	Difficulty getting to toilet in time	

The nurse used several other significant defining characteristics to rule out other urinary incontinence nursing diagnoses. Mr. Lehman is aware of the need to void so a diagnosis of Reflex Incontinence is eliminated. The observation that Mr. Lehman voids in large amounts in fairly regular 2- to 3-hour intervals is not consistent with a diagnosis of Stress Incontinence.

The plan of care for Mr. Lehman is based on the nursing diagnoses and the desired nursing-sensitive outcomes and includes the nursing interventions selected

Continued

to achieve the outcomes. Mr. Lehman and the nurse agreed that he should be able to consistently demonstrate urinary continence, have a totally adequate fluid intake, be completely independent with his toileting self-care, and be knowledgeable about his medications. The primary NOC outcome for Mr. Lehman is Urinary Continence. Nursing interventions for his plan of care are selected to resolve or ameliorate the identified etiologies of his urinary incontinence diagnoses. The establishment of a predictable pattern of urination is most important to avoid an incontinent accident due to the inability to suppress urge. It is also important to monitor the timeliness of Mr. Lehman's response to urge and the adequacy of time needed to reach the toilet in the event a predictable pattern of voiding is not attained. Assessment of dryness of undergarments during the day and of bedding at night provides data needed to determine if there are any incontinent episodes. Mr. Lehman's ability to manage clothing independently is evaluated periodically to assess whether it continues to interfere with the time it takes him to respond to the urge to urinate. His self-care with toileting is monitored to evaluate both his abilities to get to and from the toilet and to remove clothing and to determine if any interventions are needed to prevent the loss of these abilities. Fluid intake is an essential outcome indicator to measure the dilution of urine and decreased bladder irritation. The amount of oral intake and avoidance of fluids that contain caffeine are important indicators for the outcome, Urinary Continence. Knowledge: Medication is an essential outcome because of the effect of Lasix on urine output and urgency and because of its role in the treatment of Mr. Lehman's congestive heart failure and should be measured weekly until he achieves the goal of substantial understanding. The other outcomes listed below for his plan of care should be assessed weekly for the first month and, depending on his progress, potentially assessed monthly or at longer agreed-on intervals.

The nurse discussed the nursing diagnoses of Urge, Iatrogenic, and Functional Incontinence with Mr. Lehman, explaining the factors that contributed to each, including the action of his medication. Mr. Lehman agreed that he desired to be continent and to increase his knowledge of his medication and improve his self-care in toileting in order to be continent. He and the nurse established the following plan to achieve the primary goal of reducing his incidents of incontinence.

NOC Outcomes and Indicators	Nursing Interventions and Activities
Urinary Continence	**Urinary Habit Training**
Scale:	Establish toileting interval not >2 hours
Never demonstrated (1) to	Maintain scheduled toileting
consistently demonstrated (5)	**Urinary Incontinence Care**
Responds in timely manner to urge	Instruct to drink not <1500 mL daily
Predictable pattern of voiding	Limit ingestion of bladder irritants
Ingests adequate amount of fluid	**Pelvic Muscle Exercise**
Free of fluid intake containing caffeine	Instruct patient to tighten, then relax, the
	ring of muscle around the urethra and anus

CASE STUDY 3–3—cont'd

Scale:
Consistently demonstrated (1) to
  never demonstrated (5)
Underclothing dry during day
Underclothing/bedding dry at night
Free of urine leakage between voidings

Instruct patient to avoid contracting the
  abdomen, thighs, and buttocks, and holding
  breath or straining down during the exercise
Perform exercises 50-100 times each day,
  holding contractions for 10 seconds each
Inform patient that it takes 6-12 weeks for
  exercise to be effective
Discuss daily record of continence with
  patient to provide reinforcement

Knowledge: Medication
Scale:
None (1) to extensive (5)
Description of action of medications

Teaching: Prescribed Medication
Instruct on purpose/action of each medicine
Instruct criteria to alter dose/schedule

Self-Care: Toileting
Scale:
Severely compromised (1) to not
  compromised (5)
Removes clothing
Gets to and from toilet

Self-Care Assistance: Toileting
Modify clothing
Provide rails and riser for bathroom stool
Monitor ambulation ability
Prescribe strengthening exercises

After Mr. Lehman understood the roles of caffeine and reduced fluid intake in causing his bladder to be irritated, he agreed to limit his coffee intake to 2 to 3 cups each day and to increase his total fluid intake to at least 1500 mL daily. He volunteered to try decaffeinated coffee and to drink noncitric juices and a beer with his evening meal. With his approval, the nurse sent a pair of his trousers to the local laundry to have Velcro fasteners placed on the fly instead of a zipper. Mr. Lehman also agreed to toilet himself at least every 2 hours in an attempt to avoid urgency and precipitance of urination. The nurse also trained Mr. Lehman to regularly perform pelvic floor exercises each time he toileted. The nurse reviewed Mr. Lehman's outcomes and indicators with him and together they rated his progress at each weekly visit. They agreed to monitor his progress monthly thereafter.

DISCUSSION OF CASE

This case study illustrates the decision-making process involved in arriving at a diagnosis. The indicators Underclothing dry during the day and during the night are reworded to fit the scale never demonstrated (1) to consistently demonstrated (5) rather than as a negative symptom that is scaled the opposite way. An additional indicator specific for this case is added: free of fluid intake containing caffeine. The case represents the use of three interventions with selected specific activities for one outcome.

Howard Butcher, R.N., Ph.D.

Constance R. is a 57-year-old married woman who was admitted to the inpatient psychiatric unit after being seen initially in an outpatient clinic by her primary care Advanced Practice Psychiatric Nurse Practitioner. Joan S., the ARNP-PMH had been seeing Constance once a week in the clinic for the last 9 weeks for increasing depressive symptoms. Constance lives with her husband, Mark, and her 22 year-old son, Kevin, in their own home. Six months ago she was laid off from her job where she had worked for 12 years. She has a history of chronic depression; however, her depression was well managed and under control until she lost her job. In the outpatient clinic she admitted that she was having periodic suicidal ideation in the form of a passive desire to die and upon admission to the inpatient unit was given the DSM-IV-TR diagnosis of Major Depression. She has a history of a previous overdose 6 years ago after the loss of her mother. She admits that she still struggles with grief and guilt over the loss of her mother, feelings which have intensified since the loss of her job. She repeatedly blamed herself for her mother's death and the loss of her job. The loss of her income has contributed to financial stress for the family. Constance has expressed feelings of worthlessness and uselessness since losing her job. Her husband states that she "cries all the time" and that "she was no longer doing any of her usual activities." She has not been able to cook, eat, do any of her usual household chores, or show much interest in her usual activities outside the home. Instead, she spends long periods in bed. She has lost 15 pounds in the last 2 months. During her admission interview, she stated, "this black cloud follows me wherever I go, nothing, nothing ever turns out right." "What future?" Constance said when asked what she envisioned for herself. "There is nothing ahead of me but a void … a darkness … I just might as well be dead." There is no history of alcohol or substance abuse. A summary of the information in this case showing the linkages among NANDA, NOC, and NIC follows.

CASE STUDY 3–4—cont'd

PLAN OF CARE FOR CONSTANCE R.

Nursing Diagnosis	Nursing Outcomes	Nursing Interventions
Risk for Suicide	Suicide Self-Restraint	Suicide Prevention
Risk Factors:	**Scale:**	**Activities:**
Verbal: Desires to die when stating, "There is nothing ahead of me but a void ... a darkness ... I just might as well be dead."	Never demonstrated (1) to consistently demonstrated (5)	Determine presence and degree of suicidal risk
Behavioral: History of a prior suicide attempt.	**Indicators** Refrains from attempting suicide	Determine if patient has available means to follow through with suicide plan
Situational: Job loss contributes to loss of autonomy/ independence and economic instability	Upholds suicide contract Discloses plan for suicide if present Seeks help when feeling self-destructive	Involve patient in planning her own treatment, as appropriate Administer medications to decrease anxiety, agitation, or psychosis and to stabilize mood, as appropriate
Psychological: Expressed feelings over loss of mother and history of depression.	Expresses feelings Expresses sense of hope Seeks treatment for depression	Monitor for medication side effects and desired outcomes Conduct mouth checks following medication administration to ensure that patient is not "cheeking" the medications for later overdose attempt
Social: Disrupted family life; loss of an important relationship; feelings of hopelessness.	Uses suicide prevention resources and social support groups within the community Plans for the future	Instruct patient in coping strategies as appropriate
		Contract with patient for "no self-harm" for a specified period, re-contracting at specified time-intervals
		Identify immediate safety needs when negotiating a no-self-harm or safety contract
		Assist the individual in discussing her feelings about the contract
		Observe individual for signs of incongruence that may indicate lack of commitment to fulfilling the contract
		Interact with the patient at regular intervals to convey caring and openness and to provide an opportunity for patient to talk about feelings

Continued

CASE STUDY 3–4—cont'd

Nursing Diagnosis	Nursing Outcomes	Nursing Interventions
Risk for Suicide	Suicide Self-Restraint	Suicide Prevention

Use direct, nonjudgmental approach in discussing suicide

Encourage patient to seek out care providers to talk as urge to harm self occurs

Avoid repeated discussion of suicide history by keeping discussions present and future oriented

Assist patient to identify network of supportive persons and resources (e.g., clergy, family, providers)

Initiate suicide precautions for the patient who is at serious risk of suicide

Place patient in least restrictive environment that allows for necessary level of observation

Continue regular assessment of suicidal risk (at least daily) in order to adjust suicide precautions appropriately

Consult with treatment team before modifying suicide precautions

Explain suicide precautions and relevant safety issues to the patient/family/significant others

Facilitate support of patient by family and friends

Refer patient to mental health care provider (e.g., psychiatrist or psychiatric/mental health advanced practice nurse) for evaluation and treatment of suicide ideation and behavior, as needed

Provide information about what community resources and outreach programs are available

Nursing Outcomes	Nursing Interventions
Depression Level	**Mood Management**
Scale:	Activities:
Severe (1) to none (5)	Administer self-report questionnaires
Indicators:	(e.g., Beck Depression Inventory,
Depressed mood	functional status scales) as
Loss of interest in	appropriate
activities	Monitor self-care ability
Negative life events	(e.g., grooming, hygiene, food/fluid
Lack of pleasure in	intake, elimination)
activities	Assist with self-care, as needed
Excessive guilt	Encourage patient to engage in
Feelings of	increasingly more complex decision-
worthlessness	making as he or she is able
Weight loss	Encourage patient to take an active
Recurrent thoughts of	role in treatment and rehabilitation,
death or suicide	as appropriate
Crying spells	Provide or refer for psychotherapy
Hopelessness	(e.g., cognitive behavioral,
Low self-esteem	interpersonal, marital, family,
Decreased activity level	group), when appropriate
	Interact with the patient at regular
	intervals to convey caring and/or
	to provide an opportunity for
	patient to talk about feelings
	Assist patient in identifying thoughts
	and feelings underlying the
	dysfunctional mood
	Limit amount of time that patient is
	allowed to express negative feelings
	and/or accounts of past failures
	Teach new coping and problem-
	solving skills
	Provide illness teaching to
	patient/significant others, if
	dysfunctional mood is illness based
	Provide guidance about development
	and maintenance of support
	systems (e.g., family, friends,
	spiritual resources, support
	groups, and counseling)

Continued

CASE STUDY 3–4—cont'd

Nursing Outcomes	Nursing Interventions
Depression Level	**Mood Management**
	Assist patient to anticipate and cope with life changes (e.g., job loss)
	Provide outpatient follow-up at appropriate intervals, as needed

DISCUSSION OF CASE

The primary concern and reason for Constance R.'s admission to the inpatient psychiatric unit is suicidal ideation. She has a number of strong risk factors including a past suicide attempt, increasing levels of depression, major losses, and decreased functioning. In addition to Risk for Suicide, other Nursing Diagnoses that should be included in her plan of care include Chronic Low Self-Esteem, Dysfunctional Grieving, and Ineffective Coping. However, the underlying issues of her depression can also be addressed by selecting the following Nursing Outcomes and indicators, which relate to the Risk for Suicide risk factors. In addition to more immediate and higher priority nursing interventions of Suicide Prevention and Mood Management, the nurse should consider Self-Esteem Enhancement, Coping Enhancement, and Grief Work Resolution as interventions to address the psychodynamic issues underlying her depression.

Nursing Outcomes	
Coping	Grief Resolution
Scale:	**Scale:**
Never demonstrated (1) to consistently demonstrated (5)	Never demonstrated (1) to consistently demonstrated (5)
Indicators:	**Indicators:**
Identifies effective coping	Resolves feeling about loss
Identifies ineffective coping patterns	Verbalizes acceptance of loss
Verbalizes sense of control	Discusses unresolved conflict(s)
Modifies lifestyle as needed	Reports decreased preoccupation with loss
Adapts to life changes	Maintains living environment
Uses effective coping strategies	Maintains grooming and hygiene
Reports decrease in negative feelings	Reports absence of sleep disturbance
Reports increase in psychological comfort	Reports adequate nutritional intake
	Reports involvement in social activities
	Progresses through stages of grief

Case Study 3–5

Mary Ann Tapper Strawhacker, R.N., B.S.N., M.P.H.

Ethan is an 8-year-old second grader attending public schools. He demonstrates above average aptitude on standardized testing. In just one semester, Ethan has missed 26 days of school due to complications of Cystic Fibrosis (CF). Unable to consume adequate calories, Ethan recently had a gastrostomy tube placed for night-time feedings. The site has healed well. Ethan requires pancreatic enzyme tablets with meals and snacks. Pulmonary treatments are usually performed at home; however, albuterol nebulizer treatments are required as needed. Ethan has spent the last 3 weeks hospitalized for a pseudomonas infection. He is recovering at home but is expected to return to school Monday. Ethan's mother recently quit her job as a clerk to care for Ethan full-time. His father is employed seasonally in construction. Ethan is the youngest of three children.

Discussion of Case

Ethan depicts a student with a medical disability who requires school health services to access public education. The severity of his CF affects his attendance, putting him at risk for school failure. His ongoing struggle to orally consume adequate calories has left him with little energy to expend for learning, interacting with peers, or fighting off infection. The intensity of his lung involvement adds to his fatigue and further weakens his immune response. The nursing diagnoses, outcomes, and interventions selected for this individual health care plan (IHP) address critical physiological needs. At the point at which this IHP was written, Ethan's survival was in question. Until these basic needs are met, Ethan cannot attain optimal health status or academic achievement. What makes caring for Ethan challenging is that his desire to attend school can often overshadow the severity of his disease. Unlike other students who want to go home when they feel ill, Ethan denies symptoms so he can stay in school. This can seriously jeopardize both his health and safety.

Ethan also presents with a host of potential psychological concerns related to altered body image, coping, and student role performance, to list a few examples. Unfortunately, in many schools, the reality of student-to-school nurse ratios is that potential concerns often do not become part of a student's formal IHP. Also, psychosocial concerns often must be referred to other practitioners within the school and private sector. They then assume the primary intervention role, and the school nurse becomes a consultant. Despite the fact that an IHP is the appropriate place to document referrals, consultations, and collaborations, as part of the comprehensive management plan, often this information is documented exclusively in progress notes.

Continued

CASE STUDY 3–5—cont'd

INDIVIDUAL HEALTH CARE PLAN

Name: Ethan M.

Building: Prairie Rose Elementary

Teacher: Mrs. F.

Parent/Guardian: Susan and Todd M.

Primary Physician: Dr. C.

Specialists: Dr. Z.

IHP Date: 09/17/03

Date of Birth: 01/08/95

Grade: 2nd

Day Phone: 1-555-555-8874 (Mom)

Cell Phone: 1-555-8823 (Dad)

Phone: 1-555-555-9997

Phone: 1-555-555-6000

Written by: Linda S., R.N, B.S.N.

Summary of Health Concerns: Ethan was born with a genetic defect that causes his body to produce thick sticky mucus and his pancreas not to function properly. Due to his health condition, Ethan coughs frequently to expel excess mucus, needs access to a private restroom, and requires medication prior to meals. Ethan is also susceptible to respiratory tract infections and may have absences due to illnesses and treatment.

CASE STUDY 3-5—cont'd

Assessment	Nursing Diagnosis	Goal	Nursing Interventions	Nursing Outcomes
• Ethan says he is hungry and takes adequate food and snacks but, after a few bites, says he is full. • Ethan has difficulty remembering to come to the health office to take his pancreatic enzymes. Teacher often forgets to remind him until after lunch. • Mother reports difficulty with both fluid and caloric intake at home. Tube feeding times have been adjusted. Currently feeding starts at 9 P.M. and runs until 7:30 A.M. Ethan is not hungry in the morning at home.	*Imbalanced Nutrition: Less Than Body Requirements (NANDA)* related to inadequate absorption of nutrients and inadequate intake	Ethan will consume half of his minimum recommended oral caloric and fluid intake during the school day, improving his rating (NOC 1008) from one to three by June 6, 2003	*Nutrition Therapy 1120 (NIC)* 1. Obtain a signed release(s) of information to facilitate communication between physician, clinical dietitian, and school nurse. 2. Request written dietary recommendation from the dietitian/physician. 3. Collaborate with student, parent, and and dietitian/physician to identify preferential, high calorie, nutritious snacks that may be consumed without leaving the classroom. 4. Facilitate monitoring classroom snack supplies weekly, storing perishable foods/beverages in health office refrigerator, and notifying parents when supplies need restocking at school.	*Nutritional Status: Food & Fluid Intake 1008 (NOC)* Oral food intake (100801) [1] Not adequate [2] Slightly adequate [3] Moderately adequate [4] Substantially adequate [5] Totally adequate Oral fluid intake (100803) [1] Not adequate [2] Slightly adequate [3] Moderately adequate [4] Substantially adequate [5] Totally adequate

Continued

CASE STUDY 3–5—cont'd

Assessment	Nursing Diagnosis	Goal	Nursing Interventions	Nursing Outcomes
• Parents provide snacks and high calorie beverages for use at school • Ethan continues to lose weight despite tube feedings. • Ethan willingly records his intake if asked.			5. In collaboration with Ethan and his parents, design and implement an incentive program to promote healthy behaviors. Target behaviors include, coming to the health office daily to take pancreatic enzymes, checking off his food and fluid intake on CF clinic's log, and refilling his water bottle once during the school day. 6. Provide information to family about new school breakfast program starting next month. *Nutritional Monitoring 1160 (NIC)* 1. Assist parent and clinic staff by weighing Ethan at school weekly. 2. Monthly, fax intake log and weekly weights to clinic, call parent to discuss progress, and send copy of log home to parent.	

CASE STUDY 3–5—cont'd

Assessment	Nursing Diagnosis	Goal	Nursing Interventions	Nursing Outcomes
• Ethan usually does well using his inhaler but occasionally needs reminders to wait 15 seconds between puffs. • Teachers report peers have asked many questions about his illness during Ethan's absence. Parents have agreed to allow general information regarding his condition to be shared with his class.	*Ineffective Airway Clearance (NANDA)* related to excessive mucus production North American Nursing Diagnosis Association (NANDA, 2003).	Ethan will be able to participate in physical activities with minimal signs of dyspnea, improving his rating (NOC 040204) from two to four by June 6, 2003 (Johnson, Maas, & Moorhead, 2000).	3. Monitor snack preferences and report to parent when preferences change. 4. Notify clinic for weekly weight loss greater than one pound. 5. Weekly tally fluid and caloric intake Ethan records on log to determine progress toward goal. *Airway Management 3140 (NIC)* 1 Perform chest percussion at school, per parent request, as needed after acute exacerbations. 2. Encourage Ethan to cough as needed throughout the school day to expel excess mucus (Ethan will continue to expectorate into a tissue and is encouraged to wash his hands in the room sink as needed afterwards.)	*Respiratory Status: Gas Exchange 0402 (NOC)* Dyspnea with exertion (040204) [1] Severe [2] Substantial [3] Moderate [4] Mild [5] None (Johnson, Maas, & Moorhead, 2000)

Continued

CASE STUDY 3–5—cont'd

Assessment	Nursing Diagnosis	Goal	Nursing Interventions	Nursing Outcomes
			3. Administer medications as ordered and monitor Ethan's inhaler technique to ensure proper use.	
			4. Encourage adequate fluid intake (see above).	
			5. With parental permission, peers will be given age-appropriate information regarding his condition and its implications at school.	
			6. Designated staff will be given information regarding his condition, need for accommodations, and potential implications for learning.	
			7. Designated staff will be trained to recognize Ethan's signs and symptoms of respiratory distress and to notify the school nurse immediately should these be observed at school (McCloskey & Bulechek, 2000).	

Johnson, M., Maas, M., & Moorhead, S. (Eds.). (2000). *Nursing Outcomes Classification (NOC)*. (2nd ed). St. Louis, MO: Mosby.
McCloskey, J. C., & Bulechek, G. M. (Eds.). (2000). *Nursing Interventions Classification (NIC)*. *(3rd ed)*. St. Louis, MO: Mosby.
NANDA International. (2003). *Nursing Diagnosis: Definitions & Classification 2003–2004*. Philadephia: Author.
Strawhacker, M., & Wellendorf, J. (2004). Caring for children with cystic fibrosis: A collaborative clinical and school approach. *Journal of School Nursing, 20*(1), 5-15.

PART II

NANDA, NOC, AND NIC LINKAGES

Introduction

This section of the book contains the linkages described in the preceding chapters. The most convenient entry to the linkages is through a NANDA diagnosis. The user will locate the diagnosis of interest, and the suggested NOC outcomes and NIC interventions will appear with that diagnosis. The diagnoses are in alphabetical order; however, the first word represents the major concept in the diagnosis. For example, when looking for the diagnosis *Impaired Gas Exchange*, look for *Gas Exchange, Impaired*. When the NANDA diagnosis begins with impaired, ineffective, or imbalanced, those terms will appear at the end of the label name rather than at the beginning. The diagnoses that capture the risk for developing a problem are not included in the alphabetical list of diagnoses that represent an altered patient/client state but, instead, appear as a group following those diagnoses that capture existing patient problems or the potential for improvement.

The "risk for" diagnoses are also listed in alphabetical order, with the major concept at the beginning and the term *risk for* following. For example, *Risk for Imbalanced Fluid Volume* is presented as *Fluid Volume, Risk for Imbalanced*. The NANDA diagnoses that capture risk do not include the same elements as the diagnoses that capture existing problem states or the potential to enhance patient states. Diagnoses that represent existing problems include a definition, defining characteristics, and related factors; *risk for* diagnoses include a definition and risk factors. In general, the outcomes linked with the risk diagnoses are the outcomes that would be evaluated to determine if the state that the patient/client is at risk for has occurred. For example, the suggested outcomes for *Activity Intolerance, Risk for* include *Activity Tolerance, Endurance,* and *Energy Conservation*. The interventions that are linked to the outcome are those associated with promoting the patient state represented by the outcome. The major interventions for *Activity Tolerance* include *Energy Management* and *Exercise Promotion: Strength Training*. However, the authors recognize that to address the risk, interventions that treat the underlying risk factors must be selected. Because the risk factors associated with each diagnosis vary from a few to a lengthy list, the authors chose not to address each of the risk factors when providing linkages in this book. To assist the user, NANDA diagnoses that represent specific risk factors are identified at the end of each linkage. Outcomes and interventions linked to those diagnoses can be found by looking up the diagnosis of interest. NANDA diagnoses suggested for *Activity Intolerance, Risk for* include *Breathing Pattern, Ineffective*; *Cardiac Output, Decreased*; *Failure to Thrive, Adult*; *Fatigue*; *Gas Exchange, Impaired*; and *Health Maintenance, Ineffective*. The authors used the list of risk factors to identify NANDA diagnoses that, in their opinion, reflected the identified risk factors. It is important to note that in some instances the suggested diagnoses may not encompass all of the risk factors if there is not a NANDA diagnosis for a particular risk factor. For example, *Impaired Parenting, Risk for* includes a number of patient characteristics that the nurse must consider, but for which NANDA does not propose a specific diagnosis. Some of the characteristics identified as risk factors include legal difficulties, single parent, low educational level, and multiple births.

Diagnoses Linked to NOC and NIC

NURSING DIAGNOSIS: Activity Intolerance

DEFINITION: Insufficient physiologic or psychological energy to endure or complete required or desired daily activities.

Outcome	Major Interventions	Suggested Interventions	Optional Interventions

Activity Tolerance
 	
DEFINITION:
Physiologic response to energy-consuming movements with daily activities
	Activity Therapy
	Exercise Promotion:
	  Strength Training
	Exercise Therapy:
	  Joint Mobility
	Exercise Therapy:
	  Muscle Control
		Asthma Management
		Body Mechanics
		  Promotion
		Cardiac Care:
		  Rehabilitative
		Energy Management
		Environmental
		  Management
		Exercise Promotion
		Exercise Promotion:
		  Stretching
		Exercise Therapy:
		  Ambulation
		Exercise Therapy:
		  Balance
		Pain Management
		Teaching: Prescribed
		  Activity/Exercise
			Autogenic Training
			Biofeedback
			Dysrhythmia
			  Management
			Medication
			  Management
			Mutual Goal Setting
			Nutrition Management
			Oxygen Therapy
			Sleep Enhancement
			Smoking Cessation
			  Assistance
			Weight Management

Continued

Outcome	Major Interventions	Suggested Interventions	Optional Interventions
Endurance			
DEFINITION: Capacity to sustain activity	Activity Therapy Energy Management Exercise Promotion: Strength Training	Exercise Promotion Nutrition Management Sleep Enhancement Teaching: Prescribed Activity/Exercise	Asthma Management Cardiac Care: Rehabilitative Eating Disorders Management Environmental Management Environmental Management: Comfort Exercise Therapy: Ambulation Exercise Therapy: Balance Exercise Therapy: Joint Mobility Exercise Therapy: Muscle Control Mutual Goal Setting Oxygen Therapy Pain Management Weight Management
Energy Conservation			
DEFINITION: Personal actions to manage energy for initiating and sustaining activity	Energy Management Environmental Management	Activity Therapy Body Mechanics Promotion Environmental Management: Comfort Exercise Promotion Nutrition Management Sleep Enhancement Teaching: Prescribed Activity/Exercise	Exercise Therapy: Ambulation Exercise Therapy: Balance Exercise Therapy: Joint Mobility Exercise Therapy: Muscle Control Weight Management

Outcome	Major Interventions	Suggested Interventions	Optional Interventions
Physical Fitness			
DEFINITION: Performance of physical activities with vigor	Activity Therapy Energy Management Exercise Promotion: Strength Training	Body Mechanics Promotion Exercise Therapy: Ambulation Exercise Therapy: Balance Exercise Therapy: Joint Mobility Exercise Therapy: Muscle Control Self-Care Assistance: IADL Teaching: Prescribed Activity/Exercise Vital Signs Monitoring	Cardiac Care: Rehabilitative Therapeutic Play Weight Management
Psychomotor Energy			
DEFINITION: Personal drive and energy to maintain activities of daily living, nutrition, and personal safety	Energy Management Mood Management	Animal-Assisted Therapy Counseling Emotional Support Exercise Promotion Hope Instillation Medication Management Recreation Therapy Therapy Group	Art Therapy Music Therapy Grief Work Facilitation Guilt Work Facilitation Self-Esteem Enhancement Spiritual Support Visitation Facilitation

Continued

A

Outcome	Major Interventions	Suggested Interventions	Optional Interventions
Self-Care: Activities of Daily Living (ADL)			
DEFINITION: Ability to perform the most basic physical tasks and personal care activities independently with or without assistive device	Exercise Promotion: Strength Training Self-Care Assistance	Energy Management Exercise Promotion: Stretching Exercise Therapy: Ambulation Exercise Therapy: Balance Exercise Therapy: Joint Mobility Self-Care Assistance: Bathing/Hygiene Self-Care Assistance: Dressing/Grooming Self-Care Assistance: Feeding Self-Care Assistance: Toileting Self-Care Assistance: Transfer Teaching: Prescribed Activity/Exercise	Body Mechanics Promotion Case Management Exercise Promotion Exercise Therapy: Muscle Control
Self-Care: Instrumental Activities of Daily Living (IADL)			
DEFINITION: Ability to perform activities needed to function in the home or community independently with or without assistive device	Home Maintenance Assistance Self-Care Assistance: IADL	Consultation Energy Management Environmental Management Environmental Management: Home Preparation Referral	Body Mechanics Promotion Exercise Promotion: Strength Training Financial Resource Assistance

NURSING DIAGNOSIS: Adjustment, Impaired

DEFINITION: Inability to modify life style/behavior in a manner consistent with a change in health status.

Outcome	Major Interventions	Suggested Interventions	Optional Interventions
Acceptance: Health Status DEFINITION: Reconciliation to significant change in health circumstances	Anticipatory Guidance Coping Enhancement Emotional Support	Body Image Enhancement Counseling Decision-Making Support Grief Work Facilitation Hope Instillation Self-Awareness Enhancement Self-Modification Assistance Support Group Support System Enhancement Teaching: Disease Process Truth Telling	Anxiety Reduction Behavior Modification Presence Spiritual Support Values Clarification
Adaptation to Physical Disability DEFINITION: Adaptive response to a significant functional challenge due to a physical disability	Anticipatory Guidance Coping Enhancement	Body Image Enhancement Counseling Emotional Support Learning Facilitation Self-Care Assistance Self-Modification Assistance Self-Responsibility Facilitation	Grief Work Facilitation Home Maintenance Assistance Hope Instillation Pass Facilitation Self-Awareness Enhancement Self-Care Assistance: IADL Support Group Support System Enhancement Values Clarification

Continued

A

Outcome	Major Interventions	Suggested Interventions	Optional Interventions
Compliance Behavior DEFINITION: Personal actions to promote wellness, recovery, and rehabilitation based on professional advice	Behavior Modification Mutual Goal Setting Patient Contracting	Coping Enhancement Counseling Decision-Making Support Health System Guidance Learning Readiness Enhancement Self-Modification Assistance Self-Responsibility Facilitation Support System Enhancement Teaching: Disease Process Teaching: Individual Values Clarification	Case Management Culture Brokerage Family Involvement Promotion Family Mobilization Family Support Patient Rights Protection Teaching: Prescribed Activity/Exercise Teaching: Prescribed Diet Teaching: Prescribed Medication Teaching: Procedure/ Treatment Teaching: Psychomotor Skill
Coping DEFINITION: Personal actions to manage stressors that tax an individual's resources	Coping Enhancement Counseling Crisis Intervention	Anticipatory Guidance Anxiety Reduction Decision-Making Support Emotional Support Family Support Grief Work Facilitation Health System Guidance Hope Instillation Mutual Goal Setting Pain Management Role Enhancement Spiritual Support Support Group Values Clarification	Behavior Modification Body Image Enhancement Caregiver Support Family Therapy Mood Management Reminiscence Therapy Sibling Support Simple Relaxation Therapy Support System Enhancement Surveillance Therapy Group Truth Telling

Outcome	Major Interventions	Suggested Interventions	Optional Interventions
Health Seeking Behavior			
DEFINITION: Personal actions to promote optimal wellness, recovery, and rehabilitation	Decision-Making Support Health Education Values Clarification	Anticipatory Guidance Counseling Health System Guidance Learning Facilitation Learning Readiness Enhancement Mutual Goal Setting Patient Contracting Self-Awareness Enhancement Self-Modification Assistance Self-Responsibility Facilitation Smoking Cessation Assistance Substance Use Prevention Support Group Teaching: Safe Sex Weight Management	Bibliotherapy Culture Brokerage Emotional Support Teaching: Disease Process
Motivation			
DEFINITION: Inner urge that moves or prompts an individual to positive action(s)	Self-Modification Assistance Self-Responsibility Facilitation Values Clarification	Behavior Modification Coping Enhancement Counseling Decision-Making Support Mutual Goal Setting Patient Contracting	Family Involvement Promotion Humor Meditation Facilitation Role Enhancement Self-Awareness Enhancement Spiritual Support

Continued

Outcome	Major Interventions	Suggested Interventions	Optional Interventions
Psychosocial Adjustment: Life Change DEFINITION: Adaptive psychosocial response of an individual to a significant life change	Anticipatory Guidance Coping Enhancement	Behavior Modification Cognitive Restructuring Complex Relationship Building Counseling Emotional Support Role Enhancement Self-Awareness Enhancement Self-Esteem Enhancement	Decision-Making Support Dying Care Health Education Humor Relocation Stress Reduction Spiritual Support Support System Enhancement

A

NURSING DIAGNOSIS: Airway Clearance, Ineffective

DEFINITION: Inability to clear secretions or obstructions from the respiratory tract to maintain a clear airway.

Outcome	Major Interventions	Suggested Interventions	Optional Interventions
Aspiration Prevention			
DEFINITION: Personal actions to prevent the passage of fluid and solid particles into the lung	Airway Suctioning Aspiration Precautions Positioning	Airway Management Cough Enhancement Respiratory Monitoring Resuscitation: Neonate Surveillance Swallowing Therapy	Chest Physiotherapy Emergency Care Endotracheal Extubation
Respiratory Status: Airway Patency			
DEFINITION: Open, clear tracheobronchial passages for air exchange	Airway Management Airway Suctioning Asthma Management Cough Enhancement	Airway Insertion and Stabilization Anxiety Reduction Artificial Airway Management Aspiration Precautions Chest Physiotherapy Positioning Respiratory Monitoring Surveillance	Allergy Management Anaphylaxis Management Emergency Care Vital Signs Monitoring
Respiratory Status: Ventilation			
DEFINITION: Movement of air in and out of the lungs	Airway Management Respiratory Monitoring Ventilation Assistance	Airway Insertion and Stabilization Airway Suctioning Allergy Management Artificial Airway Management Aspiration Precautions Energy Management Infection Control Mechanical Ventilation Medication Administration: Inhalation Positioning	Acid-Base Monitoring Anxiety Reduction Asthma Management Chest Physiotherapy Cough Enhancement Fluid Monitoring Mechanical Ventilatory Weaning Oxygen Therapy Smoking Cessation Assistance Tube Care: Chest

NURSING DIAGNOSIS: Anxiety

DEFINITION: Vague uneasy feeling of discomfort or dread accompanied by an autonomic response (the source often nonspecific or unknown to the individual); a feeling of apprehension caused by anticipation of danger. It is an altering signal that warns of impending danger and enables the individual to take measures to deal with threat.

Outcome	Major Interventions	Suggested Interventions	Optional Interventions
Anxiety Level			
DEFINITION: Severity of manifested apprehension, tension, or uneasiness arising from an unidentifiable source	Anxiety Reduction Calming Technique	Active Listening Animal-Assisted Therapy Anticipatory Guidance Aromatherapy Coping Enhancement Dementia Management Dementia Management: Bathing Distraction Medication Administration Progressive Muscle Relaxation Security Enhancement Simple Guided Imagery Simple Relaxation Therapy Therapy Group	Anger Control Assistance Asthma Management Autogenic Training Counseling Crisis Intervention Emotional Support Humor Hypnosis Music Therapy Relocation Stress Reduction Support Group

Outcome	Major Interventions	Suggested Interventions	Optional Interventions
Anxiety Self-Control			
DEFINITION: Personal actions to eliminate or reduce feelings of apprehension, tension, or uneasiness from an unidentifiable source	Anxiety Reduction	Active Listening Anticipatory Guidance Autogenic Training Behavior Management Calming Technique Childbirth Preparation Coping Enhancement Counseling Dementia Management Examination Assistance Exercise Promotion Medication Administration Medication Prescribing Preparatory Sensory Information Presence Progressive Muscle Relaxation Security Enhancement Simple Guided Imagery Simple Relaxation Therapy Telephone Consultation	Animal-Assisted Therapy Art Therapy Biofeedback Distraction Environmental Management Guilt Work Facilitation Humor Hypnosis Meditation Facilitation Music Therapy Premenstrual Syndrome (PMS) Management Support Group Teaching: Preoperative Therapeutic Play Therapy Group
Concentration			
DEFINITION: Ability to focus on a specific stimulus	Anxiety Reduction Calming Technique	Anticipatory Guidance Behavior Management: Overactivity/ Inattention Learning Facilitation Learning Readiness Enhancement Reminiscence Therapy Simple Guided Imagery Simple Relaxation Therapy	Animal-Assisted Therapy Childbirth Preparation Cognitive Restructuring Relocation Stress Reduction Teaching: Individual

Continued

A

Outcome	Major Interventions	Suggested Interventions	Optional Interventions
Coping			
DEFINITION: Personal actions to manage stressors that tax an individual's resources	Anticipatory Guidance Coping Enhancement Emotional Support	Anxiety Reduction Calming Technique Counseling Crisis Intervention Grief Work Facilitation Grief Work Facilitation: Perinatal Death Guilt Work Facilitation Hope Instillation Humor Meditation Facilitation Presence Progressive Muscle Relaxation Simple Relaxation Therapy Spiritual Support Support Group	Animal-Assisted Therapy Art Therapy Childbirth Preparation Distraction Genetic Counseling Preparatory Sensory Information Recreation Therapy Reminiscence Therapy Self-Awareness Enhancement Sibling Support Therapeutic Play Therapy Group

NURSING DIAGNOSIS: Autonomic Dysreflexia

DEFINITION: Life-threatening, uninhibited sympathetic response of the nervous system to a noxious stimulus after a spinal cord injury at T7 or above.

Outcome	Major Interventions	Suggested Interventions	Optional Interventions
Neurological Status DEFINITION: Ability of the peripheral and central nervous system to receive, process, and respond to internal and external stimuli	Dysreflexia Management Vital Signs Monitoring	Emergency Care Medication Administration Neurologic Monitoring Respiratory Monitoring Seizure Precautions Surveillance Temperature Regulation	Code Management Teaching: Disease Process Teaching: Prescribed Medication Teaching: Procedure/ Treatment
Neurological Status: Autonomic DEFINITION: Ability of the autonomic nervous system to coordinate visceral and homeostatic function	Dysreflexia Management Vital Signs Monitoring	Bowel Management Emergency Care Medication Administration Medication Management Neurologic Monitoring Positioning Respiratory Monitoring Surveillance Urinary Elimination Management	Code Management Fever Treatment Infection Control Infection Protection Intravenous (IV) Insertion Intravenous (IV) Therapy Technology Management Temperature Regulation Urinary Catheterization Urinary Catheterization: Intermittent

Continued

A

Outcome	Major Interventions	Suggested Interventions	Optional Interventions
Sensory Function: Cutaneous			
DEFINITION: Extent to which stimulation of the skin is correctly sensed	Dysreflexia Management Skin Surveillance	Bowel Management Lower Extremity Monitoring Infection Control Neurologic Monitoring Pain Management Positioning Pressure Management Pressure Ulcer Care Temperature Regulation Urinary Elimination Management	Infection Protection Pressure Ulcer Prevention Pruritus Management Vital Signs Monitoring
Vital Signs			
DEFINITION: Extent to which temperature, pulse, respiration, and blood pressure are within normal range	Dysreflexia Management Vital Signs Monitoring	Airway Management Anxiety Reduction Environmental Management Fluid Management Fluid Monitoring Medication Administration Medication Management Medication Prescribing Shock Prevention	Cough Enhancement Emergency Care Infection Protection Pain Management Teaching: Individual Teaching: Prescribed Medication

NURSING DIAGNOSIS: Body Image, Disturbed

DEFINITION: Confusion in mental picture of one's physical self.

Outcome	Major Interventions	Suggested Interventions	Optional Interventions
Adaptation to Physical Disability			
DEFINITION: Adaptive response to a significant functional challenge due to a physical disability	Body Image Enhancement Self-Esteem Enhancement	Active Listening Anticipatory Guidance Coping Enhancement Counseling Grief Work Facilitation Support Group	Anxiety Reduction Emotional Support Home Maintenance Assistance Pain Management Self-Care Assistance: IADL Socialization Enhancement Support System Enhancement Teaching: Disease Process
Body Image			
DEFINITION: Perception of own appearance and body functions	Body Image Enhancement	Active Listening Amputation Care Coping Enhancement Counseling Emotional Support Grief Work Facilitation Self-Awareness Enhancement Self-Care Assistance Self-Esteem Enhancement Support Group Support System Enhancement Therapy Group Values Clarification Weight Management	Anticipatory Guidance Anxiety Reduction Cognitive Restructuring Eating Disorders Management Nutritional Counseling Ostomy Care Pain Management Postpartal Care Prenatal Care Truth Telling Unilateral Neglect Management

Continued

Outcome	Major Interventions	Suggested Interventions	Optional Interventions
Child Development: 2 Years			
DEFINITION: Milestones of physical, cognitive, and psychosocial progression by 2 years of age	Developmental Enhancement: Child Parent Education: Childrearing Family	Anticipatory Guidance Family Involvement Promotion Nutrition Management Security Enhancement Socialization Enhancement	Abuse Protection Support: Child Behavior Management Bowel Training Nutritional Counseling Nutritional Monitoring Sibling Support Support System Enhancement Therapeutic Play Urinary Habit Training
Child Development: 3 Years			
DEFINITION: Milestones of physical, cognitive, and psychosocial progression by 3 years of age	Developmental Enhancement: Child Parent Education: Childrearing Family	Anticipatory Guidance Bowel Incontinence Care: Encopresis Bowel Management Bowel Training Family Involvement Promotion Nutrition Management Security Enhancement Socialization Enhancement Urinary Habit Training	Abuse Protection Support: Child Behavior Management Nutritional Counseling Nutritional Monitoring Sibling Support Therapeutic Play

Outcome	Major Interventions	Suggested Interventions	Optional Interventions
Child Development: 4 Years			
DEFINITION: Milestones of physical, cognitive, and psychosocial progression by 4 years of age	Developmental Enhancement: Child Parent Education: Childrearing Family	Anticipatory Guidance Family Involvement Promotion Nutrition Management Security Enhancement Self-Care Assistance Socialization Enhancement Therapeutic Play	Abuse Protection Support: Child Behavior Management Behavior Modification Bowel Incontinence Care: Encopresis Counseling Nutritional Counseling Nutritional Monitoring Sibling Support Urinary Habit Training Urinary Incontinence Care: Enuresis
Child Development: 5 Years			
DEFINITION: Milestones of physical, cognitive, and psychosocial progression by 5 years of age	Developmental Enhancement: Child Parent Education: Childrearing Family	Anticipatory Guidance Body Image Enhancement Family Involvement Promotion Nutrition Management Security Enhancement Self-Care Assistance Socialization Enhancement Therapeutic Play	Abuse Protection Support: Child Behavior Management Behavior Modification Counseling Nutritional Counseling Nutritional Monitoring Sibling Support Urinary Habit Training Urinary Incontinence Care: Enuresis

Continued

Outcome	Major Interventions	Suggested Interventions	Optional Interventions
Child Development: Middle Childhood DEFINITION: Milestones of physical, cognitive, and psychosocial progression from 6 years through 11 years of age	Developmental Enhancement: Child Parent Education: Childrearing Family Risk Identification	Abuse Protection Support: Child Anticipatory Guidance Body Image Enhancement Exercise Promotion Family Involvement Promotion Mutual Goal Setting Nutrition Management Nutritional Monitoring Patient Contracting Self-Awareness Enhancement Self-Esteem Enhancement Self-Modification Assistance Self-Responsibility Facilitation Substance Use Prevention Teaching: Sexuality Urinary Incontinence Care: Enuresis Values Clarification Weight Management	Behavior Management Behavior Modification Counseling Eating Disorders Management Nutritional Counseling Sibling Support Therapeutic Play

Outcome	Major Interventions	Suggested Interventions	Optional Interventions
Child Development: Adolescence			
DEFINITION: Milestones of physical, cognitive, and psychosocial progression from 12 years through 17 years of age	Developmental Enhancement: Adolescent Parent Education: Adolescent Risk Identification Self-Esteem Enhancement	Anticipatory Guidance Body Image Enhancement Eating Disorders Management Exercise Promotion Family Involvement Promotion Mutual Goal Setting Nutrition Management Nutritional Counseling Nutritional Monitoring Self-Awareness Enhancement Self-Modification Assistance Self-Responsibility Facilitation Socialization Enhancement Substance Use Prevention Teaching: Individual Teaching: Safe Sex Teaching: Sexuality Values Clarification Weight Management	Abuse Protection Support Behavior Management Behavior Modification Counseling Role Enhancement Sexual Counseling Sibling Support Spiritual Support Support System Enhancement

Continued

Outcome	Major Interventions	Suggested Interventions	Optional Interventions
Psychosocial Adjustment: Life Change			
DEFINITION: Adaptive psychosocial response of an individual to a significant life change	Anticipatory Guidance Coping Enhancement	Childbirth Preparation Counseling Developmental Enhancement: Adolescent Developmental Enhancement: Child Dying Care Emotional Support Grief Work Facilitation Health Education	Cognitive Restructuring Decision-Making Support Family Process Maintenance Humor Lactation Counseling Presence Spiritual Support
Self-Esteem			
DEFINITION: Personal judgment of self-worth	Self-Esteem Enhancement	Active Listening Body Image Enhancement Counseling Developmental Enhancement: Adolescent Developmental Enhancement: Child Eating Disorders Management Emotional Support Self-Awareness Enhancement Socialization Enhancement Support Group Weight Management	Assertiveness Training Behavior Modification Behavior Modification: Social Skills Bibliotherapy Complex Relationship Building Coping Enhancement Family Mobilization Parent Education: Adolescent Parent Education: Childrearing Family Security Enhancement Self-Modification Assistance Spiritual Support

NURSING DIAGNOSIS: Bowel Incontinence

DEFINITION: Change in normal bowel habits characterized by involuntary passage of stool.

Outcome	Major Interventions	Suggested Interventions	Optional Interventions
Bowel Continence			
DEFINITION: Control of passage of stool from the bowel	Bowel Incontinence Care Bowel Training	Bowel Incontinence Care: Encopresis Bowel Irrigation Bowel Management Diarrhea Management Flatulence Reduction Fluid Management Medication Management Nutrition Management Rectal Prolapse Management Self-Care Assistance: Toileting	Emotional Support Environmental Management Exercise Promotion Exercise Therapy: Ambulation Teaching: Prescribed Activity/Exercise Teaching: Prescribed Diet Teaching: Prescribed Medication Teaching: Procedure/ Treatment
Bowel Elimination			
DEFINITION: Formation and evacuation of stool	Bowel Incontinence Care Bowel Management Bowel Training	Bowel Incontinence Care: Encopresis Diarrhea Management Medication Management Nutrition Management Nutritional Monitoring Rectal Prolapse Management	Exercise Promotion Fluid Monitoring Medication Administration: Rectal Ostomy Care Teaching: Toilet Training
Tissue Integrity: Skin & Mucous Membranes			
DEFINITION: Structural intactness and normal physiologic function of skin and mucous membranes	Bowel Incontinence Care Perineal Care Skin Surveillance	Bathing Diarrhea Management Nutrition Management Ostomy Care Self-Care Assistance: Toileting	Medication Administration: Skin Medication Management

NURSING DIAGNOSIS: Breastfeeding, Effective

DEFINITION: Mother-infant dyad/family exhibits adequate proficiency and satisfaction with breastfeeding process.

Outcome	Major Interventions	Suggested Interventions	Optional Interventions
Breastfeeding Establishment: Infant			
DEFINITION: Infant attachment to and sucking from the mother's breast for nourishment during the first 3 weeks of breastfeeding	Breastfeeding Assistance Lactation Counseling	Attachment Promotion Calming Technique Newborn Care Parent Education: Infant Presence Teaching: Infant Stimulation	Infant Care Teaching: Infant Safety
Breastfeeding Establishment: Maternal			
DEFINITION: Maternal establishment of proper attachment of an infant to and sucking from the breast for nourishment during the first 3 weeks of breastfeeding	Breastfeeding Assistance Lactation Counseling	Anticipatory Guidance Fluid Management Infection Protection Nutrition Management Nutritional Counseling Positioning Skin Surveillance	Heat/Cold Application Support Group Teaching: Individual Teaching: Psychomotor Skill Weight Management

Outcome	Major Interventions	Suggested Interventions	Optional Interventions
Breastfeeding Maintenance			
DEFINITION: Continuation of breastfeeding for nourishment of an infant/toddler	Lactation Counseling	Energy Management Family Involvement Promotion Family Support Fluid Management Infant Care Infection Protection Nutrition Management Simple Relaxation Therapy Skin Care: Topical Treatments Skin Surveillance Sleep Enhancement Teaching: Infant Nutrition	Nutrition Therapy Support Group Teaching: Infant Stimulation Weight Management
Breastfeeding Weaning			
DEFINITION: Progressive discontinuation of breastfeeding	Lactation Suppression	Active Listening Anticipatory Guidance Emotional Support Family Involvement Promotion Family Support Skin Surveillance Teaching: Infant Nutrition	Breast Examination Heat/Cold Application Infection Protection Pain Management

NURSING DIAGNOSIS: Breastfeeding, Ineffective

DEFINITION: Dissatisfaction or difficulty a mother, infant, or child experiences with the breastfeeding process.

Outcome	Major Interventions	Suggested Interventions	Optional Interventions
Breastfeeding Establishment: Infant DEFINITION: Infant attachment to and sucking from the mother's breast for nourishment during the first 3 weeks of breastfeeding	Breastfeeding Assistance Lactation Counseling	Attachment Promotion Calming Technique Newborn Monitoring Parent Education: Infant Positioning Presence Surveillance Teaching: Infant Stimulation	Bottle Feeding Infant Care Kangaroo Care Nonnutritive Sucking Teaching: Infant Nutrition

Outcome	Major Interventions	Suggested Interventions	Optional Interventions
Breastfeeding Establishment: Maternal			
DEFINITION: Maternal establishment of proper attachment of an infant to and sucking from the breast for nourishment during the first 3 weeks of breastfeeding	Breastfeeding Assistance Lactation Counseling	Active Listening Analgesic Administration Anticipatory Guidance Anxiety Reduction Discharge Planning Emotional Support Environmental Management: Attachment Process Family Involvement Promotion Family Support Fluid Management Infection Protection Nutrition Management Parent Education: Infant Positioning Skin Care: Topical Treatments Skin Surveillance Teaching: Infant Nutrition Teaching: Infant Stimulation Teaching: Prescribed Diet	Cesarean Section Care Coping Enhancement Heat/Cold Application Pain Management Simple Relaxation Therapy Sleep Enhancement Support Group Teaching: Individual Telephone Consultation

B

Continued

Outcome	Major Interventions	Suggested Interventions	Optional Interventions
Breastfeeding Maintenance DEFINITION: Continuation of breastfeeding for nourishment of an infant/toddler	Breastfeeding Assistance Lactation Counseling	Active Listening Emotional Support Energy Management Family Involvement Promotion Family Support Fluid Management Infection Protection Nutrition Management Skin Care: Topical Treatments Skin Surveillance Sleep Enhancement Surveillance Teaching: Individual	Attachment Promotion Simple Relaxation Therapy Support Group Teaching: Infant Safety Teaching: Psychomotor Skill Weight Management
Breastfeeding Weaning DEFINITION: Progressive discontinuation of breastfeeding	Lactation Suppression	Active Listening Anticipatory Guidance Emotional Support Family Involvement Promotion Family Support Skin Surveillance Teaching: Infant Nutrition	Family Mobilization Heat/Cold Application Infection Protection Pain Management
Knowledge: Breastfeeding DEFINITION: Extent of understanding conveyed about lactation and nourishment of an infant through breastfeeding	Lactation Counseling	Breastfeeding Assistance Learning Facilitation Learning Readiness Enhancement Parent Education: Infant Teaching: Individual Teaching: Infant Nutrition Teaching: Infant Stimulation	Anticipatory Guidance Bottle Feeding Environmental Management: Attachment Process Nonnutritive Sucking

NURSING DIAGNOSIS: Breastfeeding, Interrupted

DEFINITION: Break in the continuity of the breastfeeding process as a result of inability or inadvisability to put baby to breast for feeding.

Outcome	Major Interventions	Suggested Interventions	Optional Interventions
Breastfeeding Maintenance DEFINITION: Continuation of breastfeeding for nourishment of an infant/toddler	Bottle Feeding Emotional Support Lactation Counseling	Coping Enhancement Family Support Fluid Management Health System Guidance Infection Protection Lactation Suppression Medication Management Nonnutritive Sucking Skin Care: Topical Treatments Skin Surveillance Teaching: Individual Teaching: Infant Nutrition	Active Listening Anticipatory Guidance Anxiety Reduction Attachment Promotion Behavior Modification Nutritional Counseling Pain Management Referral Simple Relaxation Therapy Support Group Wound Care
Breastfeeding Weaning DEFINITION: Progressive discontinuation of breastfeeding	Bottle Feeding Lactation Suppression	Anticipatory Guidance Anxiety Reduction Coping Enhancement Lactation Counseling Pain Management Skin Care: Topical Treatments Skin Surveillance Teaching: Infant Nutrition	Breast Examination Infection Protection Medication Management Nonnutritive Sucking

Continued

Outcome	Major Interventions	Suggested Interventions	Optional Interventions
Knowledge: Breastfeeding			
DEFINITION: Extent of understanding conveyed about lactation and nourishment of an infant through breastfeeding	Lactation Counseling Lactation Suppression	Bottle Feeding Learning Facilitation Learning Readiness Enhancement Parent Education: Infant Teaching: Individual Teaching: Infant Nutrition Teaching: Infant Stimulation	Anticipatory Guidance Environmental Management: Attachment Process Health System Guidance Nonnutritive Sucking
Parent-Infant Attachment			
DEFINITION: Parent and infant behaviors that demonstrate an enduring affectionate bond	Attachment Promotion Environmental Management: Attachment Process	Bottle Feeding Family Integrity Promotion Infant Care Kangaroo Care Parent Education: Infant	Anticipatory Guidance Anxiety Reduction Coping Enhancement Emotional Support Role Enhancement

NURSING DIAGNOSIS: Breathing Pattern, Ineffective

DEFINITION: Inspiration and/or expiration that does not provide adequate ventilation.

Outcome	Major Interventions	Suggested Interventions	Optional Interventions
Allergic Response: Systemic			
DEFINITION: Severity of systemic hypersensitive immune response to a specific environmental (exogenous) antigen	Airway Management Anaphylaxis Management Asthma Management	Airway Insertion and Stabilization Airway Suctioning Allergy Management Anxiety Reduction Emergency Care Medication Administration Medication Administration: Nasal Respiratory Monitoring Ventilation Assistance	Fluid Monitoring Mechanical Ventilation Presence Resuscitation Vital Signs Monitoring
Mechanical Ventilation Response: Adult			
DEFINITION: Alveolar exchange and tissue perfusion are supported by mechanical ventilation	Artificial Airway Management Mechanical Ventilation	Acid-Base Monitoring Airway Suctioning Anxiety Reduction Aspiration Precautions Mechanical Ventilatory Weaning Medication Management Neurologic Monitoring Pain Management Positioning Respiratory Monitoring	Emergency Care Emotional Support Endotracheal Extubation Energy Management Phlebotomy: Arterial Blood Sample Phlebotomy: Venous Blood Sample

Continued

Outcome	Major Interventions	Suggested Interventions	Optional Interventions
Mechanical Ventilation Weaning Response: Adult			
DEFINITION: Respiratory and psychological adjustment to progressive removal of mechanical ventilation	Mechanical Ventilation Mechanical Ventilatory Weaning	Acid-Base Monitoring Airway Suctioning Anxiety Reduction Emotional Support Medication Management Oxygen Therapy Positioning Respiratory Monitoring Vital Signs Monitoring	Aspiration Precautions Cough Management Energy Management Pain Management
Respiratory Status: Airway Patency			
DEFINITION: Open, clear tracheobronchial passages for air exchange	Airway Management Airway Suctioning	Airway Insertion and Stabilization Artificial Airway Management Aspiration Precautions Chest Physiotherapy Cough Enhancement Positioning Respiratory Monitoring Surveillance	Allergy Management Anaphylaxis Management Emergency Care Resuscitation Smoking Cessation Assistance

Outcome	Major Interventions	Suggested Interventions	Optional Interventions
Respiratory Status: Ventilation			
DEFINITION: Movement of air in and out of the lungs	Airway Management Respiratory Monitoring Ventilation Assistance	Airway Insertion and Stabilization Airway Suctioning Anxiety Reduction Artificial Airway Management Aspiration Precautions Cough Enhancement Oxygen Therapy Positioning Progressive Muscle Relaxation Vital Signs Monitoring	Acid-Base Monitoring Allergy Management Analgesic Administration Chest Physiotherapy Energy Management Exercise Promotion Pain Management Mechanical Ventilatory Weaning Tube Care: Chest
Vital Signs			
DEFINITION: Extent to which temperature, pulse, respiration, and blood pressure are within normal range	Respiratory Monitoring Vital Signs Monitoring	Acid-Base Management Airway Management Anxiety Reduction Fluid Management Intravenous (IV) Insertion Intravenous (IV) Therapy Medication Management Surveillance Ventilation Assistance	Allergy Management Emergency Care Oxygen Therapy Pain Management Postanesthesia Care Resuscitation Teaching: Prescribed Activity/Exercise Teaching: Prescribed Medication Teaching: Procedure/ Treatment

B

NURSING DIAGNOSIS: Cardiac Output, Decreased

DEFINITION: Inadequate blood pumped by the heart to meet metabolic demands of the body.

Outcome	Major Interventions	Suggested Interventions	Optional Interventions
Blood Loss Severity			
DEFINITION: Severity of internal or external bleeding/hemorrhage	Bleeding Reduction Hemorrhage Control Shock Management: Volume	Bleeding Reduction: Antepartum Uterus Bleeding Reduction: Gastrointestinal Bleeding Reduction: Nasal Bleeding Reduction: Postpartum Uterus Bleeding Reduction: Wound Fluid Management Fluid Monitoring Fluid Resuscitation Hemodynamic Regulation Shock Management Shock Management: Cardiac Shock Prevention Vital Signs Monitoring	Dysrhythmia Management Intravenous (IV) Therapy Invasive Hemodynamic Monitoring Pneumatic Tourniquet Precautions Resuscitation

Outcome	Major Interventions	Suggested Interventions	Optional Interventions

Cardiac Pump Effectiveness
 	
DEFINITION:
Adequacy of blood volume ejected from the left ventricle to support systemic perfusion pressure
	Cardiac Care
	Cardiac Care: Acute
	Hemodynamic
	  Regulation
	Shock Management:
	  Cardiac
		Acid-Base
		  Management
		Acid-Base Monitoring
		Airway Management
		Cardiac Care:
		  Rehabilitative
		Cardiac Precautions
		Code Management
		Electrolyte
		  Management
		Electrolyte Monitoring
		Fluid/Electrolyte
		  Management
		Fluid Management
		Fluid Monitoring
		Invasive Hemodynamic
		  Monitoring
		Medication
		  Administration
		Medication
		  Management
		Temporary Pacemaker
		  Management
		Vital Signs Monitoring
			Bleeding Reduction
			Blood Products
			  Administration
			Dysrhythmia
			  Management
			Electronic Fetal
			  Monitoring:
			  Antepartum
			Electronic Fetal
			  Monitoring:
			  Intrapartum
			Energy Management
			Fluid Monitoring
			Intravenous (IV)
			  Insertion
			Intravenous (IV)
			  Therapy
			Patient Rights
			  Protection
			Phlebotomy: Arterial
			  Blood Sample
			Phlebotomy:
			  Cannulated Vessel
			Phlebotomy: Venous
			  Blood Sample
			Resuscitation
			Resuscitation: Fetus
			Resuscitation: Neonate

Continued

Outcome	Major Interventions	Suggested Interventions	Optional Interventions
Circulation Status			
DEFINITION: Unobstructed, unidirectional blood flow at an appropriate pressure through large vessels of the systemic and pulmonary circuits	Circulatory Care: Arterial Insufficiency Circulatory Care: Mechanical Assist Device Circulatory Care: Venous Insufficiency	Bleeding Precautions Fluid Monitoring Fluid Resuscitation Hemodynamic Regulation Hypovolemia Management Laboratory Data Interpretation Shock Prevention	Autotransfusion Bedside Laboratory Testing Blood Products Administration Circulatory Precautions Intravenous (IV) Insertion Intravenous (IV) Therapy Invasive Hemodynamic Monitoring Peripherally Inserted Central (PIC) Catheter Care Pneumatic Tourniquet Precautions Shock Management: Vasogenic

Outcome	Major Interventions	Suggested Interventions	Optional Interventions
Tissue Perfusion: Abdominal Organs			
DEFINITION: Adequacy of blood flow through the small vessels of the abdominal viscera to maintain organ function	Circulatory Care: Arterial Insufficiency Circulatory Care: Venous Insufficiency Intravenous (IV) Therapy	Acid-Base Management Acid-Base Management: Metabolic Acidosis Acid-Base Management: Metabolic Alkalosis Acid-Base Monitoring Bedside Laboratory Testing Bleeding Precautions Electrolyte Management Electrolyte Monitoring Fluid Management Fluid Monitoring Hypovolemia Management Laboratory Data Interpretation Shock Prevention Surveillance Vital Signs Monitoring	Bleeding Reduction: Antepartum Uterus Bleeding Reduction: Gastrointestinal Bleeding Reduction: Postpartum Uterus Bleeding Reduction: Wound Blood Products Administration Emergency Care Fluid Resuscitation Hemodialysis Therapy Intravenous (IV) Insertion Intravenous (IV) Therapy

Continued

Outcome	Major Interventions	Suggested Interventions	Optional Interventions
Tissue Perfusion: Cardiac			
DEFINITION: Adequacy of blood flow through the coronary vasculature to maintain heart function	Circulatory Care: Arterial Insufficiency Shock Management: Cardiac	Anxiety Reduction Cardiac Care: Acute Circulatory Care: Venous Insufficiency Code Management Dysrhythmia Management Electrolyte Management Fluid Management Fluid Monitoring Medication Management Oxygen Therapy Pain Management	Bleeding Precautions Invasive Hemodynamic Monitoring Patient Rights Protection Shock Management: Vasogenic Shock Management: Volume Sleep Enhancement Temporary Pacemaker Management Visitation Facilitation Vital Signs Monitoring
Tissue Perfusion: Cerebral			
DEFINITION: Adequacy of blood flow through the cerebral vasculature to maintain brain function	Cerebral Perfusion Promotion Neurologic Monitoring	Fluid Management Fluid Monitoring Fluid Resuscitation Hypovolemia Management Positioning: Neurologic Seizure Precautions Shock Prevention	Cerebral Edema Management Code Management Seizure Management Vital Signs Monitoring

Outcome	Major Interventions	Suggested Interventions	Optional Interventions
Tissue Perfusion: Peripheral			
DEFINITION: Adequacy of blood flow through the small vessels of the extremities to maintain tissue function	Circulatory Care: Arterial Insufficiency Circulatory Care: Venous Insufficiency Embolus Care: Peripheral	Bleeding Precautions Bleeding Reduction Blood Products Administration Cardiac Care: Acute Circulatory Care: Mechanical Assist Device Circulatory Precautions Fluid Management Hemodynamic Regulation Hypovolemia Management Pneumatic Tourniquet Precautions Shock Prevention	Blood Products Administration Fluid Resuscitation Intravenous (IV) Insertion Intravenous (IV) Therapy Resuscitation Resuscitation: Fetus Resuscitation: Neonate Skin Surveillance
Tissue Perfusion: Pulmonary			
DEFINITION: Adequacy of blood flow through pulmonary vasculature to perfuse alveoli/ capillary unit	Circulatory Care: Arterial Insufficiency Embolus Care: Pulmonary	Acid-Base Management: Respiratory Acidosis Acid-Base Management: Respiratory Alkalosis Anxiety Reduction Fluid Management Fluid Monitoring Oxygen Therapy Respiratory Monitoring	Airway Management Code Management Pain Management Resuscitation Shock Management Vital Signs Monitoring

Continued

Outcome	Major Interventions	Suggested Interventions	Optional Interventions
Vital Signs			
DEFINITION: Extent to which temperature, pulse, respiration, and blood pressure are within normal range	Hemodynamic Regulation Vital Signs Monitoring	Acid-Base Management Anxiety Reduction Cardiac Care Dysrhythmia Management Electrolyte Management Fluid Management Hypovolemia Management Intravenous (IV) Therapy Medication Administration Medication Management Medication Prescribing Shock Prevention	Blood Products Administration Emergency Care Fluid Resuscitation Hemorrhage Control Malignant Hyperthermia Precautions Postanesthesia Care Postpartal Care Resuscitation Shock Management Surveillance

NURSING DIAGNOSIS: Caregiver Role Strain

DEFINITION: Difficulty in performing caregiver role.

Outcome	Major Interventions	Suggested Interventions	Optional Interventions
Caregiver Emotional Health DEFINITION: Emotional well-being of a family care provider while caring for a family member	Caregiver Support Coping Enhancement Respite Care	Anticipatory Guidance Counseling Decision-Making Support Emotional Support Family Integrity Promotion Hope Instillation Mood Management Presence Resiliency Promotion Self-Awareness Enhancement Spiritual Support Support System Enhancement	Anxiety Reduction Crisis Intervention Grief Work Facilitation Guilt Work Facilitation Humor Meditation Facilitation Recreation Therapy Substance Use Prevention

Continued

Outcome	Major Interventions	Suggested Interventions	Optional Interventions
Caregiver Lifestyle Disruption			
DEFINITION: Severity of disturbances in the lifestyle of a family member due to caregiving	Caregiver Support Coping Enhancement Respite Care	Assertiveness Training Decision-Making Support Emotional Support Family Support Health System Guidance Home Maintenance Assistance Mutual Goal Setting Role Enhancement Support Group Support System Enhancement Telephone Consultation	Case Management Family Integrity Promotion Family Involvement Promotion Family Process Maintenance Insurance Authorization Referral Resiliency Promotion
Caregiver-Patient Relationship			
DEFINITION: Positive interactions and connections between the caregiver and care recipient	Coping Enhancement Presence Role Enhancement	Active Listening Caregiver Support Complex Relationship Building Humor Mutual Goal Setting Reminiscence Therapy Socialization Enhancement Touch	Anger Control Assistance Conflict Mediation Forgiveness Facilitation Guilt Work Facilitation Teaching: Individual Visitation Facilitation

Outcome	Major Interventions	Suggested Interventions	Optional Interventions
Caregiver Performance: Direct Care DEFINITION: Provision by family care provider of appropriate personal and health care for a family member	Anticipatory Guidance Role Enhancement	Caregiver Support Dementia Management: Bathing Family Involvement Promotion Infant Care Learning Facilitation Medication Management Newborn Care Nutrition Management Pain Management Parent Education: Infant Parenting Promotion Teaching: Disease Process Teaching Prescribed Activity/Exercise Teaching: Prescribed Diet Teaching: Prescribed Medication Teaching: Procedure/ Treatment Teaching: Psychomotor Skill	Abuse Protection Support: Child Abuse Protection Support: Elder Infection Protection Lactation Counseling Respite Care Self-Care Assistance Self-Care Assistance: Bathing/Hygiene Self-Care Assistance: Dressing/Grooming Self-Care Assistance: Feeding Self-Care Assistance: IADL Self-Care Assistance: Toileting Self-Care Assistance: Transfer Teaching: Foot Care Teaching: Infant Nutrition Teaching: Infant Safety Teaching: Infant Stimulation Teaching: Toddler Nutrition Teaching: Toddler Safety Teaching: Toileting Training

Continued

Outcome	Major Interventions	Suggested Interventions	Optional Interventions
Caregiver Performance: Indirect Care			
DEFINITION: Arrangement and oversight by family care provider of appropriate care for a family member	Consultation Health System Guidance	Anticipatory Guidance Coping Enhancement Decision-Making Support Environmental Management Environmental Management: Comfort Environmental Management: Home Preparation Environmental Management: Safety Family Involvement Promotion Financial Resource Assistance Mutual Goal Setting	Assertiveness Training Culture Brokerage Family Presence Facilitation Family Process Maintenance Insurance Authorization Parenting Promotion Referral Respite Care Teaching: Individual Telephone Consultation
Caregiver Physical Health			
DEFINITION: Physical well-being of a family care provider while caring for a family member	Energy Management Nutrition Management	Body Mechanics Promotion Exercise Promotion Fluid Management Health Screening Oral Health Maintenance Respite Care Teaching: Individual Sleep Enhancement Weight Management	Anxiety Reduction Caregiver Support Premenstrual Syndrome (PMS) Management Progressive Muscle Relaxation Temperature Regulation Substance Use Prevention

Outcome	Major Interventions	Suggested Interventions	Optional Interventions
Caregiver Well-Being DEFINITION: Extent of positive perception of primary care provider's health status and life circumstances	Caregiver Support Respite Care Teaching: Individual	Coping Enhancement Family Involvement Promotion Family Mobilization Family Support Home Maintenance Assistance Hope Instillation Support Group Support System Enhancement	Active Listening Anticipatory Guidance Counseling Emotional Support Family Integrity Promotion Normalization Promotion Presence Resiliency Promotion

Continued

Outcome	Major Interventions	Suggested Interventions	Optional Interventions
Parenting Performance DEFINITION: Parental actions to provide a child a nurturing and constructive physical, emotional, and social environment	Attachment Promotion Parenting Promotion Role Enhancement	Developmental Care Developmental Enhancement: Adolescent Developmental Enhancement: Child Family Integrity Promotion: Childbearing Family Family Support Infant Care Normalization Promotion Parent Education: Adolescent Parent Education: Childrearing Family Parent Education: Infant Resiliency Promotion Teaching: Infant Nutrition Teaching: Infant Safety Teaching: Infant Stimulation Teaching: Toddler Nutrition Teaching: Toddler Safety Teaching: Toilet Training	Abuse Protection Support: Child Behavior Management: Overactivity/ Inattention Bowel Incontinence Care: Encopresis Breastfeeding Assistance Kangaroo Care Lactation Counseling Sibling Support Urinary Incontinence Care: Enuresis

Outcome	Major Interventions	Suggested Interventions	Optional Interventions
Role Performance			
DEFINITION: Congruence of an individual's role behavior with role expectations	Role Enhancement	Abuse Protection Support: Child Abuse Protection Support: Domestic Partner Abuse Protection Support: Elder Anger Control Assistance Anticipatory Guidance Behavior Modification Cognitive Restructuring Coping Enhancement Counseling Emotional Support Mood Management Substance Use Prevention Substance Use Treatment Support Group Values Clarification	Active Listening Decision-Making Support Family Integrity Promotion Family Therapy Financial Resource Assistance Home Maintenance Assistance Parenting Promotion Support System Enhancement Teaching: Individual

NURSING DIAGNOSIS: Communication, Impaired Verbal

DEFINITION: Decreased, delayed, or absent ability to receive, process, transmit, and use a system of symbols.

Outcome	Major Interventions	Suggested Interventions	Optional Interventions
Communication			
DEFINITION: Reception, interpretation, and expression of spoken, written, and non-verbal messages	Active Listening Communication Enhancement: Hearing Deficit Communication Enhancement: Speech Deficit	Anxiety Reduction Communication Enhancement: Visual Deficit Environmental Management Presence Touch	Art Therapy Bibliotherapy Culture Brokerage Relocation Stress Reduction Socialization Enhancement
Communication: Expressive			
DEFINITION: Expression of meaningful verbal and/or non-verbal messages	Communication Enhancement: Speech Deficit	Active Listening Anxiety Reduction Assertiveness Training Communication Enhancement: Hearing Deficit Communication Enhancement: Visual Deficit	Bibliotherapy Socialization Enhancement
Communication: Receptive			
DEFINITION: Reception and interpretation of verbal and/or non-verbal messages	Communication Enhancement: Hearing Deficit Communication Enhancement: Visual Deficit	Communication Enhancement: Speech Deficit Learning Readiness Enhancement	Active Listening Cognitive Stimulation Culture Brokerage Ear Care Environmental Management Eye Care Reality Orientation

Outcome	Major Interventions	Suggested Interventions	Optional Interventions
Information Processing DEFINITION: Ability to acquire, organize, and use information	Anxiety Reduction Memory Training	Cognitive Stimulation Decision-Making Support Dementia Management Learning Facilitation Learning Readiness Enhancement Reality Orientation Reminiscence Therapy	Cerebral Perfusion Promotion Cognitive Restructuring Fluid/Electrolyte Management Hallucination Management

NURSING DIAGNOSIS: Communication, Readiness for Enhanced

DEFINITION: A pattern of exchanging information and ideas with others that is sufficient for meeting one's needs and life goals and can be strengthened.

Outcome	Major Interventions	Suggested Interventions	Optional Interventions
Communication DEFINITION: Reception, interpretation, and expression of spoken, written, and non-verbal messages	Assertiveness Training Complex Relationship Building Socialization Enhancement	Active Listening Anxiety Reduction Culture Brokerage Development Enhancement: Adolescent Development Enhancement: Child Forgiveness Facilitation Humor	Bibliotherapy Environmental Management Family Integrity Promotion Mutual Goal Setting Self-Awareness Enhancement
Communication: Expressive DEFINITION: Expression of meaningful verbal and/or non-verbal messages	Assertiveness Training Communication Enhancement: Speech Deficit	Anxiety Reduction Complex Relationship Building Socialization Enhancement	Culture Brokerage Development Enhancement: Adolescent Development Enhancement: Child Self-Awareness Enhancement
Communication: Receptive DEFINITION: Reception and interpretation of verbal and/or non-verbal messages	Anxiety Reduction Communication Enhancement: Hearing Deficit	Communication Enhancement: Visual Deficit Environmental Management Learning Facilitation Presence Self-Awareness Enhancement	Culture Brokerage Development Enhancement: Adolescent Development Enhancement: Child Family Integrity Promotion

NURSING DIAGNOSIS: Community Coping, Ineffective

DEFINITION: Pattern of community activities (for adaptation and problem solving) that is unsatisfactory for meeting the demands or needs of the community.

Outcome	Major Interventions	Suggested Interventions	Optional Interventions
Community Competence			
DEFINITION: Capacity of a community to collectively problem solve to achieve community goals	Bioterrorism Preparedness Community Disaster Preparedness Community Health Development Environmental Management: Community	Conflict Mediation Environmental Management: Safety Environmental Management: Violence Prevention Environmental Risk Protection Fiscal Resource Management Health Policy Monitoring Program Development Risk Identification Surveillance: Community	Consultation Documentation Health Education Resiliency Promotion Sustenance Support Triage: Disaster Vehicle Safety Promotion
Community Disaster Readiness			
DEFINITION: Community preparedness to respond to a natural or man-made calamitous event	Bioterrorism Preparedness Community Disaster Preparedness	Environmental Risk Protection Program Development Surveillance: Community Triage: Disaster	Environmental Management: Safety Health Policy Monitoring Immunization/ Vaccination Management Risk Identification

Continued

Outcome	Major Interventions	Suggested Interventions	Optional Interventions
Community Health Status			
DEFINITION: General state of well-being of a community or population	Communicable Disease Management Community Health Development Health Screening	Environmental Management: Safety Environmental Management: Violence Prevention Environmental Risk Protection Health Education Immunization/ Vaccination Management Infection Control Risk Identification Surveillance: Community	Documentation Health Policy Monitoring Risk Identification: Genetic Sports-Injury Prevention: Youth Vehicle Safety Promotion
Community Health Status: Immunity			
DEFINITION: Resistance of community members to the invasion and spread of an infectious agent that could threaten public health	Immunization/ Vaccination Management	Communicable Disease Management Community Health Development Environmental Risk Protection Health Education Health Screening Infection Control Risk Identification Surveillance: Community	Documentation Health Policy Monitoring Program Development

Outcome	Major Interventions	Suggested Interventions	Optional Interventions
Community Risk Control: Chronic Disease			
DEFINITION: Community actions to reduce the risk of chronic diseases and related complications	Case Management Health Education Program Development	Community Health Development Environmental Risk Protection Health Policy Monitoring Health Screening Surveillance: Community	Documentation Environmental Management: Community Risk Identification
Community Risk: Communicable Disease			
DEFINITION: Community actions to eliminate or reduce the spread of infectious agents that threaten public health	Communicable Disease Management Immunization/ Vaccination Management	Health Education Health Policy Monitoring Health Screening Program Development Risk Identification Surveillance: Community	Documentation Infection Control
Community Risk Control: Lead Exposure			
DEFINITION: Community actions to reduce lead exposure and poisoning	Environmental Management: Community Environmental Risk Protection	Case Management Community Health Development Environmental Management: Worker Safety Health Education Program Development Risk Identification Surveillance: Community	Communicable Disease Management Documentation Health Screening Referral

Continued

Outcome	Major Interventions	Suggested Interventions	Optional Interventions
Community Risk Control: Violence			
DEFINITION: Community actions to eliminate or reduce intentional violent acts resulting in serious physical or psychological harm	Environmental Management: Community Environmental Management: Violence Prevention	Environmental Management: Safety Program Development Risk Identification Surveillance: Community	Abuse Protection Support Vehicle Safety Promotion
Community Violence Level			
DEFINITION: Incidence of violent acts compared with local, state, or national values	Environmental Management: Violence Prevention Surveillance: Community	Environmental Management: Community Environmental Management: Safety Environmental Risk Protection Program Development	Abuse Protection Support Health Policy Monitoring Vehicle Safety Promotion

NURSING DIAGNOSIS: Community Coping, Readiness for Enhanced

DEFINITION: Pattern of community activities for adaptation and problem solving that is satisfactory for meeting the demands or needs of the community but can be improved for management of current and future problems/stressors.

Outcome	Major Interventions	Suggested Interventions	Optional Interventions
Community Competence DEFINITION: Capacity of a community to collectively problem solve to achieve community goals	Bioterrorism Preparedness Community Disaster Preparedness Health Policy Monitoring Program Development	Environmental Management: Community Environmental Management: Violence Prevention Environmental Management: Worker Safety Environmental Risk Protection Fiscal Resource Management Health Education Health Screening Risk Identification Sports-Injury Prevention: Youth Vehicle Safety Promotion	Communicable Disease Management Community Health Development Health Screening Immunization/ Vaccination Management Resiliency Promotion
Community Disaster Readiness DEFINITION: Community preparedness to respond to a natural or man-made calamitous event	Community Disaster Preparedness Bioterrorism Preparedness	Health Policy Monitoring Program Development Risk Identification Surveillance: Community	Fiscal Resource Management Immunization/ Vaccination Management

Continued

Outcome	Major Interventions	Suggested Interventions	Optional Interventions
Community Health Status: Immunity			
DEFINITION: Resistance of community members to the invasion and spread of an infectious agent that could threaten public health	Immunization/ Vaccination Management	Community Health Development Health Education Health Policy Monitoring Health Screening Program Development Risk Identification Surveillance: Community	Bioterrorism Preparedness Communicable Disease Management Documentation Environmental Risk Protection Infection Control
Community Risk Control: Communicable Disease			
DEFINITION: Community actions to eliminate or reduce the spread of infectious agents that threaten public health	Communicable Disease Management Program Development	Health Education Health Policy Monitoring Health Screening Immunization/ Vaccination Management Risk Identification Surveillance: Community	Documentation Infection Control
Community Risk Control: Lead Exposure			
DEFINITION: Community actions to reduce lead exposure and poisoning	Environmental Management: Community Environmental Risk Protection	Community Health Development Environmental Management: Worker Safety Health Education Program Development Risk Identification Surveillance: Community	Bioterrorism Preparedness Documentation Health Screening Referral

Outcome	Major Interventions	Suggested Interventions	Optional Interventions
Community Violence Level			
DEFINITION: Incidence of violent acts compared with local, state, or national values	Environmental Management: Violence Prevention Surveillance: Community	Environmental Management: Community Environmental Management: Safety Health Policy Management Program Development Risk Identification	Documentation Vehicle Safety Promotion

C

NURSING DIAGNOSIS: Community Therapeutic Regimen Management, Ineffective

DEFINITION: Pattern of regulating and integrating into community processes programs for treatment of illness and the sequelae of illness that are unsatisfactory for meeting health-related goals.

Outcome	Major Interventions	Suggested Interventions	Optional Interventions
Community Competence DEFINITION: Capacity of a community to collectively problem solve to achieve community goals	Community Health Development Health Policy Monitoring Program Development	Communicable Disease Management Environmental Management: Community Environmental Risk Protection Health Education Health Screening Immunization/ Vaccination Management Risk Identification Surveillance: Community	Conflict Mediation Documentation Fiscal Resource Management Resiliency Promotion Surveillance: Safety

Outcome	Major Interventions	Suggested Interventions	Optional Interventions
Community Health Status			
DEFINITION: General state of well-being of a community or population	Community Health Development Environmental Management: Community	Communicable Disease Management Environmental Management Environmental Risk Protection Health Education Health Policy Monitoring Health Screening Immunization/ Vaccination Management Infection Control Program Development Risk Identification Surveillance: Community	Documentation Risk Identification: Genetic
Community Health Status: Immunity			
DEFINITION: Resistance of community members to the invasion and spread of an infectious agent that could threaten public health	Immunization/ Vaccination Management	Communicable Disease Management Community Health Development Environmental Risk Protection Health Education Health Screening Infection Control Risk Identification Surveillance: Community	Documentation Health Policy Monitoring Infection Protection Program Development

Continued

Outcome	Major Interventions	Suggested Interventions	Optional Interventions
Community Risk Control: Chronic Disease			
DEFINITION: Community actions to reduce the risk of chronic diseases and related complications	Health Education Program Development	Community Health Development Health Policy Monitoring Health Screening Risk Identification Surveillance: Community	Case Management Documentation Environmental Management: Community Environmental Risk Protection
Community Risk Control: Communicable Disease			
DEFINITION: Community actions to eliminate or reduce the spread of infectious agents that threaten public health	Communicable Disease Management Program Development	Health Education Health Policy Monitoring Health Screening Immunization/ Vaccination Management Risk Identification Surveillance: Community	Bioterrorism Preparedness Documentation Infection Control
Community Risk Control: Lead Exposure			
DEFINITION: Community actions to reduce lead exposure and poisoning	Environmental Management: Community Environmental Risk Protection	Community Health Development Health Education Health Policy Monitoring Program Development Risk Identification Surveillance: Community	Documentation Health Screening Referral

NURSING DIAGNOSIS: Confusion, Acute

DEFINITION: Abrupt onset of a cluster of global, transient changes and disturbances in attention, cognition, psychomotor activity, level of consciousness, and/or sleep/wake cycle.

Outcome	Major Interventions	Suggested Interventions	Optional Interventions
Cognitive Orientation			
DEFINITION: Ability to identify person, place, and time accurately	Delirium Management Delusion Management Reality Orientation	Acid-Base Management Anxiety Reduction Environmental Management: Safety Fall Prevention Hallucination Management Medication Administration Medication Management Pain Management Sleep Enhancement Surveillance: Safety	Calming Technique Fluid/Electrolyte Management Physical Restraint Presence Seclusion Self-Care Assistance Sleep Enhancement Touch
Distorted Thought Self-Control			
DEFINITION: Self-restraint of disruptions in perception, thought processes, and thought content	Delirium Management Delusion Management Hallucination Management	Anxiety Reduction Medication Management Reality Orientation	Calming Technique Environmental Management Surveillance: Safety

Continued

Outcome	Major Interventions	Suggested Interventions	Optional Interventions
Information Processing			
DEFINITION: Ability to acquire, organize, and use information	Cognitive Stimulation	Anxiety Reduction Calming Technique Delirium Management Delusion Management Medication Management Reality Orientation	Environmental Management Fluid/Electrolyte Management Hallucination Management Oxygen Therapy Pain Management Sleep Enhancement
Neurological Status: Consciousness			
DEFINITION: Arousal, orientation, and attention to the environment	Cerebral Perfusion Promotion Cognitive Stimulation Neurologic Monitoring	Airway Management Cerebral Edema Management Delirium Management Hyperglycemia Management Hypoglycemia Management Medication Administration Medication Administration: Intramuscular (IM) Medication Administration: Intravenous (IV) Medication Management Reality Orientation Seizure Precautions Surveillance Vital Signs Monitoring	Environmental Management Intracranial Pressure (ICP) Monitoring Mechanical Ventilation Patient Rights Protection Shock Management Substance Use Treatment Substance Use Treatment: Alcohol Withdrawal Substance Use Treatment: Drug Withdrawal Substance Use Treatment: Overdose

NURSING DIAGNOSIS: Confusion, Chronic

DEFINITION: Irreversible, long-standing, and/or progressive deterioration of intellect and personality characterized by decreased ability to interpret environmental stimuli; decreased capacity for intellectual thought processes; and manifested by disturbances of memory, orientation, and behavior.

Outcome	Major Interventions	Suggested Interventions	Optional Interventions
Cognition			
DEFINITION: Ability to execute complex mental processes	Cognitive Stimulation Dementia Management	Anxiety Reduction Area Restriction Decision-Making Support Dementia Management: Bathing Family Involvement Promotion Family Support Milieu Therapy Mood Management Reality Orientation Reminiscence Therapy Sleep Enhancement Surveillance: Safety	Anger Control Assistance Calming Technique Energy Management Environmental Management Fall Prevention Patient Rights Protection Recreation Therapy
Cognitive Orientation			
DEFINITION: Ability to identify person, place, and time accurately	Dementia Management Reality Orientation	Area Restriction Calming Technique Chemical Restraint Cognitive Stimulation Environmental Management: Safety Family Involvement Promotion Humor Medication Management Memory Training Physical Restraint Surveillance: Safety	Animal-Assisted Therapy Art Therapy Milieu Therapy Music Therapy Neurologic Monitoring Patient Rights Protection Presence Recreation Therapy Reminiscence Therapy Substance Use Treatment Visitation Facilitation

Continued

Outcome	Major Interventions	Suggested Interventions	Optional Interventions
Concentration			
DEFINITION: Ability to focus on a specific stimulus	Anxiety Reduction Cognitive Stimulation Dementia Management	Emotional Support Medication Management Presence Substance Use Treatment Touch	Calming Technique Environmental Management Relocation Stress Reduction Simple Relaxation Therapy
Decision-Making			
DEFINITION: Ability to make judgments and choose between two or more alternatives	Decision-Making Support Family Involvement Promotion	Emotional Support Health System Guidance Learning Facilitation Patient Rights Protection Support System Enhancement Teaching: Individual	Caregiver Support Case Management Family Support Health Care Information Exchange Multidisciplinary Care Conference
Distorted Thought Self-Control			
DEFINITION: Self-restraint of disruptions in perception, thought processes, and thought content	Delusion Management	Anxiety Reduction Cognitive Stimulation Hallucination Management Medication Management Milieu Therapy Mood Management Reality Orientation Therapy Group	Activity Therapy Animal-Assisted Therapy Art Therapy Environmental Management Memory Training Music Therapy Recreation Therapy

Outcome	Major Interventions	Suggested Interventions	Optional Interventions
Identity			
DEFINITION: Distinguishes between self and non-self and characterizes one's essence	Cognitive Restructuring Reality Orientation	Body Image Enhancement Medication Management Self-Awareness Enhancement Self-Esteem Enhancement Socialization Enhancement Spiritual Support Values Clarification	Dementia Management Environmental Management Environmental Management: Violence Prevention Family Mobilization Hallucination Management Milieu Therapy Therapy Group
Information Processing			
DEFINITION: Ability to acquire, organize, and use information	Cognitive Stimulation Decision-Making Support	Active Listening Calming Technique Dementia Management Learning Facilitation Learning Readiness Enhancement Medication Management Memory Training Reality Orientation	Anxiety Reduction Cerebral Perfusion Promotion Environmental Management Fluid/Electrolyte Management Hallucination Management Oxygen Therapy Pain Management Reminiscence Therapy Sleep Enhancement
Memory			
DEFINITION: Ability to cognitively retrieve and report previously stored information	Memory Training	Active Listening Cognitive Stimulation Learning Facilitation Milieu Therapy Reality Orientation Reminiscence Therapy	Bibliotherapy Cognitive Restructuring Coping Enhancement Learning Readiness Enhancement Medication Management Patient Rights Protection

Continued

Outcome	Major Interventions	Suggested Interventions	Optional Interventions
Neurological Status: Consciousness DEFINITION: Arousal, orientation, and attention to the environment	Cerebral Perfusion Promotion Neurologic Monitoring Reality Orientation	Cognitive Stimulation Dementia Management Environmental Management Environmental Management: Safety Laboratory Data Interpretation Medication Administration Medication Administration: Intramuscular (IM) Medication Management Patient Rights Protection Substance Use Treatment Surveillance Vital Signs Monitoring	Family Involvement Promotion Family Support Humor Seizure Precautions

NURSING DIAGNOSIS: Constipation

DEFINITION: Decrease in normal frequency of defecation accompanied by difficult or incomplete passage of stool and/or passage of excessively hard, dry stool.

Outcome	Major Interventions	Suggested Interventions	Optional Interventions
Bowel Elimination			
DEFINITION: Formation and evacuation of stool	Bowel Management Constipation/ Impaction Management	Bowel Irrigation Bowel Training Exercise Promotion Fluid Management Fluid Monitoring Medication Management Medication Prescribing Nutrition Management Nutritional Monitoring	Diet Staging Flatulence Reduction Medication Administration Medication Administration: Oral Medication Administration: Rectal Ostomy Care Pain Management Rectal Prolapse Management Self-Care Assistance: Toileting Skin Surveillance Specimen Management
Hydration			
DEFINITION: Adequate water in the intracellular and extracellular compartments of the body	Fluid Management Fluid/Electrolyte Management	Fluid Monitoring Intravenous (IV) Insertion Intravenous (IV) Therapy Medication Management Nutrition Management	Bottle Feeding Enteral Tube Feeding Feeding Fever Treatment

Continued

Outcome	Major Interventions	Suggested Interventions	Optional Interventions
Symptom Control			
DEFINITION: Personal actions to minimize perceived adverse changes in physical and emotional functioning	Constipation/ Impaction Management	Bowel Irrigation Bowel Management Exercise Promotion Fluid Management Medication Management Nutrition Management Rectal Prolapse Management	Anxiety Reduction Flatulence Reduction Pain Management Simple Relaxation Therapy

NURSING DIAGNOSIS: Constipation, Perceived

DEFINITION: Self-diagnosis of constipation and abuse of laxatives, enemas, and suppositories to ensure a daily bowel movement.

Outcome	Major Interventions	Suggested Interventions	Optional Interventions
Bowel Elimination			
DEFINITION: Formation and evacuation of stool	Bowel Management	Counseling Exercise Promotion Fluid Management Fluid Monitoring Medication Management Nutrition Management Teaching: Individual	Distraction Simple Relaxation Therapy Teaching: Prescribed Diet
Health Beliefs			
DEFINITION: Personal convictions that influence health behaviors	Health Education Values Clarification	Active Listening Behavior Modification Counseling Risk Identification Self-Modification Assistance	Culture Brokerage Learning Facilitation Learning Readiness Enhancement Mutual Goal Setting Patient Contracting Teaching: Individual
Knowledge: Health Behavior			
DEFINITION: Extent of understanding conveyed about the promotion and protection of health	Health Education Teaching: Individual	Learning Readiness Enhancement Teaching: Prescribed Activity/Exercise Teaching: Prescribed Diet	Active Listening Anxiety Reduction Emotional Support

NURSING DIAGNOSIS: Coping, Defensive

DEFINITION: Repeated projection of falsely positive self-evaluation based on a self-protective pattern that defends against underlying perceived threats to positive self-regard.

Outcome	Major Interventions	Suggested Interventions	Optional Interventions
Acceptance: Health Status DEFINITION: Reconciliation to significant change in health circumstances	Coping Enhancement Emotional Support Self-Awareness Enhancement	Body Image Enhancement Counseling Grief Work Facilitation Hope Installation Presence Self-Esteem Enhancement Spiritual Support Support Group	Active Listening Anticipatory Guidance Cognitive Restructuring Normalization Promotion Support System Enhancement Truth Telling Values Clarification
Adaptation to Physical Disability DEFINITION: Adaptive response to a significant functional challenge due to a physical disability	Body Image Enhancement Coping Enhancement Self-Esteem Enhancement	Active Listening Anticipatory Guidance Behavior Modification Cognitive Restructuring Counseling Mutual Goal Setting Self-Awareness Enhancement Self-Modification Assistance	Activity Therapy Emotional Support Hope Installation Security Enhancement Sexual Counseling Support Group

Outcome	Major Interventions	Suggested Interventions	Optional Interventions
Child Development: Adolescence			
DEFINITION: Milestones of physical, cognitive, and psychosocial progression from 12 years through 17 years of age	Self-Esteem Enhancement Self-Responsibility Facilitation	Body Image Enhancement Environmental Management Exercise Promotion Nutrition Management Nutritional Counseling Patient Contracting Role Enhancement Self-Awareness Enhancement Self-Modification Assistance Socialization Enhancement Spiritual Support	Cognitive Restructuring Counseling Eating Disorders Management Family Support Family Therapy Sexual Counseling Sibling Support Support System Enhancement Truth Telling Values Clarification Weight Management
Coping			
DEFINITION: Personal actions to manage stressors that tax an individual's resources	Coping Enhancement Counseling	Anxiety Reduction Calming Technique Complex Relationship Building Crisis Intervention Emotional Support Exercise Promotion Patient Contracting Self-Awareness Enhancement Socialization Enhancement	Behavior Modification Medication Management Mood Management Normalization Promotion Relocation Stress Reduction Reminiscence Therapy Spiritual Support Surveillance: Safety Therapy Group

Continued

Outcome	Major Interventions	Suggested Interventions	Optional Interventions
Self-Esteem			
DEFINITION: Personal judgment of self-worth	Self-Esteem Enhancement	Active Listening Body Image Enhancement Cognitive Restructuring Counseling Developmental Enhancement: Adolescent Developmental Enhancement: Child Emotional Support Self-Awareness Enhancement Socialization Enhancement Support Group Therapy Group	Assertiveness Training Behavior Modification Behavior Modification: Social Skills Complex Relationship Building Coping Enhancement Eating Disorders Management Family Mobilization Milieu Therapy Security Enhancement Self-Modification Assistance Spiritual Support Weight Management

Outcome	Major Interventions	Suggested Interventions	Optional Interventions
Social Interaction Skills			
DEFINITION: Personal behaviors that promote effective relationships	Behavior Modification: Social Skills Complex Relationship Building	Active Listening Assertiveness Training Behavior Management Counseling Developmental Enhancement: Adolescent Developmental Enhancement: Child Family Integrity Promotion Family Process Maintenance Recreation Therapy Role Enhancement Self-Awareness Enhancement Self-Esteem Enhancement Self-Responsibility Facilitation Socialization Enhancement Touch	Anger Control Assistance Anxiety Reduction Body Image Enhancement Coping Enhancement Culture Brokerage Family Support Family Therapy Forgiveness Facilitation Guilt Work Facilitation Humor Reminiscence Therapy Therapy Group Visitation Facilitation

NURSING DIAGNOSIS: Coping, Ineffective

DEFINITION: Inability to form a valid appraisal of the stressors, inadequate choices of practiced responses, and/or inability to use available resources.

Outcome	Major Interventions	Suggested Interventions	Optional Interventions
Acceptance: Health Status DEFINITION: Reconciliation to significant change in health circumstances	Coping Enhancement Emotional Support	Body Image Enhancement Counseling Grief Work Facilitation Hope Instillation Presence Self-Awareness Enhancement Self-Esteem Enhancement Spiritual Support Support Group	Active Listening Anger Control Assistance Anticipatory Guidance Normalization Promotion Support System Enhancement Truth Telling
Adaptation to Physical Disability DEFINITION: Adaptive response to a significant functional challenge due to a physical disability	Coping Enhancement Self-Esteem Enhancement	Active Listening Anger Control Assistance Anticipatory Guidance Anxiety Reduction Behavior Modification Body Image Enhancement Counseling Environmental Management	Activity Therapy Emotional Support Hope Instillation Security Enhancement Sexual Counseling Support Group

Outcome	Major Interventions	Suggested Interventions	Optional Interventions
Caregiver Adaptation to Patient Institutionalization			
DEFINITION: Adaptive response of family caregiver when the care recipient is moved to an institution	Coping Enhancement Emotional Support	Anxiety Reduction Caregiver Support Counseling Decision-Making Support Family Integrity Promotion Family Support Guilt Work Facilitation Support Group Visitation Facilitation	Anticipatory Guidance Grief Work Facilitation Reminiscence Therapy Spiritual Support
Child Adaptation to Hospitalization			
DEFINITION: Adaptive response of a child from 3 years through 17 years of age to hospitalization	Anticipatory Guidance Coping Enhancement Emotional Support	Active Listening Anxiety Reduction Behavior Modification Calming Technique Distraction Family Involvement Promotion Family Presence Facilitation Mutual Goal Setting Presence Security Enhancement Self-Modification Assistance	Environmental Management Family Support Preparatory Sensory Information Sibling Support Sleep Enhancement Trauma Therapy: Child

Continued

Outcome	Major Interventions	Suggested Interventions	Optional Interventions
Coping			
DEFINITION: Personal actions to manage stressors that tax an individual's resources	Coping Enhancement Counseling Decision-Making Support	Anticipatory Guidance Anxiety Reduction Calming Technique Caregiver Support Complex Relationship Building Crisis Intervention Delusion Management Dementia Management Distraction Emotional Support Meditation Facilitation Mood Management Pass Facilitation Presence Progressive Muscle Relaxation Reminiscence Therapy Resiliency Promotion Sleep Enhancement Support Group Support System Enhancement Therapy Group Touch	Activity Therapy Animal-Assisted Therapy Art Therapy Autogenic Training Behavior Management: Self-Harm Behavior Modification Biofeedback Cognitive Restructuring Family Therapy Grief Work Facilitation Grief Work Facilitation: Perinatal Death Humor Hypnosis Mutual Goal Setting Rape-Trauma Treatment Self-Awareness Enhancement Self-Esteem Enhancement Sibling Support Simple Relaxation Therapy Spiritual Support Substance Use Prevention Sustenance Support Trauma Therapy: Child

Outcome	Major Interventions	Suggested Interventions	Optional Interventions
Decision-Making			
DEFINITION: Ability to make judgments and choose between two or more alternatives	Decision-Making Support	Counseling Emotional Support Genetic Counseling Learning Facilitation Patient Rights Protection Support System Enhancement Teaching: Individual Values Clarification	Culture Brokerage Family Involvement Promotion Family Support Health Care Information Exchange Parent Education: Adolescent Parent Education: Childrearing Family Parent Education: Infant Self-Responsibility Facilitation Sexual Counseling Teaching: Prescribed Medication Teaching: Safe Sex

Continued

C

Outcome	Major Interventions	Suggested Interventions	Optional Interventions
Impulse Self-Control			
DEFINITION: Self-restraint of compulsive or impulsive behaviors	Coping Enhancement Impulse Control Training	Anger Control Assistance Anxiety Reduction Area Restriction Behavior Management Behavior Management: Self-Harm Behavior Management: Sexual Behavior Modification: Social Skills Elopement Precautions Environmental Management: Safety Environmental Management: Violence Prevention Fire-Setting Precautions Limit Setting Mutual Goal Setting Patient Contracting Seclusion Self-Modification Assistance Self-Responsibility Facilitation Substance Use Prevention	Emotional Support Medication Administration Mood Management Presence Risk Identification Security Enhancement Substance Use Treatment Support Group Support System Enhancement Surveillance: Safety Teaching: Safe Sex Therapy Group

Outcome	Major Interventions	Suggested Interventions	Optional Interventions
Knowledge: Health Resources			
DEFINITION: Extent of understanding conveyed about relevant health care resources	Anticipatory Guidance Health System Guidance	Case Management Coping Enhancement Decision-Making Support Financial Resource Assistance Learning Facilitation Teaching: Individual	Discharge Planning Patient Rights Protection
Psychosocial Adjustment: Life Change			
DEFINITION: Adaptive psychosocial response of an individual to a significant life change	Anticipatory Guidance Coping Enhancement	Anxiety Reduction Counseling Decision-Making Support Emotional Support Relocation Stress Reduction Role Enhancement Security Enhancement Self-Esteem Enhancement Spiritual Support Support Group Support System Enhancement	Animal-Assisted Therapy Environmental Management Reminiscence Therapy Sleep Enhancement Substance Use Prevention

Continued

Outcome	Major Interventions	Suggested Interventions	Optional Interventions
Risk Control: Alcohol Use			
DEFINITION: Personal actions to prevent, eliminate, or reduce alcohol use that poses a threat to health	Coping Enhancement Substance Use Prevention	Anxiety Reduction Behavior Management: Self-Harm Behavior Modification Counseling Crisis Intervention Health System Guidance Risk Identification Self-Modification Assistance Self-Responsibility Facilitation Substance Use Treatment Support Group	Family Involvement Promotion Grief Work Facilitation Guilt Work Facilitation Impulse Control Training Self-Esteem Enhancement Spiritual Support Support System Enhancement
Risk Control: Drug Use			
DEFINITION: Personal actions to prevent, eliminate, or reduce drug use that poses a threat to health	Coping Enhancement Substance Use Prevention	Anxiety Reduction Behavior Management: Self-Harm Behavior Modification Counseling Crisis Intervention Health System Guidance Risk Identification Self-Modification Assistance Self-Responsibility Facilitation Substance Use Treatment Support Group	Family Involvement Promotion Grief Work Facilitation Guilt Work Facilitation Impulse Control Training Self-Esteem Enhancement Spiritual Support Support System Enhancement

Outcome	Major Interventions	Suggested Interventions	Optional Interventions
Role Performance			
DEFINITION: Congruence of an individual's role behavior with role expectations	Role Enhancement	Anticipatory Guidance Behavior Modification Caregiver Support Cognitive Restructuring Counseling Emotional Support Parenting Promotion Self-Awareness Enhancement	Childbirth Preparation Decision-Making Support Health Education Parent Education: Adolescent Parent Education: Childrearing Family Parent Education: Infant Self-Esteem Enhancement Substance Use Treatment Support Group Support System Enhancement Sustenance Support

C

NURSING DIAGNOSIS: Coping, Readiness for Enhanced

DEFINITION: A pattern of cognitive and behavioral efforts to manage demands that is sufficient for well-being and can be strengthened.

Outcome	Major Interventions	Suggested Interventions	Optional Interventions
Acceptance: Health Status DEFINITION: Reconciliation to significant change in health circumstances	Coping Enhancement Support System Enhancement Teaching: Disease Process	Assertiveness Training Behavior Modification Complex Relationship Building Decision-Making Support Self-Awareness Enhancement Self-Modification Assistance Self-Responsibility Facilitation	Counseling Family Mobilization Family Therapy Financial Resource Assistance Genetic Counseling Role Enhancement Sexual Counseling Socialization Enhancement Spiritual Growth Facilitation
Adaptation to Physical Disability DEFINITION: Adaptive response to a significant functional challenge due to a physical disability	Anticipatory Guidance Coping Enhancement	Behavior Modification Decision-Making Support Self-Modification Assistance Self-Responsibility Facilitation Teaching: Individual Teaching: Prescribed Activity/Exercise	Body Image Enhancement Energy Management Exercise Promotion Grief Work Facilitation Learning Facilitation Role Enhancement Self-Care Assistance Self-Care Assistance: Bathing/Hygiene Self-Care Assistance: Dressing/Grooming Self-Care Assistance: Feeding Self-Care Assistance: IADL Self-Care Assistance: Toileting Self-Care Assistance: Transfer

Outcome	Major Interventions	Suggested Interventions	Optional Interventions
Coping DEFINITION: Personal actions to manage stressors that tax an individual's resources	Coping Enhancement Resiliency Promotion System Support Enhancement	Assertiveness Training Behavior Modification Complex Relationship Building Counseling Decision-Making Support Religious Ritual Enhancement Role Enhancement Self-Modification Assistance Self-Responsibility Facilitation	Family Mobilization Health Education Meditation Facilitation Relocation Stress Reduction Self-Awareness Enhancement Simple Guided Imagery Simple Relaxation Therapy Values Clarification
Personal Well-Being DEFINITION: Extent of positive perception of one's health status and life circumstances	Coping Enhancement Self-Awareness Enhancement	Decision-Making Support Health Education Health System Guidance Hope Instillation Role Enhancement Self-Esteem Enhancement Self-Modification Assistance	Aromatherapy Family Integrity Promotion Hormone Replacement Therapy Meditation Facilitation Premenstrual Syndrome (PMS) Management Risk Identification Simple Relaxation Therapy Socialization Enhancement

Continued

Outcome	Major Interventions	Suggested Interventions	Optional Interventions
Role Performance			
DEFINITION: Congruence of an individual's role behavior with role expectations	Coping Enhancement Role Enhancement	Anticipatory Guidance Childbirth Preparation Counseling Decision-Making Support Self-Awareness Enhancement Self-Modification Assistance Support System Enhancement Values Clarification	Caregiver Support Family Integrity Promotion Health Education Parent Education: Adolescent Parent Education: Childrearing Family Parent Education: Infant
Stress Level			
DEFINITION: Severity of manifested physical or mental tension resulting from factors that alter an existing equilibrium	Anxiety Reduction Coping Enhancement	Behavior Modification Counseling Decision-Making Support Relocation Stress Reduction Self-Modification Assistance Simple Relaxation Therapy Support Group	Aromatherapy Distraction Emotional Support Humor Meditation Facilitation Security Enhancement Self-Hypnosis Facilitation Spiritual Support

NURSING DIAGNOSIS: Death Anxiety

DEFINITION: Apprehension, worry, or fear related to death or dying.

Outcome	Major Interventions	Suggested Interventions	Optional Interventions
Acceptance: Health Status			
DEFINITION: Reconciliation to significant change in health circumstances	Coping Enhancement Emotional Support	Anticipatory Guidance Decision-Making Support Grief Work Facilitation Hope Instillation Presence Spiritual Support Support System Enhancement Values Clarification	Active Listening Referral Truth Telling
Anxiety Self-Control			
DEFINITION: Personal actions to eliminate or reduce feelings of apprehension, tension, or uneasiness from an unidentifiable source	Anxiety Reduction Dying Care	Active Listening Calming Technique Coping Enhancement Music Therapy Presence Simple Massage Simple Relaxation Therapy Spiritual Support Touch	Animal-Assisted Therapy Aromatherapy Bibliotherapy Meditation Facilitation Sleep Enhancement

Continued

Outcome	Major Interventions	Suggested Interventions	Optional Interventions
Comfortable Death			
DEFINITION: Physical and psychological ease with the impending end of life	Dying Care Pain Management Presence	Airway Management Analgesic Administration Bed Rest Care Energy Management Environmental Management: Comfort Family Presence Facilitation Medication Management Nausea Management Nutrition Management Nutritional Monitoring Oral Health Maintenance Patient-Controlled Analgesia (PCA) Assistance Positioning Self-Care Assistance Simple Guided Imagery Simple Massage Simple Relaxation Therapy Sleep Enhancement Vomiting Management	Aspiration Precautions Bathing Bowel Management Ear Care Eye Care Feeding Hair Care Oxygen Therapy Perineal Care Pruritus Management Skin Surveillance Therapeutic Touch

Outcome	Major Interventions	Suggested Interventions	Optional Interventions
Depression Level			
DEFINITION: Severity of melancholic mood and loss of interest in life events	Hope Instillation Spiritual Support	Bibliotherapy Dying Care Emotional Support Grief Work Facilitation Medication Management Mood Management Sleep Enhancement	Animal-Assisted Therapy Music Therapy Reminiscence Therapy Support System Enhancement
Dignified Life Closure			
DEFINITION: Personal actions to maintain control during approaching end of life	Decision-Making Support Dying Care	Anticipatory Guidance Anxiety Reduction Family Involvement Promotion Family Mobilization Forgiveness Facilitation Grief Work Facilitation Patient-Controlled Analgesia (PCA) Assistance Patient Rights Protection Spiritual Support Values Clarification	Active Listening Anger Control Assistance Animal-Assisted Therapy Bibliotherapy Caregiver Support Coping Enhancement Culture Brokerage Emotional Support Family Integrity Promotion Family Process Maintenance Family Support Music Therapy Organ Procurement Presence Reminiscence Therapy Spiritual Growth Facilitation Visitation Facilitation

Continued

Outcome	Major Interventions	Suggested Interventions	Optional Interventions
Fear Self-Control			
DEFINITION: Personal actions to eliminate or reduce disabling feelings of apprehension, tension, or uneasiness from an identifiable source	Coping Enhancement	Active Listening Anxiety Reduction Calming Technique Decision-Making Support Dying Care Emotional Support Family Mobilization Presence Spiritual Support	Animal-Assisted Therapy Caregiver Support Culture Brokerage Meditation Facilitation Pain Management Resiliency Promotion Simple Guided Imagery Simple Relaxation Therapy
Hope			
DEFINITION: Optimism that is personally satisfying and life-supporting	Hope Instillation Spiritual Support	Coping Enhancement Dying Care Emotional Support Grief Work Facilitation	Family Mobilization Mutual Goal Setting Presence Touch
Spiritual Health			
DEFINITION: Connectedness with self, others, higher power, all life, nature, and the universe that transcends and empowers the self	Religious Ritual Enhancement Spiritual Support	Dying Care Forgiveness Facilitation Grief Work Facilitation Guilt Work Facilitation Spiritual Growth Facilitation Values Clarification	Anxiety Reduction Hope Instillation Meditation Facilitation Presence Self-Awareness Enhancement

NURSING DIAGNOSIS: Decisional Conflict (Specify)

DEFINITION: Uncertainty about course of action to be taken when choice among competing actions involves risk, loss, or challenge to personal life values.

Outcome	Major Interventions	Suggested Interventions	Optional Interventions
Decision-Making			
DEFINITION: Ability to make judgments and choose between two or more alternatives	Decision-Making Support Mutual Goal Setting	Coping Enhancement Counseling Emotional Support Genetic Counseling Preconception Counseling Self-Awareness Enhancement Support System Enhancement Teaching: Individual Telephone Consultation	Culture Brokerage Health Care Information Exchange Health Education Health System Guidance Patient Contracting Preparatory Sensory Information Simple Guided Imagery Teaching: Sexuality Values Clarification
Information Processing			
DEFINITION: Ability to acquire, organize, and use information	Decision-Making Support Learning Facilitation	Active Listening Coping Enhancement Counseling Teaching: Individual	Anxiety Reduction Culture Brokerage Dementia Management Developmental Enhancement: Adolescent Environmental Management Music Therapy Reminiscence Therapy Sleep Enhancement

Continued

Outcome	Major Interventions	Suggested Interventions	Optional Interventions
Participation in Health Care Decisions			
DEFINITION: Personal involvement in selecting and evaluating health care options to achieve desired outcome	Decision-Making Support Health System Guidance	Active Listening Admission Care Anticipatory Guidance Assertiveness Training Counseling Culture Brokerage Discharge Planning Patient Rights Protection Self-Responsibility Facilitation Telephone Consultation Values Clarification	Anxiety Reduction Behavior Modification Caregiver Support Coping Enhancement Family Involvement Promotion Health Care Information Exchange Insurance Authorization Referral Sustenance Support
Personal Autonomy			
DEFINITION: Personal actions of a competent individual to exercise governance in life decisions	Assertiveness Training Decision-Making Support Health System Guidance	Anticipatory Guidance Behavior Modification Coping Enhancement Emotional Support Health Education Patient Rights Protection Role Enhancement Self-Awareness Enhancement	Conflict Mediation Learning Facilitation Mutual Goal Setting Resiliency Promotion Teaching: Individual

NURSING DIAGNOSIS: Denial, Ineffective

DEFINITION: Conscious or unconscious attempt to disavow the knowledge or meaning of an event to reduce anxiety/fear, but leading to the detriment of health.

Outcome	Major Interventions	Suggested Interventions	Optional Interventions
Acceptance: Health Status DEFINITION: Reconciliation to significant change in health circumstances	Coping Enhancement Counseling Emotional Support	Body Image Enhancement Crisis Intervention Decision-Making Support Hope Instillation Spiritual Support Support Group Support System Enhancement Truth Telling Values Clarification	Cognitive Restructuring Mutual Goal Setting Normalization Promotion Reality Orientation Reminiscence Therapy Self-Awareness Enhancement Therapy Group
Anxiety Self-Control DEFINITION: Personal actions to eliminate or reduce feelings of apprehension, tension, or uneasiness from anunidentifiable source	Anxiety Reduction	Active Listening Calming Technique Coping Enhancement Counseling Medication Administration Medication Prescribing Presence Recreation Therapy Security Enhancement Spiritual Support Support System Enhancement	Childbirth Preparation Decision-Making Support Environmental Management Family Therapy Guilt Work Facilitation Humor Milieu Therapy Support Group Therapeutic Play Therapy Group Truth Telling

Continued

Outcome	Major Interventions	Suggested Interventions	Optional Interventions
Fear Self-Control			
DEFINITION: Personal actions to eliminate or reduce disabling feelings of apprehension, tension, or uneasiness from an identifiable source	Anxiety Reduction Calming Technique Security Enhancement	Active Listening Anticipatory Guidance Coping Enhancement Counseling Decision-Making Support Emotional Support Family Support Support System Enhancement Truth Telling	Dying Care Support Group Therapy Group
Health Beliefs: Perceived Threat			
DEFINITION: Personal conviction that a threatening health problem is serious and has potential negative consequences for lifestyle	Health Education Self-Awareness Enhancement Teaching: Disease Process	Active Listening Counseling Self-Modification Assistance Self-Responsibility Facilitation Teaching: Individual Truth Telling Values Clarification	Anxiety Reduction Coping Enhancement Emotional Support Genetic Counseling Smoking Cessation Assistance Substance Use Prevention Substance Use Treatment
Symptom Control			
DEFINITION: Personal actions to minimize perceived adverse changes in physical and emotional functioning	Self-Modification Assistance Self-Responsibility Facilitation	Anticipatory Guidance Behavior Modification Health Education Health System Guidance Learning Facilitation Learning Readiness Enhancement Self-Awareness Enhancement Teaching: Disease Process Teaching: Individual Teaching: Procedure/ Treatment	Coping Enhancement Counseling Emotional Support Family Involvement Promotion Mutual Goal Setting Patient Contracting

NURSING DIAGNOSIS: Dentition, Impaired

DEFINITION: Disruption in tooth development/eruption patterns or structural integrity of individual teeth.

Outcome	Major Interventions	Suggested Interventions	Optional Interventions
Oral Hygiene			
DEFINITION: Condition of the mouth, teeth, gums, and tongue	Oral Health Maintenance Oral Health Restoration	Medication Management Nutrition Management Oral Health Promotion Pain Management Referral Teaching: Individual	Health System Guidance Insurance Authorization Teaching: Psychomotor Skill
Self-Care: Oral Hygiene			
DEFINITION: Ability to care for own mouth and teeth independently with or without assistive device	Oral Health Maintenance Oral Health Restoration	Oral Health Promotion Self-Care Assistance: Bathing/Hygiene Teaching: Individual	Nutrition Management Self-Care Assistance: Feeding Teaching: Psychomotor Skill

NURSING DIAGNOSIS: Diarrhea

DEFINITION: Passage of loose, unformed stools.

Outcome	Major Interventions	Suggested Interventions	Optional Interventions
Bowel Continence			
DEFINITION: Control of passage of stool from the bowel	Bowel Management Diarrhea Management	Bowel Incontinence Care Bowel Incontinence Care: Encopresis Fluid Management Medication Management Medication Prescribing Nutrition Management Perineal Care Self-Care Assistance: Toileting Skin Surveillance	Anxiety Reduction Bathing Skin Care: Topical Treatments Specimen Management
Bowel Elimination			
DEFINITION: Formation and evacuation of stool	Bowel Management Diarrhea Management	Fluid Management Medication Management Medication Prescribing Nutrition Management Perineal Care	Anxiety Reduction Bowel Incontinence Care Bowel Incontinence Care: Encopresis Fluid Monitoring Ostomy Care Self-Care Assistance: Toileting Specimen Management

Outcome	Major Interventions	Suggested Interventions	Optional Interventions
Electrolyte & Acid/Base Balance			
DEFINITION: Balance of the electrolytes and non-electrolytes in the intracellular and extracellular compartments of the body	Electrolyte Management Fluid/Electrolyte Management	Acid-Base Management Acid-Base Monitoring Diarrhea Management Electrolyte Monitoring Fluid Monitoring Intravenous (IV) Insertion Intravenous (IV) Therapy Laboratory Data Interpretation Medication Management Vital Signs Monitoring	Electrolyte Management: Hypokalemia Electrolyte Management: Hyponatremia Specimen Management Total Parenteral Nutrition (TPN) Administration
Fluid Balance			
DEFINITION: Water balance in the intracellular and extracellular compartments of the body	Diarrhea Management Fluid/Electrolyte Management Fluid Management	Electrolyte Management Electrolyte Monitoring Fluid Monitoring Fluid Resuscitation Intravenous (IV) Insertion Intravenous (IV) Therapy Nutrition Management Nutrition Therapy Nutritional Monitoring Vital Signs Monitoring	Enteral Tube Feeding Peripherally Inserted Central (PIC) Catheter Care Total Parenteral Nutrition (TPN) Administration Tube Care: Gastrointestinal Venous Access Device (VAD) Maintenance

Continued

Outcome	Major Interventions	Suggested Interventions	Optional Interventions
Hydration			
DEFINITION: Adequate water in the intracellular and extracellular compartments of the body	Diarrhea Management Fluid Management	Bottle Feeding Electrolyte Management Electrolyte Monitoring Feeding Fluid/Electrolyte Management Fluid Monitoring Fluid Resuscitation Nutrition Management Nutritional Monitoring	Intravenous (IV) Insertion Intravenous (IV) Therapy Nausea Management Temperature Regulation Vital Signs Monitoring Vomiting Management
Ostomy Self-Care			
DEFINITION: Personal actions to maintain ostomy for elimination	Diarrhea Management Ostomy Care	Bowel Management Fluid Management Nutrition Management Skin Surveillance	Fluid Resuscitation Skin Care: Topical Treatments Teaching: Individual Teaching: Psychomotor Skill Wound Care
Symptom Severity			
DEFINITION: Severity of perceived adverse changes in physical, emotional, and social functioning	Diarrhea Management	Anxiety Reduction Bowel Management Coping Enhancement Emotional Support Energy Management Medication Administration Medication Management Medication Prescribing Pain Management	Flatulence Reduction Nausea Management Perineal Care Skin Care: Topical Treatments Surveillance Weight Management

NURSING DIAGNOSIS: Diversional Activity Deficit

DEFINITION: Decreased stimulation from (or interest or engagement in) recreational or leisure activities.

Outcome	Major Interventions	Suggested Interventions	Optional Interventions
Family Social Climate			
DEFINITION: Supportive milieu as characterized by family member relationships and goals	Family Process Maintenance Family Support	Developmental Enhancement: Adolescent Developmental Enhancement: Child Family Therapy Self-Awareness Enhancement	Family Integrity Promotion Family Integrity Promotion: Childbearing Family Recreation Therapy Security Enhancement Therapeutic Play
Leisure Participation			
DEFINITION: Use of relaxing, interesting, and enjoyable activities to promote well-being	Recreation Therapy Self-Responsibility Facilitation	Activity Therapy Exercise Promotion Socialization Enhancement Therapeutic Play	Animal-Assisted Therapy Art Therapy Bibliotherapy Exercise Promotion Family Mobilization Humor Music Therapy Reminiscence Therapy
Motivation			
DEFINITION: Inner urge that moves or prompts an individual to positive action(s)	Self-Responsibility Facilitation	Behavior Management Behavior Modification: Social Skills Mutual Goal Setting Patient Contracting Self-Esteem Enhancement Self-Modification Assistance	Assertiveness Training Self-Awareness Enhancement Socialization Enhancement

Continued

Outcome	Major Interventions	Suggested Interventions	Optional Interventions
Play Participation			
DEFINITION: Use of activities by a child from 1 year through 11 years of age to promote enjoyment, entertainment, and development	Therapeutic Play	Exercise Promotion Recreation Therapy Socialization Enhancement	Activity Therapy Animal-Assisted Therapy Art Therapy Music Therapy Surveillance: Safety
Social Involvement			
DEFINITION: Social interactions with persons, groups, or organizations	Socialization Enhancement	Activity Therapy Animal-Assisted Therapy Art Therapy Developmental Enhancement: Adolescent Developmental Enhancement: Child Milieu Therapy Mutual Goal Setting Recreation Therapy Self-Awareness Enhancement Self-Esteem Enhancement Self-Responsibility Facilitation Therapeutic Play Visitation Facilitation	Active Listening Assertiveness Training Behavior Modification: Social Skills Communication Enhancement: Hearing Deficit Communication Enhancement: Speech Deficit Communication Enhancement: Visual Deficit Complex Relationship Building Counseling Culture Brokerage Family Mobilization Family Therapy Humor Presence Support Group Support System Enhancement

NURSING DIAGNOSIS: Energy Field, Disturbed

DEFINITION: Disruption of the flow of energy surrounding a person's being that results in disharmony of the body, mind, and/or spirit.

Outcome	Major Interventions	Suggested Interventions	Optional Interventions
Comfort Level			
DEFINITION: Extent of positive perception of physical and psychological ease	Environmental Management: Comfort Therapeutic Touch	Aromatherapy Energy Management Fever Treatment Meditation Facilitation Simple Guided Imagery Spiritual Support Temperature Regulation	Anxiety Reduction Positioning Sleep Enhancement
Pain Level			
DEFINITION: Severity of observed or reported pain	Pain Management Therapeutic Touch	Acupressure Analgesic Administration Analgesic Administration: Intraspinal Environmental Management: Comfort Simple Guided Imagery Simple Massage Simple Relaxation Therapy Transcutaneous Electrical Nerve Stimulation (TENS) Vital Signs Monitoring	Energy Management Heat/Cold Application Hypnosis Music Therapy Positioning Presence Splinting Touch

Continued

Outcome	Major Interventions	Suggested Interventions	Optional Interventions
Personal Well-Being			
DEFINITION: Extent of positive perception of one's health status and life circumstances	Self-Awareness Enhancement Therapeutic Touch	Acupressure Energy Management Hope Instillation Meditation Facilitation Pain Management Self-Esteem Enhancement Simple Guided Imagery Spiritual Support Temperature Regulation Values Clarification	Aromatherapy Communication Enhancement: Hearing Deficit Communication Enhancement: Speech Deficit Communication Enhancement: Visual Deficit Counseling Environmental Management Risk Identification Security Enhancement Support System Enhancement
Spiritual Health			
DEFINITION: Connectedness with self, others, higher power, all life, nature, and the universe that transcends and empowers the self	Hope Instillation Spiritual Growth Facilitation	Forgiveness Facilitation Meditation Facilitation Spiritual Support Support Group Therapeutic Touch Values Clarification	Bibliotherapy Counseling Grief Work Facilitation Guilt Work Facilitation Touch

NURSING DIAGNOSIS: Environmental Interpretation Syndrome, Impaired

DEFINITION: Consistent lack of orientation to person, place, time, or circumstances over more than 3 to 6 months necessitating a protective environment.

Outcome	Major Interventions	Suggested Interventions	Optional Interventions
Cognitive Orientation			
DEFINITION: Ability to identify person, place, and time accurately	Dementia Management Reality Orientation	Anxiety Reduction Cognitive Stimulation Dementia Management Emotional Support Environmental Management Memory Training Milieu Therapy	Area Restriction Bathing Behavior Management Mood Management Music Therapy Patient Rights Protection Presence
Concentration			
DEFINITION: Ability to focus on a specific stimulus	Anxiety Reduction Cognitive Stimulation	Cerebral Perfusion Promotion Dementia Management Energy Management Environmental Management Medication Management Reality Orientation	Active Listening Calming Technique Communication Enhancement: Hearing Deficit Communication Enhancement: Speech Deficit Communication Enhancement: Visual Deficit Touch
Fall Prevention Behavior			
DEFINITION: Personal or family caregiver actions to minimize risk factors that might precipitate falls in the personal environment	Environmental Management: Safety Fall Prevention	Area Restriction Dementia Management Risk Identification Self-Care Assistance Surveillance: Safety	Elopement Precautions Incident Reporting Physical Restraint Presence Quality Monitoring

Continued

Outcome	Major Interventions	Suggested Interventions	Optional Interventions
Memory DEFINITION: Ability to cognitively retrieve and report previously stored information	Dementia Management Memory Training	Cognitive Stimulation Learning Facilitation Milieu Therapy Reality Orientation Reminiscence Therapy	Coping Enhancement Energy Management Medication Management Patient Rights Protection Sleep Enhancement
Neurological Status: Consciousness DEFINITION: Arousal, orientation, and attention to the environment	Cerebral Perfusion Promotion Environmental Management: Safety Neurologic Monitoring	Cognitive Stimulation Dementia Management Environmental Management Medication Administration Medication Management	Aspiration Precautions Patient Rights Protection Security Enhancement Seizure Precautions Surveillance Vital Signs Monitoring
Safe Home Environment DEFINITION: Physical arrangements to minimize environmental factors that might cause physical harm or injury in the home	Environmental Management: Safety Surveillance: Safety	Area Restriction Environmental Management: Violence Prevention Fire-Setting Precautions Home Maintenance Assistance Limit Setting Security Enhancement	Dementia Management Hallucination Management Incident Reporting Risk Identification Self-Care Assistance

NURSING DIAGNOSIS: Failure to Thrive, Adult

DEFINITION: Progressive functional deterioration of a physical and cognitive nature. The individual's ability to live with multisystem diseases, cope with ensuing problems, and manage his/her care are remarkably diminished.

Outcome	Major Interventions	Suggested Interventions	Optional Interventions
Appetite			
DEFINITION: Desire to eat when ill or receiving treatment	Nutrition Therapy Nutritional Monitoring	Diet Staging Fluid Management Fluid Monitoring Hope Instillation Mood Management Nutrition Management Oral Health Maintenance	Emotional Support Medication Management Nausea Management Vomiting Management
Cognition			
DEFINITION: Ability to execute complex mental processes	Cognitive Stimulation Hope Instillation	Active Listening Learning Facilitation Memory Training Mood Management Patient Rights Protection Reminiscence Therapy	Energy Management Medication Management Presence Reality Orientation
Nutritional Status			
DEFINITION: Extent to which nutrients are available to meet metabolic needs	Nutrition Management Nutrition Therapy	Energy Management Feeding Fluid/Electrolyte Management Fluid Monitoring Nutritional Monitoring Teaching: Prescribed Diet Weight Gain Assistance	Eating Disorders Management Enteral Tube Feeding Self-Care Assistance: Feeding Sustenance Support Total Parenteral Nutrition (TPN) Administration

Continued

Outcome	Major Interventions	Suggested Interventions	Optional Interventions
Nutritional Status: Food and Fluid Intake			
DEFINITION: Amount of food and fluid taken into the body over a 24-hour period	Fluid Monitoring Nutritional Monitoring	Diet Staging Feeding Nutrition Management Nutrition Therapy Self-Care Assistance: Feeding Teaching: Prescribed Diet Weight Gain Assistance	Enteral Tube Feeding Gastrointestinal Intubation Intravenous (IV) Insertion Intravenous (IV) Therapy Swallowing Therapy Total Parenteral Nutrition (TPN) Administration Tube Care: Gastrointestinal
Physical Aging			
DEFINITION: Normal physical changes that occur with the natural aging process	Environmental Management Home Maintenance Assistance Risk Identification	Body Mechanics Promotion Case Management Coping Enhancement Diet Staging Emotional Support Energy Management Family Involvement Promotion Family Mobilization Medication Management Nutrition Management Nutrition Therapy Nutritional Monitoring	Bathing Bowel Management Dressing Family Support Feeding Foot Care Hair Care Nail Care Skin Surveillance Urinary Elimination Management

Outcome	Major Interventions	Suggested Interventions	Optional Interventions
Self-Care: Activities of Daily Living (ADL)			
DEFINITION: Ability to perform the most basic physical tasks and personal care activities independently with or without assistive device	Self-Care Assistance	Caregiver Support Case Management Environmental Management: Comfort Self-Care Assistance: Bathing/Hygiene Self-Care Assistance: Dressing/ Grooming Self-Care Assistance: Feeding Self-Care Assistance: Toileting Self-Care Assistance: Transfer	Energy Management Environmental Management: Safety Exercise Promotion Fall Prevention Home Maintenance Assistance
Will to Live			
DEFINITION: Desire, determination, and effort to survive	Hope Installation Spiritual Support	Emotional Support Family Support Patient Rights Protection Relocation Stress Reduction Support System Enhancement	Animal-Assisted Therapy Coping Enhancement

NURSING DIAGNOSIS: Family Coping, Compromised

DEFINITION: Usually supportive primary person (family member or close friend) provides insufficient, ineffective, or compromised support, comfort, assistance, or encouragement that may be needed by the client to manage or master adaptive tasks related to his/her health challenge.

Outcome	Major Interventions	Suggested Interventions	Optional Interventions
Caregiver Emotional Health			
DEFINITION: Emotional well-being of a family care provider while caring for a family member	Emotional Support Respite Care	Anger Control Assistance Anticipatory Guidance Caregiver Support Decision-Making Support Family Involvement Promotion Grief Work Facilitation Guilt Work Facilitation Resiliency Promotion Spiritual Support Support Group Support System Enhancement	Abuse Protection Support Coping Enhancement Family Integrity Promotion Family Mobilization Family Process Maintenance Family Support Forgiveness Facilitation Health System Guidance Referral Role Enhancement Simple Relaxation Therapy
Caregiver-Patient Relationship			
DEFINITION: Positive interactions and connections between the caregiver and care recipient	Caregiver Support	Conflict Mediation Emotional Support Family Integrity Promotion Family Involvement Promotion Family Mobilization Family Support Home Maintenance Assistance Respite Care Support Group Support System Enhancement	Abuse Protection Support Anxiety Reduction Complex Relationship Building Environmental Management: Attachment Process Environmental Management: Violence Prevention Mutual Goal Setting

Outcome	Major Interventions	Suggested Interventions	Optional Interventions
Caregiver Performance: Direct Care			
DEFINITION: Provision by family care provider of appropriate personal and health care for a family member	Caregiver Support Learning Facilitation	Environmental Management: Comfort Family Involvement Promotion Respite Care Teaching: Disease Process Teaching: Individual Teaching: Prescribed Activity/Exercise Teaching: Prescribed Diet Teaching: Prescribed Medication Teaching: Procedure/Treatment Teaching: Psychomotor Skill	Case Management Health Education Health System Guidance Learning Readiness Enhancement Normalization Promotion
Caregiver Performance: Indirect Care			
DEFINITION: Arrangement and oversight by family care provider of appropriate care for a family member	Health System Guidance	Anticipatory Guidance Decision-Making Support Discharge Planning Financial Resource Assistance Insurance Authorization Patient Rights Protection Referral	Family Integrity Promotion Family Involvement Promotion Family Mobilization Support Group

Continued

Outcome	Major Interventions	Suggested Interventions	Optional Interventions
Caregiving Endurance Potential			
DEFINITION: Factors that promote family care provider continuance over an extended period of time	Caregiver Support Coping Enhancement Respite Care	Decision-Making Support Energy Management Exercise Promotion Family Involvement Promotion Health System Guidance Spiritual Support Support Group Support System Enhancement	Active Listening Anxiety Reduction Emotional Support Environmental Management: Home Preparation Family Mobilization Financial Resource Assistance Recreation Therapy
Family Coping			
DEFINITION: Family actions to manage stressors that tax family resources	Coping Enhancement Family Involvement Promotion Family Mobilization	Caregiver Support Complex Relationship Building Conflict Mediation Counseling Family Integrity Promotion Family Presence Facilitation Family Process Maintenance Family Support Grief Work Facilitation Grief Work Facilitation: Perinatal Death Normalization Promotion Resiliency Promotion Spiritual Support	Abuse Protection Support: Child Abuse Protection Support: Domestic Partner Abuse Protection Support: Elder Anger Control Assistance Bowel Incontinence Care: Encopresis Case Management Consultation Crisis Intervention Decision-Making Support Family Therapy Financial Resource Assistance Guilt Work Facilitation Mutual Goal Setting Respite Care Sibling Support Trauma Therapy: Child Urinary Incontinence Care: Enuresis

Outcome	Major Interventions	Suggested Interventions	Optional Interventions
Family Normalization			
DEFINITION: Capacity of the family system to maintain routines and develop strategies for optimal functioning when a member has a chronic illness or disability	Family Process Maintenance Family Support Normalization Promotion	Caregiver Support Coping Enhancement Counseling Decision-Making Support Family Integrity Promotion Family Involvement Promotion Family Mobilization Respite Care Sibling Support Spiritual Support	Complex Relationship Building Consultation Mutual Goal Setting Reminiscence Therapy Role Enhancement Sustenance Support

NURSING DIAGNOSIS: Family Coping, Disabled

DEFINITION: Behavior of significant person (family member or other primary person) that disables his/her capacities and the client's capacities to effectively address tasks essential to either person's adaptation to the health challenge.

Outcome	Major Interventions	Suggested Interventions	Optional Interventions
Caregiver-Patient Relationship DEFINITION: Positive interactions and connections between the caregiver and care recipient	Caregiver Support	Abuse Protection Support: Child Abuse Protection Support: Domestic Partner Abuse Protection Support: Elder Emotional Support Family Integrity Promotion Family Involvement Promotion Family Mobilization Family Support Home Maintenance Assistance Respite Care Support Group Support System Enhancement	Abuse Protection Support Anger Control Assistance Complex Relationship Building Counseling Environmental Management: Violence Prevention Mutual Goal Setting Self-Modification Assistance

Outcome	Major Interventions	Suggested Interventions	Optional Interventions
Caregiver Performance: Direct Care			
DEFINITION: Provision by family care provider of appropriate personal and health care for a family member	Caregiver Support Learning Facilitation	Environmental Management: Comfort Family Involvement Promotion Respite Care Teaching: Disease Process Teaching: Individual Teaching: Prescribed Activity/Exercise Teaching: Prescribed Diet Teaching: Prescribed Medication Teaching: Procedure/ Treatment Teaching: Psychomotor Skill	Case Management Health Education Health System Guidance Learning Readiness Enhancement Normalization Promotion
Caregiver Performance: Indirect Care			
DEFINITION: Arrangement and oversight by family care provider of appropriate care for a family member	Health System Guidance	Anticipatory Guidance Decision-Making Support Discharge Planning Financial Resource Assistance Insurance Authorization Patient Rights Protection Referral	Family Integrity Promotion Family Involvement Promotion Family Mobilization Support Group

Continued

Outcome	Major Interventions	Suggested Interventions	Optional Interventions
Caregiver Well-Being			
DEFINITION: Extent of positive perception of primary care provider's health status and life circumstances	Caregiver Support Respite Care	Anger Control Assistance Decision-Making Support Emotional Support Family Involvement Promotion Family Mobilization Family Support Grief Work Facilitation Guilt Work Facilitation Hope Instillation Self-Esteem Enhancement Socialization Enhancement Spiritual Support	Assertiveness Training Coping Enhancement Family Integrity Promotion Family Process Maintenance Referral Role Enhancement Simple Relaxation Therapy Support Group Support System Enhancement
Caregiving Endurance Potential			
DEFINITION: Factors that promote family care provider continuance over an extended period of time	Caregiver Support Coping Enhancement	Decision-Making Support Energy Management Exercise Promotion Family Involvement Promotion Respite Care Spiritual Support Support Group Support System Enhancement	Assertiveness Training Emotional Support Family Mobilization Family Support Mutual Goal Setting Recreation Therapy Simple Relaxation Therapy

Outcome	Major Interventions	Suggested Interventions	Optional Interventions
Family Coping			
DEFINITION: Family actions to manage stressors that tax family resources	Coping Enhancement Family Support Family Therapy	Abuse Protection Support: Child Abuse Protection Support: Domestic Partner Abuse Protection Support: Elder Complex Relationship Building Conflict Mediation Counseling Crisis Intervention Family Integrity Promotion Family Mobilization Normalization Promotion Resiliency Promotion Spiritual Support Sustenance Support	Abuse Protection Support Anger Control Assistance Case Management Consultation Environmental Management: Violence Prevention Family Involvement Promotion Family Presence Facilitation Family Process Maintenance Financial Resource Assistance Grief Work Facilitation Grief Work Facilitation: Perinatal Death
Family Normalization			
DEFINITION: Capacity of the family system to maintain routines and develop strategies for optimal functioning when a member has a chronic illness or disability	Family Support Family Therapy Normalization Promotion	Coping Enhancement Counseling Family Integrity Promotion Family Involvement Promotion Family Mobilization Family Process Maintenance Spiritual Support	Abuse Protection Support Anxiety Reduction Case Management Consultation Decision-Making Support Environmental Management: Home Preparation Mutual Goal Setting

NURSING DIAGNOSIS: Family Coping, Readiness for Enhanced

DEFINITION: Effective management of adaptive tasks by family member involved with the client's health challenge, who now exhibits desire and readiness for enhanced health and growth in regard to self and in relation to the client.

Outcome	Major Interventions	Suggested Interventions	Optional Interventions
Caregiver Well-Being DEFINITION: Extent of positive perception of primary care provider's health status and life circumstances	Caregiver Support Respite Care	Coping Enhancement Emotional Support Family Involvement Promotion Family Mobilization Family Support Support Group Support System Enhancement	Counseling Family Integrity Promotion Home Maintenance Assistance Normalization Promotion Role Enhancement
Family Coping DEFINITION: Family actions to manage stressors that tax family resources	Family Involvement Promotion Family Support	Consultation Counseling Family Integrity Promotion Family Mobilization Financial Resource Assistance Normalization Promotion Resiliency Promotion	Coping Enhancement Grief Work Facilitation Grief Work Facilitation: Perinatal Death High-Risk Pregnancy Care Mutual Goal Setting Preconception Counseling Role Enhancement

Outcome	Major Interventions	Suggested Interventions	Optional Interventions
Family Functioning			
DEFINITION: Capacity of the family system to meet the needs of its members during developmental transitions	Family Support Normalization Promotion	Anticipatory Guidance Developmental Care Developmental Enhancement: Adolescent Developmental Enhancement: Child Family Involvement Promotion Family Planning: Contraception Family Integrity Promotion Parent Education: Adolescent Parent Education: Childrearing Family Preconception Counseling Sibling Support	Family Planning: Infertility Family Planning: Unplanned Pregnancy High Risk Pregnancy Care Prenatal Care Teaching: Infant Nutrition Teaching: Infant Stimulation Teaching: Infant Safety Teaching: Toddler Safety Teaching: Toilet Training
Family Normalization			
DEFINITION: Capacity of the family system to maintain routines and develop strategies for optimal functioning when a member has a chronic illness or disability	Family Support Normalization Promotion	Anticipatory Guidance Consultation Developmental Care Developmental Enhancement: Adolescent Developmental Enhancement: Child Family Integrity Promotion Family Involvement Promotion Family Mobilization Role Enhancement	Complex Relationship Building Counseling Genetic Counseling Pass Facilitation Respite Care Sibling Support

Continued

Outcome	Major Interventions	Suggested Interventions	Optional Interventions
Health Promoting Behavior			
DEFINITION: Personal actions to sustain or increase wellness	Health Education Self-Modification Assistance	Behavior Modification Coping Enhancement Counseling Emotional Support Exercise Promotion Health Screening Mutual Goal Setting Risk Identification Self-Awareness Enhancement Support Group Support System Enhancement	Developmental Enhancement: Adolescent Developmental Enhancement: Child Family Mobilization Family Planning: Contraception Nutrition Management Prenatal Care Smoking Cessation Assistance Substance Use Prevention Teaching: Safe Sex Weight Management
Health Seeking Behavior			
DEFINITION: Personal actions to promote optimal wellness, recovery, and rehabilitation	Health Education Learning Facilitation	Anticipatory Guidance Counseling Decision-Making Support Developmental Enhancement: Adolescent Developmental Enhancement: Child Family Integrity Promotion Health Screening Health System Guidance Self-Awareness Enhancement Self-Modification Assistance Support Group	Exercise Promotion Nutrition Management Parenting Promotion Smoking Cessation Assistance Substance Use Prevention Weight Management

Outcome	Major Interventions	Suggested Interventions	Optional Interventions
Participation in Health Care Decisions			
DEFINITION: Personal involvement in selecting and evaluating health care options to achieve desired outcome	Decision-Making Support Health System Guidance	Active Listening Anticipatory Guidance Assertiveness Training Counseling Culture Brokerage Patient Rights Protection Self-Responsibility Facilitation	Behavior Modification Caregiver Support Coping Enhancement Family Involvement Promotion Health Care Information Exchange Referral

F

NURSING DIAGNOSIS: Family Processes, Dysfunctional: Alcoholism

DEFINITION: Psychosocial, spiritual, and physiological functions of the family unit are chronically disorganized, which leads to conflict, denial of problems, resistance to change, ineffective problem solving, and a series of self-perpetuating crises.

Outcome	Major Interventions	Suggested Interventions	Optional Interventions
Family Coping			
DEFINITION: Family actions to manage stressors that tax family resources	Coping Enhancement Family Process Maintenance Substance Use Treatment	Abuse Protection Support Abuse Protection Support: Child Abuse Protection Support: Domestic Partner Abuse Protection Support: Elder Conflict Mediation Counseling Crisis Intervention Family Integrity Promotion Family Support Family Therapy Normalization Promotion Spiritual Support Support Group	Anger Control Assistance Anxiety Reduction Behavior Management Impulse Control Training Referral Self-Awareness Enhancement Self-Responsibility Facilitation Teaching: Group
Family Functioning			
DEFINITION: Capacity of the family system to meet the needs of its members during developmental transitions	Family Integrity Promotion Family Process Maintenance Substance Use Treatment	Anger Control Assistance Behavior Management Counseling Family Mobilization Family Support Family Therapy Mutual Goal Setting Normalization Promotion Substance Use Prevention Support System Enhancement	Abuse Protection Support Coping Enhancement Decision-Making Support Impulse Control Training Referral Self-Responsibility Facilitation Spiritual Support Support Group Teaching: Group

Outcome	Major Interventions	Suggested Interventions	Optional Interventions
Family Resiliency DEFINITION: Capacity of the family system to successfully adapt and function competently following significant adversity or crises	Family Process Maintenance Resiliency Promotion Substance Use Treatment	Coping Enhancement Crisis Intervention Family Integrity Promotion Family Support Family Therapy Spiritual Support	Counseling Decision-Making Support Sibling Support Support System Enhancement
Family Social Climate DEFINITION: Supportive milieu as characterized by family member relationships and goals	Family Therapy Substance Use Treatment	Abuse Protection Support Abuse Protection Support: Child Abuse Protection Support: Domestic Partner Abuse Protection Support: Elder Conflict Mediation Counseling Family Integrity Promotion Family Support Support Group	Anger Control Assistance Behavior Modification Coping Enhancement Decision-Making Support Support System Enhancement

Continued

Outcome	Major Interventions	Suggested Interventions	Optional Interventions
Parenting Performance			
DEFINITION: Parental actions to provide a child a nurturing and constructive physical, emotional, and social environment	Family Integrity Promotion: Childbearing Family Parenting Promotion Substance Use Treatment	Abuse Protection Support: Child Caregiver Support Family Involvement Promotion Family Support Parent Education: Adolescent Parent Education: Childrearing Family Parent Education: Infant	Counseling Home Maintenance Assistance Impulse Control Training Respite Care Self-Responsibility Facilitation
Role Performance			
DEFINITION: Congruence of an individual's role behavior with role expectations	Role Enhancement Self-Responsibility Facilitation Substance Use Treatment	Behavior Modification Caregiver Support Counseling Family Involvement Promotion Family Support Self-Awareness Enhancement Values Clarification	Decision-Making Support Family Integrity Promotion Support System Enhancement

Outcome	Major Interventions	Suggested Interventions	Optional Interventions
Substance Addiction Consequences			
DEFINITION: Severity of change in health status and social functioning due to substance addiction	Substance Use Prevention Substance Use Treatment	Anxiety Reduction Behavior Management Behavior Management: Self-Harm Behavior Modification Behavior Modification: Social Skills Coping Enhancement Counseling Crisis Intervention Emotional Support Family Involvement Promotion Family Mobilization Family Support Impulse Control Training Limit Setting Mutual Goal Setting Patient Contracting Self-Awareness Enhancement Self-Esteem Enhancement Self-Modification Assistance Self-Responsibility Facilitation Spiritual Support Support Group Support System Enhancement Teaching: Disease Process Therapy Group	Active Listening Anger Control Assistance Body Image Enhancement Complex Relationship Building Decision-Making Support Environmental Management Family Therapy Mood Management Progressive Muscle Relaxation Socialization Enhancement

NURSING DIAGNOSIS: Family Processes, Interrupted

DEFINITION: Change in family relationships and/or functioning.

Outcome	Major Interventions	Suggested Interventions	Optional Interventions
Family Coping DEFINITION: Family actions to manage stressors that tax family resources	Coping Enhancement Family Support	Conflict Mediation Counseling Decision-Making Support Emotional Support Family Mobilization Family Process Maintenance Family Therapy Financial Resource Assistance Grief Work Facilitation Grief Work Facilitation: Perinatal Death Respite Care Support Group Support System Enhancement	Behavior Management Behavior Modification Caregiver Support Dementia Management Family Integrity Promotion Guilt Work Facilitation Home Maintenance Assistance Labor Suppression Newborn Care Parent Education: Adolescent Parent Education: Childrearing Family Reproductive Technology Management Trauma Therapy: Child

Outcome	Major Interventions	Suggested Interventions	Optional Interventions
Family Functioning			
DEFINITION: Capacity of the family system to meet the needs of its members during developmental transitions	Family Integrity Promotion Family Process Maintenance	Assertiveness Training Conflict Mediation Counseling Developmental Enhancement: Adolescent Developmental Enhancement: Child Family Involvement Promotion Family Mobilization Family Support Family Therapy Financial Resource Assistance Normalization Promotion Role Enhancement Support System Enhancement	Attachment Promotion Behavior Management Coping Enhancement Decision-Making Support Family Integrity Promotion: Childbearing Family Family Planning: Contraception Family Planning: Infertility Family Planning: Unplanned Pregnancy Parent Education: Adolescent Parent Education: Childrearing Family Spiritual Support Support Group
Family Normalization			
DEFINITION: Capacity of the family system to maintain routines and develop strategies for optimal functioning when a member has a chronic illness or disability	Family Process Maintenance Normalization Promotion	Caregiver Support Coping Enhancement Counseling Emotional Support Family Mobilization Family Support Financial Resource Assistance Home Maintenance Assistance Respite Care Role Enhancement Support System Enhancement	Behavior Management Behavior Modification Dementia Management Developmental Enhancement: Adolescent Developmental Enhancement: Child Family Integrity Promotion Family Therapy Grief Work Facilitation Guilt Work Facilitation Trauma Therapy: Child

Continued

Outcome	Major Interventions	Suggested Interventions	Optional Interventions
Family Resiliency			
DEFINITION: Capacity of the family system to successfully adapt and function competently following significant adversity or crises	Family Process Maintenance Resiliency Promotion	Coping Enhancement Counseling Decision-Making Support Family Process Maintenance Family Support Normalization Promotion Support Group Support System Enhancement	Conflict Mediation Emotional Support Family Therapy Financial Resource Assistance Family Planning: Unplanned Pregnancy Home Maintenance Assistance
Family Social Climate			
DEFINITION: Supportive milieu as characterized by family member relationships and goals	Family Integrity Promotion Family Process Maintenance	Behavior Management Conflict Mediation Counseling Decision-Making Support Family Involvement Promotion Family Support Home Maintenance Assistance Mutual Goal Setting Role Enhancement	Behavior Modification Caregiver Support Developmental Enhancement: Adolescent Developmental Enhancement: Child Family Therapy Financial Resource Assistance

Outcome	Major Interventions	Suggested Interventions	Optional Interventions
Family Support During Treatment			
DEFINITION: Family presence and emotional support for an individual undergoing treatment	Family Involvement Promotion Family Presence Facilitation	Case Management Family Integrity Promotion Family Integrity Promotion: Childbearing Family Family Mobilization Family Process Maintenance Health Care Information Exchange Teaching: Disease Process Teaching: Procedure/ Treatment Visitation Facilitation	Caregiver Support Chemotherapy Management Pass Facilitation Radiation Therapy Management Spiritual Support Support Group Touch

Continued

Outcome	Major Interventions	Suggested Interventions	Optional Interventions
Parenting Performance			
DEFINITION: Parental actions to provide a child a nurturing and constructive physical, emotional, and social environment	Parent Education: Adolescent Parent Education: Childrearing Family Parent Education: Infant Parenting Promotion	Abuse Protection Support: Child Anticipatory Guidance Coping Enhancement Counseling Developmental Enhancement: Adolescent Developmental Enhancement: Child Family Integrity Promotion: Childbearing Family Family Involvement Promotion Family Process Maintenance Family Support Normalization Promotion Respite Care Role Enhancement Sibling Support Support System Enhancement	Breastfeeding Assistance Emotional Support Family Integrity Promotion Family Therapy Guilt Work Facilitation Health System Guidance Home Maintenance Assistance Prenatal Care Security Enhancement Self-Esteem Enhancement Socialization Enhancement Support Group Sustenance Support Telephone Consultation

NURSING DIAGNOSIS: Family Processes, Readiness for Enhanced

DEFINITION: A pattern of family functioning that is sufficient to support the well-being of family members and can be strengthened.

Outcome	Major Interventions	Suggested Interventions	Optional Interventions
Family Coping			
DEFINITION: Family actions to manage stressors that tax family resources	Coping Enhancement Family Mobilization	Decision-Making Support Family Support Humor Religious Ritual Enhancement Role Enhancement Spiritual Growth Facilitation Support System Enhancement	Grief Work Facilitation Guilt Work Facilitation Relocation Stress Reduction
Family Functioning			
DEFINITION: Capacity of the family system to meet the needs of its members during developmental transitions	Family Integrity Promotion Family Integrity Promotion: Childbearing Family	Family Process Maintenance Family Support Financial Resource Assistance Developmental Enhancement: Adolescent Developmental Enhancement: Child Parenting Promotion Resiliency Promotion	Home Maintenance Assistance Parent Education: Childrearing Family Parent Education: Adolescent Role Enhancement Sibling Support

Continued

Outcome	Major Interventions	Suggested Interventions	Optional Interventions
Family Health Status DEFINITION: Overall health and social competence of family unit	Family Integrity Promotion Health System Guidance	Childbirth Preparation Family Integrity Promotion: Childbearing Family Family Planning: Infertility Family Process Maintenance Family Support Genetic Counseling Health Education Parent Education: Adolescent Parent Education: Childrearing Family Risk Identification: Childbearing Family Role Enhancement Support System Enhancement	Activity Therapy Attachment Promotion Caregiver Support Exercise Promotion Family Involvement Promotion Family Mobilization Family Therapy Grief Work Facilitation: Perinatal Death Respite Care Home Maintenance Assistance
Family Integrity DEFINITION: Family members' behaviors that collectively demonstrate cohesion, strength, and emotional bonding	Family Integrity Promotion Family Integrity Promotion: Childbearing Family	Attachment Promotion Developmental Enhancement: Adolescent Developmental Enhancement: Child Environmental Management: Attachment Process Family Process Maintenance Family Support Parenting Promotion	Childbirth Preparation Parent Education: Adolescent Parent Education: Childrearing Family Parent Education: Infant Resiliency Promotion Sibling Support Role Enhancement

Outcome	Major Interventions	Suggested Interventions	Optional Interventions
Family Resiliency			
DEFINITION: Capacity of the family system to successfully adapt and function competently following significant adversity or crises	Resiliency Promotion	Coping Enhancement Family Integrity Promotion Family Process Maintenance Family Support Support System Enhancement Values Clarification	Family Mobilization Decision-Making Support Grief Work Facilitation
Family Social Climate			
DEFINITION: Supportive milieu as characterized by family member relationships and goals	Family Integrity Promotion Socialization Enhancement	Complex Relationship Building Emotional Support Developmental Enhancement: Adolescent Developmental Enhancement: Child Family Support	Forgiveness Facilitation Grief Work Facilitation Resiliency Promotion Sibling Support

NURSING DIAGNOSIS: Family Therapeutic Regimen Management, Ineffective

DEFINITION: Pattern of regulating and integrating into family processes a program for treatment of illness and the sequelae of illness that is unsatisfactory for meeting specific health goals.

Outcome	Major Interventions	Suggested Interventions	Optional Interventions
Family Coping			
DEFINITION: Family actions to manage stressors that tax family resources	Coping Enhancement Family Process Maintenance	Counseling Decision-Making Support Emotional Support Family Integrity Promotion Family Mobilization Family Process Maintenance Family Support Family Therapy Financial Resource Assistance Normalization Promotion Support System Enhancement	Family Involvement Promotion Home Maintenance Assistance Respite Care Role Enhancement Support Group
Family Functioning			
DEFINITION: Capacity of the family system to meet the needs of its members during developmental transitions	Family Integrity Promotion Family Involvement Promotion Family Process Maintenance	Conflict Mediation Counseling Family Mobilization Family Support Family Therapy Financial Resource Assistance Normalization Promotion Role Enhancement Sibling Support	Abuse Protection Support Caregiver Support Health System Guidance Home Maintenance Assistance Referral Respite Care Support System Enhancement

Outcome	Major Interventions	Suggested Interventions	Optional Interventions
Family Normalization			
DEFINITION: Capacity of the family system to maintain routines and develop strategies for optimal functioning when a member has a chronic illness or disability	Family Involvement Promotion Family Mobilization Normalization Promotion	Case Management Coping Enhancement Counseling Family Integrity Promotion Family Process Maintenance Family Support Family Therapy Health System Guidance Home Maintenance Assistance Respite Care Role Enhancement Sibling Support Support System Enhancement Sustenance Support	Caregiver Support Culture Brokerage Referral Respite Care Risk Identification Support Group
Family Participation in Professional Care			
DEFINITION: Family involvement in decision-making, delivery, and evaluation of care provided by health care personnel	Decision-Making Support Health System Guidance	Active Listening Anticipatory Guidance Assertiveness Training Counseling Culture Brokerage Discharge Planning Patient Rights Protection Self-Responsibility Facilitation Telephone Consultation	Anxiety Reduction Behavior Modification Caregiver Support Coping Enhancement Family Involvement Promotion Health Care Information Exchange Referral Sustenance Support

Continued

Outcome	Major Interventions	Suggested Interventions	Optional Interventions
Family Resiliency			
DEFINITION: Capacity of the family system to successfully adapt and function competently following significant adversity or crises	Coping Enhancement Resiliency Promotion	Decision-Making Support Family Integrity Promotion Family Involvement Promotion Family Process Maintenance Family Support Normalization Promotion Sibling Support Support System Enhancement	Caregiver Support Counseling Financial Resource Assistance Home Maintenance Assistance Respite Care Support Group
Knowledge: Treatment Regimen			
DEFINITION: Extent of understanding conveyed about a specific treatment regimen	Teaching: Disease Process Teaching: Procedure/ Treatment	Anticipatory Guidance Learning Facilitation Learning Readiness Enhancement Medication Management Nutrition Management Teaching: Group Teaching: Individual Teaching: Prescribed Activity/Exercise Teaching: Prescribed Diet Teaching: Prescribed Medication Teaching: Psychomotor Skill	Family Involvement Promotion Health System Guidance Prenatal Care Telephone Follow-up Weight Management

NURSING DIAGNOSIS: Fatigue

DEFINITION: An overwhelming sustained sense of exhaustion and decreased capacity for physical and mental work at usual level.

Outcome	Major Interventions	Suggested Interventions	Optional Interventions
Activity Tolerance			
DEFINITION: Physiologic response to energy-consuming movements with daily activities	Energy Management	Environmental Management Exercise Promotion Exercise Promotion: Strength Training Teaching: Prescribed Activity/Exercise	Asthma Management Cardiac Care: Rehabilitative Exercise Promotion: Stretching Exercise Therapy: Ambulation Self-Care Assistance
Endurance			
DEFINITION: Capacity to sustain activity	Activity Therapy Energy Management	Exercise Promotion Health Screening Mutual Goal Setting Nutrition Management Risk Identification Sleep Enhancement Teaching: Prescribed Activity/Exercise Teaching: Prescribed Diet	Exercise Promotion: Strength Training Exercise Therapy: Ambulation Exercise Therapy: Balance Exercise Therapy: Joint Mobility Exercise Therapy: Muscle Control Mood Management Self-Care Assistance Support System Enhancement Weight Management

Continued

Outcome	Major Interventions	Suggested Interventions	Optional Interventions
Energy Conservation DEFINITION: Personal actions to manage energy for initiating and sustaining activity	Energy Management Environmental Management	Body Mechanics Promotion Exercise Promotion Nutrition Management Sleep Enhancement Teaching: Prescribed Activity/Exercise	Dementia Management Dying Care Exercise Therapy: Ambulation Exercise Therapy: Balance Exercise Therapy: Joint Mobility Exercise Therapy: Muscle Control Simple Guided Imagery Simple Relaxation Therapy Weight Management
Nutritional Status: Energy DEFINITION: Extent to which nutrients and oxygen provide cellular energy	Energy Management Nutrition Management	Feeding Nutrition Therapy Nutritional Counseling Nutritional Monitoring Self-Care Assistance: Feeding Teaching: Prescribed Diet	Diet Staging Eating Disorders Management Enteral Tube Feeding Sustenance Support Total Parenteral Nutrition (TPN) Administration Weight Management

Outcome	Major Interventions	Suggested Interventions	Optional Interventions
Psychomotor Energy DEFINITION: Personal drive and energy to maintain activities of daily living, nutrition, and personal safety	Energy Management Mood Management	Coping Enhancement Counseling Crisis Intervention Grief Work Facilitation Guilt Work Facilitation Medication Management Self-Esteem Enhancement	Animal-Assisted Therapy Art Therapy Bibliotherapy Exercise Promotion Music Therapy Pain Management Progressive Muscle Relaxation Simple Guided Imagery Simple Massage Simple Relaxation Therapy Sleep Enhancement

NURSING DIAGNOSIS: Fear

DEFINITION: Response to a perceived threat that is consciously recognized as a danger.

Outcome	Major Interventions	Suggested Interventions	Optional Interventions
Fear Level			
DEFINITION: Severity of manifested apprehension, tension, or uneasiness arising from an identifiable source	Anxiety Reduction Calming Technique Presence	Abuse Protection Support: Domestic Partner Abuse Protection Support: Elder Active Listening Anticipatory Guidance Behavior Modification Coping Enhancement Emotional Support Environmental Management Preparatory Sensory Information Relocation Stress Reduction Security Enhancement Teaching: Disease Process Teaching: Preoperative Teaching: Procedure/ Treatment	Animal-Assisted Therapy Childbirth Preparation Crisis Intervention Distraction Simple Guided Imagery Support Group Therapy Group

Outcome	Major Interventions	Suggested Interventions	Optional Interventions
Fear Level: Child			
DEFINITION: Severity of manifested apprehension, tension, or uneasiness arising from an identifiable source in a child from 1 year through 17 years of age	Calming Technique Presence Security Enhancement	Abuse Protection Support: Child Active Listening Animal-Assisted Therapy Emotional Support Environmental Management Family Presence Facilitation Preparatory Sensory Information Teaching: Individual Therapeutic Play Truth Telling	Art Therapy Distraction Examination Assistance Music Therapy Pain Management

Continued

Outcome	Major Interventions	Suggested Interventions	Optional Interventions
Fear Self-Control			
DEFINITION: Personal actions to eliminate or reduce disabling feelings of apprehension, tension, or uneasiness from an identifiable source	Coping Enhancement Security Enhancement	Active Listening Anticipatory Guidance Anxiety Reduction Calming Technique Counseling Crisis Intervention Decision-Making Support Emotional Support Environmental Management Examination Assistance Family Involvement Promotion Preparatory Sensory Information Presence Support System Enhancement Teaching: Preoperative Teaching: Procedure/Treatment Therapeutic Touch Truth Telling	Abuse Protection Support Abuse Protection Support: Child Abuse Protection Support: Elder Autogenic Training Biofeedback Childbirth Preparation Culture Brokerage Dying Care Meditation Facilitation Pain Management Progressive Muscle Relaxation Rape-Trauma Treatment Self-Esteem Enhancement Self-Hypnosis Facilitation Simple Guided Imagery Simple Relaxation Therapy Support Group Therapy Group

NURSING DIAGNOSIS: Fluid Balance, Readiness for Enhanced

DEFINITION: A pattern of equilibrium between fluid volume and chemical composition of body fluids that is sufficient for meeting physical needs and can be strengthened.

Outcome	Major Interventions	Suggested Interventions	Optional Interventions
Fluid Balance			
DEFINITION: Water balance in the intracellular and extracellular compartments of the body	Fluid Management	Fluid/Electrolyte Management Fluid Monitoring Medication Management Nutritional Counseling Urinary Elimination Management Weight Management	Hemodynamic Regulation Vital Signs Monitoring
Hydration			
DEFINITION: Adequate water in the intracellular and extracellular compartments of the body	Fluid Management Fluid Monitoring	Electrolyte Management Fluid/Electrolyte Management Medication Management Nutritional Counseling Weight Management	Urinary Elimination Management
Kidney Function			
DEFINITION: Filtration of blood and elimination of metabolic waste products through the formation of urine	Fluid Management Urinary Elimination Management	Fluid/Electrolyte Management Health Education Nutritional Counseling Teaching: Individual Teaching: Prescribed Diet	Hemodialysis Therapy Peritoneal Dialysis Therapy Self-Care Assistance: Toileting Urinary Bladder Training Urinary Retention Care

NURSING DIAGNOSIS: Fluid Volume, Deficient

DEFINITION: Decreased intravascular, interstitial, and/or intracellular fluid. This refers to dehydration, water loss alone without change in sodium.

Outcome	Major Interventions	Suggested Interventions	Optional Interventions
Electrolyte and Acid/Base Balance			
DEFINITION: Balance of the electrolytes and non-electrolytes in the intracellular and extracellular compartments of the body	Acid-Base Management Electrolyte Management Fluid/Electrolyte Management	Acid-Base Monitoring Electrolyte Monitoring Fluid Management Fluid Monitoring Hemodynamic Regulation Intravenous (IV) Insertion Intravenous (IV) Therapy Laboratory Data Interpretation Neurologic Monitoring Surveillance Vital Signs Monitoring	Electrolyte Management: Hypercalcemia Electrolyte Management: Hyperkalemia Electrolyte Management: Hypermagnesemia Electrolyte Management: Hypernatremia Electrolyte Management: Hyperphosphatemia Electrolyte Management: Hypocalcemia Electrolyte Management: Hypokalemia Electrolyte Management: Hypomagnesemia Electrolyte Management: Hyponatremia Electrolyte Management: Hypophosphatemia Phlebotomy: Arterial Blood Sample Phlebotomy: Venous Blood Sample Total Parenteral Nutrition (TPN) Administration

Outcome	Major Interventions	Suggested Interventions	Optional Interventions
Fluid Balance DEFINITION: Water balance in the intracellular and extracellular compartments of the body	Fluid Management Fluid Monitoring Hypovolemia Management	Diarrhea Management Electrolyte Management Electrolyte Monitoring Fluid Resuscitation Intravenous (IV) Insertion Intravenous (IV) Therapy Laboratory Data Interpretation Medication Administration Medication Management Medication Prescribing Nutrition Management Shock Management: Volume Total Parenteral Nutrition (TPN) Administration Urinary Elimination Management Vital Signs Monitoring	Bleeding Reduction Blood Products Administration Cardiac Care: Acute Dysrhythmia Management Eating Disorders Management Enteral Tube Feeding Hemodynamic Regulation Hemorrhage Control Invasive Hemodynamic Monitoring Peripherally Inserted Central (PIC) Catheter Care Shock Management Shock Prevention Venous Access Devices (VAD) Maintenance

Continued

Outcome	Major Interventions	Suggested Interventions	Optional Interventions
Hydration			
DEFINITION: Adequate water in the intracellular and extracellular compartments of the body	Fluid Management Hypovolemia Management Intravenous (IV) Therapy	Bottle Feeding Diarrhea Management Electrolyte Management Electrolyte Monitoring Feeding Fever Treatment Fluid/Electrolyte Management Fluid Monitoring Fluid Resuscitation Intravenous (IV) Insertion Nutrition Management Shock Management: Volume Urinary Elimination Management Vital Signs Monitoring Vomiting Management	Amnioinfusion Bleeding Precautions Bleeding Reduction Bleeding Reduction: Antepartum Uterus Bleeding Reduction: Gastrointestinal Bleeding Reduction: Postpartum Uterus Hemorrhage Control Gastrointestinal Intubation Peripherally Inserted Central (PIC) Catheter Care Temperature Regulation Venous Access Devices (VAD) Maintenance
Nutritional Status: Food and Fluid Intake			
DEFINITION: Amount of food and fluid taken into the body over a 24-hour period	Fluid Management Fluid Monitoring Nutrition Management Nutritional Monitoring	Bottle Feeding Enteral Tube Feeding Feeding Nutrition Therapy Self-Care Assistance: Feeding Total Parenteral Nutrition (TPN) Administration	Breastfeeding Assistance Intravenous (IV) Therapy Lactation Counseling Oral Health Restoration Swallowing Therapy Teaching: Prescribed Diet

NURSING DIAGNOSIS: Fluid Volume, Excess

DEFINITION: Increased isotonic fluid retention.

Outcome	Major Interventions	Suggested Interventions	Optional Interventions
Electrolyte and Acid/Base Balance DEFINITION: Balance of the electrolytes and non-electrolytes in the intracellular and extracellular compartments of the body	Fluid/Electrolyte Management Fluid Management Fluid Monitoring	Acid-Base Management Electrolyte Management Electrolyte Monitoring Hemodialysis Therapy Hemodynamic Regulation Invasive Hemodynamic Monitoring Laboratory Data Interpretation Vital Signs Monitoring	Electrolyte Management: Hypocalcemia Electrolyte Management: Hypokalemia Electrolyte Management: Hypomagnesemia Electrolyte Management: Hyponatremia Electrolyte Management: Hypophosphatemia Phlebotomy: Arterial Blood Sample Phlebotomy: Cannulated Vessel Phlebotomy: Venous Blood Sample

Continued

Outcome	Major Interventions	Suggested Interventions	Optional Interventions
Fluid Balance DEFINITION: Water balance in the intracellular and extracellular compartments of the body	Fluid Management Fluid Monitoring Hypervolemia Management	Bedside Laboratory Testing Electrolyte Management Electrolyte Monitoring Fluid/Electrolyte Management Intravenous (IV) Therapy Laboratory Data Interpretation Medication Administration Medication Management Nutrition Management Urinary Elimination Management Vital Signs Monitoring	Cardiac Care: Acute Hemodynamic Regulation Intracranial Pressure (ICP) Monitoring Invasive Hemodynamic Monitoring Neurologic Monitoring Peritoneal Dialysis Therapy Respiratory Monitoring Weight Management

Outcome	Major Interventions	Suggested Interventions	Optional Interventions
Fluid Overload Severity DEFINITION: Severity of excess fluids in the intracellular and extracellular compartments of the body	Fluid/Electrolyte Management Hypervolemia Management	Cerebral Edema Management Electrolyte Management Electrolyte Monitoring Fluid Management Fluid Monitoring Hemodialysis Therapy Medication Administration Medication Management Neurologic Monitoring Peritoneal Dialysis Therapy Urinary Elimination Management Vital Signs Monitoring	Cardiac Care: Acute Dialysis Access Maintenance Intracranial Pressure (ICP) Monitoring Nutrition Management Nutritional Monitoring Temperature Regulation

Continued

Outcome	Major Interventions	Suggested Interventions	Optional Interventions
Kidney Function DEFINITION: Filtration of blood and elimination of metabolic waste products through the formation of urine	Fluid/Electrolyte Management Fluid Management Urinary Elimination Management	Acid-Base Management Bedside Laboratory Testing Electrolyte Monitoring Fluid Monitoring Hemodialysis Therapy Laboratory Data Interpretation Nutrition Therapy Nutritional Counseling Peritoneal Dialysis Therapy Specimen Management Teaching: Prescribed Diet	Dialysis Access Maintenance Self-Care Assistance: Toileting Urinary Catheterization Urinary Retention Care

NURSING DIAGNOSIS: Gas Exchange, Impaired

DEFINITION: Excess or deficit in oxygenation and/or carbon dioxide elimination at the alveolar-capillary membrane.

Outcome	Major Interventions	Suggested Interventions	Optional Interventions
Allergic Response: Systemic DEFINITION: Severity of systemic hypersensitive immune response to a specific environmental (exogenous) antigen	Anaphylaxis Management Asthma Management	Airway Insertion and Stabilization Airway Management Airway Suctioning Anxiety Reduction Oxygen Therapy Respiratory Monitoring Ventilation Assistance	Artificial Airway Management Chest Physiotherapy Cough Enhancement Fever Treatment Mechanical Ventilation Medication Administration

Continued

Outcome	Major Interventions	Suggested Interventions	Optional Interventions
Electrolyte and Acid/Base Balance			
DEFINITION: Balance of the electrolytes and non-electrolytes in the intracellular and extracellular compartments of the body	Acid-Base Management Electrolyte Management Laboratory Data Interpretation	Acid-Base Management: Respiratory Acidosis Acid-Base Management: Respiratory Alkalosis Acid-Base Monitoring Electrolyte Monitoring Fluid/Electrolyte Management Fluid Management Hemodynamic Regulation Intravenous (IV) Therapy Peripherally Inserted Central (PIC) Catheter Care Respiratory Monitoring Vital Signs Monitoring	Electrolyte Management: Hypercalcemia Electrolyte Management: Hyperkalemia Electrolyte Management: Hypermagnesemia Electrolyte Management: Hypernatremia Electrolyte Management: Hypocalcemia Electrolyte Management: Hypomagnesemia Electrolyte Management: Hyponatremia Specimen Management

Outcome	Major Interventions	Suggested Interventions	Optional Interventions
Mechanical Ventilation Response: Adult			
DEFINITION: Alveolar exchange and tissue perfusion are supported by mechanical ventilation	Mechanical Ventilation	Airway Insertion and Stabilization Airway Management Airway Suctioning Anxiety Reduction Artificial Airway Management Aspiration Precautions Mechanical Ventilatory Weaning Oxygen Therapy Respiratory Monitoring	Bedside Laboratory Testing Chest Physiotherapy Family Presence Facilitation Laboratory Data Interpretation Ventilation Assistance
Respiratory Status: Gas Exchange			
DEFINITION: Alveolar exchange of carbon dioxide and oxygen to maintain arterial blood gas concentrations	Acid-Base Management Oxygen Therapy Ventilation Assistance	Acid-Base Management: Respiratory Acidosis Acid-Base Management: Respiratory Alkalosis Acid-Base Monitoring Airway Management Anxiety Reduction Bedside Laboratory Testing Chest Physiotherapy Energy Management Positioning Respiratory Monitoring	Airway Insertion and Stabilization Airway Suctioning Artificial Airway Management Aspiration Precautions Cough Enhancement Embolus Care: Pulmonary Laboratory Data Interpretation Mechanical Ventilation Phlebotomy: Arterial Blood Sample

Continued

Outcome	Major Interventions	Suggested Interventions	Optional Interventions
Respiratory Status: Ventilation DEFINITION: Movement of air in and out of the lungs	Airway Management Respiratory Monitoring Ventilation Assistance	Airway Insertion and Stabilization Airway Suctioning Allergy Management Artificial Airway Management Aspiration Precautions Asthma Management Chest Physiotherapy Cough Enhancement Mechanical Ventilation Pain Management Positioning	Acid-Base Monitoring Anxiety Reduction Energy Management Embolus Care: Pulmonary Intrapartal Care: High-Risk Delivery Mechanical Ventilatory Weaning Medication Administration: Intrapleural Oxygen Therapy Postanesthesia Care Resuscitation Resuscitation: Neonate Smoking Cessation Assistance

Outcome	Major Interventions	Suggested Interventions	Optional Interventions
Tissue Perfusion: Pulmonary			
DEFINITION: Adequacy of blood flow through pulmonary vasculature to perfuse alveoli/ capillary unit	Acid-Base Management: Respiratory Acidosis	Acid-Base Monitoring	Chest Physiotherapy
	Acid Base Management: Respiratory Alkalosis	Bedside Laboratory Testing	Cough Enhancement
		Fluid Management	Emergency Care
	Embolus Care: Pulmonary	Fluid Monitoring	Mechanical Ventilation
	Hemodynamic Regulation	Intravenous (IV) Insertion	Resuscitation
		Intravenous (IV) Therapy	Resuscitation: Fetus
		Invasive Hemodynamic Monitoring	Specimen Management
		Laboratory Data Interpretation	Tube Care: Chest
		Medication Administration	Ventilation Assistance
		Medication Management	
		Oxygen Therapy	
		Respiratory Monitoring	
		Surveillance	
		Vital Signs Monitoring	

Continued

Outcome	Major Interventions	Suggested Interventions	Optional Interventions
Vital Signs			
DEFINITION: Extent to which temperature, pulse, respiration, and blood pressure are within normal range	Airway Management Respiratory Monitoring Vital Signs Monitoring	Acid-Base Management Acid-Base Monitoring Anxiety Reduction Electrolyte Management Fluid Management Hemodynamic Regulation Intravenous (IV) Insertion Intravenous (IV) Therapy Medication Administration Medication Management Medication Prescribing Oxygen Therapy Ventilation Assistance	Biofeedback Emergency Care Pain Management Resuscitation

G

NURSING DIAGNOSIS: Grieving, Anticipatory

DEFINITION: Intellectual and emotional responses and behaviors by which individuals, families, communities work through the process of modifying self-concept based on the perception of potential loss.

Outcome	Major Interventions	Suggested Interventions	Optional Interventions
Adaptation to Physical Disability			
DEFINITION: Adaptive response to a significant functional challenge due to a physical disability	Body Image Enhancement Coping Enhancement Emotional Support	Active Listening Anticipatory Guidance Grief Work Facilitation Hope Instillation Self-Esteem Enhancement Support Group Truth Telling	Amputation Care Decision-Making Support Mood Management Relocation Stress Reduction Role Enhancement Spiritual Support Support System Enhancement
Coping			
DEFINITION: Personal actions to manage stressors that tax an individual's resources	Coping Enhancement Grief Work Facilitation Grief Work Facilitation: Perinatal Death	Anticipatory Guidance Anxiety Reduction Caregiver Support Counseling Emotional Support Family Integrity Promotion Family Support Forgiveness Facilitation Hope Instillation Meditation Facilitation Presence Resiliency Promotion Spiritual Support Support Group Support System Enhancement Touch	Animal-Assisted Therapy Body Image Enhancement Genetic Counseling Mood Management Normalization Promotion Reminiscence Therapy Sibling Support Therapeutic Play Therapy Group Truth Telling

Continued

Outcome	Major Interventions	Suggested Interventions	Optional Interventions
Family Coping			
DEFINITION: Family actions to manage stressors that tax family resources	Family Support Grief Work Facilitation Grief Work Facilitation: Perinatal Death	Coping Enhancement Counseling Family Integrity Promotion Family Process Maintenance Family Therapy Normalization Promotion Resiliency Promotion Spiritual Support Support System Enhancement	Caregiver Support Culture Brokerage Sibling Support Support Group
Family Social Climate			
DEFINITION: Supportive milieu as characterized by family member relationships and goals	Family Integrity Promotion Family Support Grief Work Facilitation	Emotional Support Family Therapy Support Group Support System Enhancement	Counseling Spiritual Support

Outcome	Major Interventions	Suggested Interventions	Optional Interventions
Grief Resolution			
DEFINITION: Adjustment to actual or impending loss	Grief Work Facilitation Grief Work Facilitation: Perinatal Death	Active Listening Anger Control Assistance Anticipatory Guidance Coping Enhancement Counseling Dying Care Emotional Support Hope Instillation Reminiscence Therapy Spiritual Support Support Group Support System Enhancement	Animal-Assisted Therapy Bibliotherapy Guilt Work Facilitation Music Therapy Organ Procurement Pregnancy Termination Care Presence Sibling Support Touch Visitation Facilitation
Psychosocial Adjustment: Life Change			
DEFINITION: Adaptive psychosocial response of an individual to a significant life change	Anticipatory Guidance Coping Enhancement	Active Listening Counseling Dying Care Emotional Support Reminiscence Therapy Truth Telling	Decision-Making Support Family Integrity Promotion Family Mobilization Family Process Maintenance Humor Self-Modification Assistance Spiritual Support

NURSING DIAGNOSIS: Grieving, Dysfunctional

DEFINITION: Extended, unsuccessful use of intellectual and emotional responses by which individuals, families, and communities attempt to work through the process of modifying self-concept based upon the perception of loss.

Outcome	Major Interventions	Suggested Interventions	Optional Interventions
Coping			
DEFINITION: Personal actions to manage stressors that tax an individual's resources	Coping Enhancement Grief Work Facilitation Grief Work Facilitation: Perinatal Death	Anxiety Reduction Calming Technique Caregiver Support Counseling Crisis Intervention Decision-Making Support Emotional Support Family Support Forgiveness Facilitation Guilt Work Facilitation Hope Instillation Presence Support Group	Animal-Assisted Therapy Art Therapy Behavior Management: Self-Harm Body Image Enhancement Cognitive Restructuring Family Therapy Normalization Promotion Reminiscence Therapy Sibling Support Simple Relaxation Therapy Spiritual Growth Facilitation Spiritual Support Support System Enhancement Therapeutic Play Therapy Group Touch Truth Telling Values Clarification Visitation Facilitation

Outcome	Major Interventions	Suggested Interventions	Optional Interventions
Family Coping			
DEFINITION: Family actions to manage stressors that tax family resources	Coping Enhancement Family Integrity Promotion Family Support	Active Listening Counseling Crisis Intervention Emotional Support Family Process Maintenance Family Therapy Grief Work Facilitation Grief Work Facilitation: Perinatal Death Role Enhancement Sibling Support	Decision-Making Support Normalization Promotion Support Group Support System Enhancement Values Clarification
Family Resiliency			
DEFINITION: Capacity of the family system to successfully adapt and function competently following significant adversity or crises	Grief Work Facilitation Grief Work Facilitation: Perinatal Death Resiliency Promotion	Coping Enhancement Counseling Crisis Intervention Family Integrity Promotion Family Support Normalization Promotion	Guilt Work Facilitation Support Group Support System Enhancement

Continued

Outcome	Major Interventions	Suggested Interventions	Optional Interventions
Grief Resolution			
DEFINITION: Adjustment to actual or impending loss	Grief Work Facilitation Grief Work Facilitation: Perinatal Death	Active Listening Anger Control Assistance Coping Enhancement Counseling Culture Brokerage Emotional Support Family Integrity Promotion Spiritual Support Support Group Support System Enhancement	Guilt Work Facilitation Hope Instillation Mutual Goal Setting Presence Sibling Support Suicide Prevention Touch Visitation Facilitation
Psychosocial Adjustment: Life Changes			
DEFINITION: Adaptive psychosocial response of an individual to a significant life change	Coping Enhancement	Anger Control Assistance Anxiety Reduction Counseling Crisis Intervention Emotional Support Grief Work Facilitation Role Enhancement	Decision-Making Support Family Integrity Promotion Family Mobilization Family Process Maintenance Relocation Stress Reduction Spiritual Growth Facilitation Spiritual Support Values Clarification
Role Performance			
DEFINITION: Congruence of an individual's role behavior with role expectations	Grief Work Facilitation Role Enhancement Self-Awareness Enhancement	Behavior Modification Counseling Emotional Support Parenting Promotion Resiliency Promotion	Family Integrity Promotion Self-Esteem Enhancement Sibling Support Support Group

NURSING DIAGNOSIS: Growth and Development, Delayed

DEFINITION: Deviations from age-group norms.

Outcome	Major Interventions	Suggested Interventions	Optional Interventions
Child Development: 1 Month DEFINITION: Milestones of physical, cognitive, and psychosocial progression by 1 month of age	Newborn Care Nutritional Monitoring Teaching: Infant Stimulation	Anticipatory Guidance Attachment Promotion Bottle Feeding Breastfeeding Assistance Infant Car Kangaroo Care Parent Education: Infant Parenting Promotion Touch	Developmental Care Environmental Management: Attachment Process Lactation Counseling Nonnutritive Sucking
Child Development: 2 Months DEFINITION: Milestones of physical, cognitive, and psychosocial progression by 2 months of age	Developmental Enhancement: Child Infant Care Parenting Promotion	Anticipatory Guidance Attachment Promotion Bottle Feeding Breastfeeding Assistance Family Integrity Promotion: Childbearing Family Family Support Parent Education: Infant Teaching: Infant Nutrition Touch	Abuse Protection Support: Child Caregiver Support Health System Guidance Lactation Counseling Nutritional Monitoring Support System Enhancement Sustenance Support

Continued

Outcome	Major Interventions	Suggested Interventions	Optional Interventions
Child Development: 4 Months			
DEFINITION: Milestones of physical, cognitive, and psychosocial progression by 4 months of age	Developmental Enhancement: Child Infant Care Parenting Promotion	Anticipatory Guidance Bottle Feeding Family Integrity Promotion: Childbearing Family Family Process Maintenance Family Support Lactation Counseling Parent Education: Infant Teaching: Infant Nutrition Teaching: Infant Safety Touch	Abuse Protection Support: Child Attachment Promotion Caregiver Support Health System Guidance Health Screening Lactation Counseling Nonnutritive Sucking Nutrition Management Nutritional Counseling Nutritional Monitoring Respite Care Support System Enhancement Sustenance Support
Child Development: 6 Months			
DEFINITION: Milestones of physical, cognitive, and psychosocial progression by 6 months of age	Developmental Enhancement: Child Health Screening Parenting Promotion	Anticipatory Guidance Family Integrity Promotion: Childbearing Family Family Process Maintenance Family Support Infant Care Nutritional Counseling Parent Education: Infant Security Enhancement Teaching: Infant Nutrition Teaching: Infant Safety	Abuse Protection Support: Child Attachment Promotion Caregiver Support Environmental Management: Safety Health System Guidance Nutrition Management Nutritional Monitoring Support System Enhancement Surveillance: Safety Sustenance Support

Outcome	Major Interventions	Suggested Interventions	Optional Interventions
Child Development: 12 Months			
DEFINITION: Milestones of physical, cognitive, and psychosocial progression by 12 months of age	Developmental Enhancement: Child Health Screening Parenting Promotion	Anticipatory Guidance Family Integrity Promotion: Childbearing Family Family Process Maintenance Family Support Nutritional Counseling Parent Education: Childrearing Family Security Enhancement Socialization Enhancement Teaching: Toddler Nutrition Teaching: Toddler Safety	Abuse Protection Support: Child Attachment Promotion Caregiver Support Environmental Management: Safety Health System Guidance Nutrition Management Nutritional Monitoring Support System Enhancement Surveillance: Safety Sustenance Support Therapeutic Play

Continued

Outcome	Major Interventions	Suggested Interventions	Optional Interventions
Child Development: 2 Years			
DEFINITION: Milestones of physical, cognitive, and psychosocial progression by 2 years of age	Developmental Enhancement: Child Health Screening Parent Education: Childrearing Family	Anticipatory Guidance Family Integrity Promotion Family Support Family Therapy Nutrition Management Parenting Promotion Security Enhancement Socialization Enhancement Teaching: Toddler Nutrition Teaching: Toddler Safety Teaching: Toilet Training	Abuse Protection Support: Child Activity Therapy Behavior Management Behavior Management: Overactivity/ Inattention Bowel Training Family Process Maintenance Health System Guidance Nutritional Counseling Support System Enhancement Surveillance: Safety Therapeutic Play Trauma Therapy: Child Urinary Habit Training

Outcome	Major Interventions	Suggested Interventions	Optional Interventions
Child Development: 3 Years			
DEFINITION: Milestones of physical, cognitive, and psychosocial progression by 3 years of age	Developmental Enhancement: Child Health Screening Parent Education: Childrearing Family	Anticipatory Guidance Behavior Management Behavior Management: Overactivity/ Inattention Bowel Incontinence Care: Encopresis Bowel Management Bowel Training Family Integrity Promotion Family Support Family Therapy Nutrition Management Parenting Promotion Security Enhancement Socialization Enhancement Support System Enhancement Teaching: Toddler Nutrition Teaching: Toddler Safety Teaching: Toilet Training Urinary Habit Training Urinary Incontinence Care: Enuresis	Abuse Protection Support: Child Activity Therapy Behavior Modification Family Process Maintenance Health System Guidance Nutritional Counseling Nutritional Monitoring Sleep Enhancement Surveillance: Safety Sustenance Support Therapeutic Play Trauma Therapy: Child

Continued

Outcome	Major Interventions	Suggested Interventions	Optional Interventions
Child Development: 4 Years			
DEFINITION: Milestones of physical, cognitive, and psychosocial progression by 4 years of age	Developmental Enhancement: Child Health Screening Parent Education: Childrearing Family	Activity Therapy Anticipatory Guidance Behavior Management Behavior Management: Overactivity/ Inattention Behavior Modification Nutrition Management Nutrition Therapy Parenting Promotion Security Enhancement Socialization Enhancement Support System Enhancement Teaching: Psychomotor Skill Urinary Incontinence Care: Enuresis	Abuse Protection Support: Child Family Integrity Promotion Family Process Maintenance Family Support Family Therapy Health System Guidance Nutritional Counseling Nutritional Monitoring Sleep Enhancement Sustenance Support Therapeutic Play Urinary Habit Training

Outcome	Major Interventions	Suggested Interventions	Optional Interventions
Child Development: 5 Years			
DEFINITION: Milestones of physical, cognitive, and psychosocial progression by 5 years of age	Developmental Enhancement: Child Health Screening	Activity Therapy Anticipatory Guidance Behavior Management: Overactivity/ Inattention Behavior Modification Learning Facilitation Nutrition Management Nutrition Therapy Parent Education: Childrearing Family Parenting Promotion Security Enhancement Socialization Enhancement Support System Enhancement Teaching: Psychomotor Skill Therapeutic Play Urinary Incontinence Care: Enuresis	Abuse Protection Support: Child Behavior Management Family Integrity Promotion Family Support Family Therapy Health System Guidance Nutritional Monitoring Sleep Enhancement Sustenance Support Urinary Habit Training

Continued

Outcome	Major Interventions	Suggested Interventions	Optional Interventions
Child Development: Middle Childhood			
DEFINITION: Milestones of physical, cognitive, and psychosocial progression from 6 years through 11 years of age	Developmental Enhancement: Child Health Screening	Anticipatory Guidance Behavior Management Behavior Management: Sexual Behavior Modification Behavior Modification: Social Skills Exercise Promotion Impulse Control Training Learning Facilitation Mutual Goal Setting Nutrition Management Nutrition Therapy Parent Education: Childrearing Family Parenting Promotion Patient Contracting Self-Awareness Enhancement Self-Responsibility Facilitation Socialization Enhancement Urinary Incontinence: Enuresis Weight Management	Abuse Protection Support: Child Body Image Enhancement Counseling Family Integrity Promotion Family Support Family Therapy Health System Guidance Nutritional Counseling Nutritional Monitoring Self-Awareness Enhancement Self-Esteem Enhancement Spiritual Support Substance Use Prevention Teaching: Individual Teaching: Safe Sex Teaching: Sexuality Values Clarification

Outcome	Major Interventions	Suggested Interventions	Optional Interventions
Child Development: Adolescence			
DEFINITION: Milestones of physical, cognitive, and psychosocial progression from 12 years through 17 years of age	Developmental Enhancement: Adolescent Health Screening Risk Identification Self-Responsibility Facilitation	Anticipatory Guidance Behavior Management Behavior Management: Sexual Behavior Modification Behavior Modification: Social Skills Counseling Eating Disorders Management Exercise Promotion Health System Guidance Impulse Control Training Learning Readiness Enhancement Mutual Goal Setting Nutrition Therapy Nutritional Monitoring Parent Education: Adolescent Parenting Promotion Self-Esteem Enhancement Socialization Enhancement Substance Use Prevention	Abuse Protection Support Bibliotherapy Body Image Enhancement Environmental Management: Violence Prevention Family Integrity Promotion Family Support Family Therapy Nutrition Management Nutritional Counseling Role Enhancement Self-Awareness Enhancement Self-Modification Assistance Sexual Counseling Spiritual Support Sports-Injury Prevention: Youth Support System Enhancement Sustenance Support Teaching: Safe Sex Teaching: Sexuality Values Clarification Weight Management

G

Continued

Outcome	Major Interventions	Suggested Interventions	Optional Interventions
Growth			
DEFINITION: Normal increase in bone size and body weight during growth years	Health Screening Nutrition Management Nutrition Therapy	Anticipatory Guidance Eating Disorders Management Energy Management Health Education Nutritional Counseling Nutritional Monitoring Teaching: Infant Nutrition Teaching: Prescribed Diet Teaching: Toddler Nutrition Weight Gain Assistance Weight Management	Bottle Feeding Breastfeeding Assistance Feeding Lactation Counseling Referral

G

Outcome	Major Interventions	Suggested Interventions	Optional Interventions
Physical Aging			
DEFINITION: Normal physical changes that occur with the natural aging process	Health Screening Risk Identification	Anticipatory Guidance Behavior Modification Communication Enhancement: Hearing Deficit Communication Enhancement: Visual Deficit Energy Management Exercise Promotion Nutrition Management Nutrition Therapy Patient Contracting Self-Modification Assistance Self-Responsibility Facilitation Teaching: Prescribed Activity/Exercise Teaching: Prescribed Diet Teaching: Prescribed Medication Weight Management	Body Mechanics Promotion Bowel Management Coping Enhancement Emotional Support Exercise Promotion: Strength Training Exercise Therapy: Joint Mobility Medication Management Medication Prescribing Nutritional Counseling Nutritional Monitoring Resiliency Promotion Sexual Counseling Urinary Elimination Management Vital Signs Monitoring

Continued

Outcome	Major Interventions	Suggested Interventions	Optional Interventions
Physical Maturation: Female			
DEFINITION: Normal physical changes in the female that occur with the transition from childhood to adulthood	Developmental Enhancement: Adolescent Health Screening	Anticipatory Guidance Behavior Management: Sexual Body Image Enhancement Impulse Control Training Nutrition Management Risk Identification Self-Awareness Enhancement Self-Esteem Enhancement Teaching: Sexuality	Eating Disorders Management Health System Guidance Nutrition Therapy Nutritional Counseling Nutritional Monitoring Parent Education: Adolescent
Physical Maturation: Male			
DEFINITION: Normal physical changes in the male that occur with the transition from childhood to adulthood	Developmental Enhancement: Adolescent Health Screening	Anticipatory Guidance Behavior Management: Sexual Body Image Enhancement Impulse Control Training Nutrition Management Risk Identification Self-Awareness Enhancement Self-Esteem Enhancement Teaching: Sexuality	Eating Disorders Management Health System Guidance Nutrition Therapy Nutritional Counseling Nutritional Monitoring Parent Education: Adolescent

NURSING DIAGNOSIS: Health Maintenance, Ineffective

DEFINITION: Inability to identify, manage, and/or seek out help to maintain health.

Outcome	Major Interventions	Suggested Interventions	Optional Interventions
Health Beliefs: Perceived Resources			
DEFINITION: Personal conviction that one has adequate means to carry out a health behavior	Financial Resource Assistance Health System Guidance Support System Enhancement	Family Mobilization Family Support Insurance Authorization Sustenance Support	Energy Management Referral Self-Care Assistance
Health Promoting Behavior			
DEFINITION: Personal actions to sustain or increase wellness	Health Education Self-Modification Assistance	Behavior Modification Coping Enhancement Counseling Exercise Promotion Health Screening Risk Identification Self-Awareness Enhancement Self-Responsibility Facilitation Support System Enhancement	Family Mobilization Nutrition Management Oral Health Promotion Referral Sleep Enhancement Smoking Cessation Assistance Sports-Injury Prevention: Youth Substance Use Prevention Teaching: Safe Sex Values Clarification Weight Management
Health Seeking Behavior			
DEFINITION: Personal actions to promote optimal wellness, recovery, and rehabilitation	Decision-Making Support Self-Responsibility Facilitation	Anticipatory Guidance Counseling Health Education Health Screening Health System Guidance Learning Facilitation Mutual Goal Setting Patient Contracting Self-Modification Assistance	Culture Brokerage Exercise Promotion Nutrition Management Referral Smoking Cessation Assistance Substance Use Prevention Support Group Teaching: Safe Sex Values Clarification Weight Management

Continued

Outcome	Major Interventions	Suggested Interventions	Optional Interventions
Knowledge: Health Behavior			
DEFINITION: Extent of understanding conveyed about the promotion and protection of health	Health Education	Anticipatory Guidance Learning Facilitation Teaching: Foot Care Teaching: Group Teaching: Individual Teaching: Infant Nutrition Teaching: Prescribed Activity/Exercise Teaching: Prescribed Diet Teaching: Prescribed Medication Teaching: Toddler Nutrition Teaching: Toddler Safety	Health System Guidance Learning Readiness Enhancement Parent Education: Adolescent Parent Education: Childrearing Family Parent Education: Infant Preconception Counseling Risk Identification Risk Identification: Childbearing Family Teaching: Psychomotor Skill Teaching: Safe Sex Teaching: Sexuality Telephone Consultation Values Clarification
Knowledge: Health Promotion			
DEFINITION: Extent of understanding conveyed about information needed to obtain and maintain optimal health	Health Education Teaching: Individual	Learning Facilitation Nutritional Counseling Oral Health Promotion Preconception Counseling Risk Identification Teaching: Safe Sex	Childbirth Preparation Health System Guidance Learning Readiness Facilitation Parent Education: Childrearing Family
Knowledge: Health Resources			
DEFINITION: Extent of understanding conveyed about relevant health care resources	Health System Guidance	Discharge Planning Health Education Learning Facilitation Teaching: Individual	Health Care Information Exchange Learning Readiness Enhancement Teaching: Group Telephone Consultation

Outcome	Major Interventions	Suggested Interventions	Optional Interventions
Knowledge: Treatment Regimen			
DEFINITION: Extent of understanding conveyed about a specific treatment regimen	Teaching: Procedure/ Treatment	Chemotherapy Management Learning Facilitation Radiation Therapy Management Surgical Preparation Teaching: Disease Process Teaching: Foot Care Teaching: Individual Teaching: Preoperative Teaching: Prescribed Activity/Exercise Teaching: Prescribed Diet Teaching: Prescribed Medication	Family Involvement Promotion Health System Guidance Learning Readiness Enhancement Prenatal Care Teaching: Group Weight Gain Assistance Weight Management Weight Reduction Assistance
Participation in Health Care Decisions			
DEFINITION: Personal involvement in selecting and evaluating health care options to achieve desired outcome	Decision-Making Support Health System Guidance	Active Listening Admission Care Anticipatory Guidance Assertiveness Training Counseling Culture Brokerage Discharge Planning Patient Rights Protection Self-Responsibility Facilitation Values Clarification	Anxiety Reduction Coping Enhancement Family Involvement Promotion Health Care Information Exchange Insurance Authorization Referral Telephone Consultation

Continued

Outcome	Major Interventions	Suggested Interventions	Optional Interventions
Personal Health Status			
DEFINITION: Overall physical, psychological, social, and spiritual functioning of an adult 18 years or older	Health Education Health Screening	Coping Enhancement Exercise Promotion Medication Management Mood Management Nutrition Management Self-Awareness Enhancement Self-Modification Assistance Self-Responsibility Facilitation Smoking Cessation Assistance Substance Use Prevention Weight Management	Health System Guidance Nutritional Counseling Patient Contracting Support System Enhancement
Risk Detection			
DEFINITION: Personal actions to identify personal health threats	Health Screening Risk Identification Risk Identification: Childbearing Family	Breast Examination Environmental Management: Safety Health System Guidance Learning Facilitation Self-Responsibility Facilitation Surveillance: Safety Teaching: Disease Process Teaching: Group Teaching: Individual Values Clarification	Abuse Protection Support Abuse Protection Support: Child Abuse Protection Support: Elder Health Education Smoking Cessation Assistance

Outcome	Major Interventions	Suggested Interventions	Optional Interventions
Self-Care Status			
DEFINITION: Ability to perform basic personal care activities and household tasks	Self-Care Assistance Self-Care Assistance: IADL	Body Mechanics Promotion Energy Management Exercise Promotion Medication Management Oral Health Maintenance Self-Care Assistance: Bathing/Hygiene Self-Care Assistance: Dressing/Grooming Self-Care Assistance: Feeding Self-Care Assistance: Toileting Self-Care Assistance: Transfer	Environmental Management: Safety Exercise Promotion: Strength Training Exercise Promotion: Stretching Exercise Therapy: Ambulation Exercise Therapy: Balance Exercise Therapy: Joint Mobility Exercise Therapy: Muscle Control Fall Prevention Oral Health Promotion Swallowing Therapy
Self-Direction of Care			
DEFINITION: Care recipient actions taken to direct others who assist with or perform physical tasks and personal health care	Self-Responsibility Facilitation	Assertiveness Training Coping Enhancement Culture Brokerage Decision-Making Support Values Clarification	Family Support Health System Guidance Medication Management Nutrition Management Role Enhancement Self-Awareness Enhancement Self-Esteem Enhancement

Continued

Outcome	Major Interventions	Suggested Interventions	Optional Interventions
Social Support			
DEFINITION: Perceived availability and actual provision of reliable assistance from others	Family Involvement Promotion Support Group Support System Enhancement	Emotional Support Family Support Financial Resource Assistance Referral Socialization Enhancement Telephone Consultation	Caregiver Support Coping Enhancement Insurance Authorization Role Enhancement Spiritual Support Sustenance Support Therapy Group
Student Health Status			
DEFINITION: Physical, cognitive/ emotional, and social status of school age children that contribute to school attendance, participation in school activities, and ability to learn	Developmental Enhancement: Adolescent Developmental Enhancement: Child Health Education Health Screening	Coping Enhancement Counseling Exercise Promotion Mood Management Nutrition Management Self-Awareness Enhancement Self-Esteem Enhancement Self-Responsibility Facilitation Spiritual Growth Facilitation Substance Use Prevention Teaching: Safe Sex Weight Management	Abuse Protection Support: Child Financial Resource Assistance Mutual Goal Setting Parent Education: Adolescent Parent Education: Childrearing Family Parenting Promotion Religious Addiction Prevention

Outcome	Major Interventions	Suggested Interventions	Optional Interventions
Treatment Behavior: Illness or Injury DEFINITION: Personal actions to palliate or eliminate pathology	Self-Responsibility Facilitation Teaching: Disease Process	Allergy Management Asthma Management Behavior Management Behavior Modification Chemotherapy Management Health System Guidance Medication Management Mutual Goal Setting Nutrition Management Patient Contracting Radiation Therapy Management Self-Modification Assistance Support System Enhancement Teaching: Foot Care Teaching: Prescribed Activity/Exercise Teaching: Prescribed Diet Teaching: Prescribed Medication Teaching: Procedure/Treatment Teaching: Psychomotor Skill	Coping Enhancement Self-Awareness Enhancement Self-Care Assistance Smoking Cessation Assistance Substance Use Treatment Support Group Telephone Consultation Weight Gain Assistance Weight Reduction Assistance

NURSING DIAGNOSIS: Health-Seeking Behaviors (Specify)

DEFINITION: Active seeking (by a person in stable health) of ways to alter personal health habits, and/or the environment in order to move toward a higher level of health.

Outcome	Major Interventions	Suggested Interventions	Optional Interventions
Adherence Behavior DEFINITION: Self-initiated actions to promote wellness, recovery, and rehabilitation	Health Education Self-Modification Assistance	Coping Enhancement Decision-Making Support Emotional Support Exercise Promotion Health System Guidance Support System Enhancement Telephone Consultation Values Clarification	Assertiveness Training Counseling Health Screening Risk Identification Teaching: Individual
Health Beliefs DEFINITION: Personal convictions that influence health behaviors	Self-Awareness Enhancement Values Clarification	Counseling Culture Brokerage Health Education Risk Identification Self-Esteem Enhancement	Bibliotherapy Health System Guidance Teaching: Individual Truth Telling
Health Orientation DEFINITION: Personal commitment to health behaviors as lifestyle priorities	Health Education Values Clarification	Counseling Culture Brokerage Decision-Making Support Self-Awareness Enhancement Self-Modification Assistance Self-Responsibility Facilitation	Active Listening Bibliotherapy Teaching: Group Teaching: Individual

Outcome	Major Interventions	Suggested Interventions	Optional Interventions
Health Promoting Behavior DEFINITION: Personal actions to sustain or increase wellness	Health Education Self-Modification Assistance	Behavior Modification Breast Examination Coping Enhancement Emotional Support Exercise Promotion Exercise Promotion: Strength Training Exercise Promotion: Stretching Health Screening Immunization/ Vaccination Management Preconception Counseling Risk Identification Self-Responsibility Facilitation Smoking Cessation Assistance Spiritual Growth Facilitation Substance Use Prevention Weight Management	Fertility Preservation Meditation Facilitation Nutrition Management Oral Health Promotion Sexual Counseling Simple Guided Imagery Simple Relaxation Therapy Sleep Enhancement Socialization Enhancement Spiritual Support Support Group Support System Enhancement

Continued

H

Outcome	Major Interventions	Suggested Interventions	Optional Interventions
Health-Seeking Behavior			
DEFINITION: Personal actions to promote optimal wellness, recovery, and rehabilitation	Decision-Making Support Health Education Values Clarification	Activity Therapy Developmental Enhancement: Adolescent Developmental Enhancement: Child Emotional Support Family Integrity Promotion Health System Guidance Learning Facilitation Self-Modification Assistance Self-Responsibility Facilitation Support Group	Bibliotherapy Culture Brokerage Exercise Promotion Mutual Goal Setting Nutrition Management Patient Contracting Self-Awareness Enhancement Smoking Cessation Assistance Substance Use Prevention Teaching: Safe Sex Weight Management
Knowledge: Health Promotion			
DEFINITION: Extent of understanding conveyed about information needed to obtain and maintain optimal health	Health Education Teaching: Individual	Learning Facilitation Nutritional Counseling Oral Health Promotion Preconception Counseling Risk Identification Teaching: Safe Sex Teaching: Sexuality	Childbirth Preparation Genetic Counseling Health System Guidance Learning Readiness Enhancement Parent Education: Childrearing Family Sexual Counseling
Knowledge: Health Resources			
DEFINITION: Extent of understanding conveyed about relevant health care resources	Health System Guidance	Discharge Planning Health Education Learning Facilitation Learning Readiness Enhancement Teaching: Individual	Financial Resource Assistance Health Care Information Exchange Teaching: Group Telephone Consultation

Outcome	Major Interventions	Suggested Interventions	Optional Interventions
Personal Health Status			
DEFINITION: Overall physical, psychological, social, and spiritual functioning of an adult 18 years or older	Health Education Health Screening	Coping Enhancement Energy Maintenance Exercise Promotion Mood Management Nutrition Management Resiliency Promotion Risk Identification Self-Awareness Enhancement Self-Modification Assistance Socialization Enhancement Spiritual Growth Facilitation Teaching: Prescribed Medication Weight Management	Anger Control Assistance Bowel Management Complex Relationship Building Decision-Making Support Learning Facilitation Medication Management Meditation Facilitation Nausea Management Nutritional Counseling Pain Management Smoking Cessation Assistance Substance Use Prevention Vehicle Safety Promotion

Continued

Outcome	Major Interventions	Suggested Interventions	Optional Interventions
Personal Well-Being DEFINITION: Extent of positive perception of one's health status and life circumstances	Risk Identification Self-Awareness Enhancement Values Clarification	Coping Enhancement Counseling Decision-Making Support Emotional Support Family Integrity Promotion Family Support Health Education Health Screening Meditation Facilitation Role Enhancement Security Enhancement Self-Esteem Enhancement Self-Modification Assistance Self-Responsibility Facilitation Socialization Enhancement Spiritual Growth Facilitation Support System Enhancement	Communication Enhancement: Hearing Deficit Communication Enhancement: Speech Deficit Communication Enhancement: Visual Deficit Exercise Promotion Health System Guidance Pain Management Substance Use Prevention Surveillance: Safety

Outcome	Major Interventions	Suggested Interventions	Optional Interventions
Prenatal Health Behavior			
DEFINITION: Personal actions to promote a healthy pregnancy and a healthy newborn	Health Education Preconception Counseling Prenatal Care	Electronic Fetal Monitoring: Antepartum Electronic Fetal Monitoring: Intrapartum Exercise Promotion Family Planning: Unplanned Pregnancy Nutrition Management Risk Identification Risk Identification: Genetic Self-Modification Assistance Smoking Cessation Assistance Substance Use Prevention Substance Use Treatment Substance Use Treatment: Alcohol Withdrawal Weight Management	Body Mechanics Promotion Culture Brokerage Fertility Preservation Genetic Counseling

Continued

Outcome	Major Interventions	Suggested Interventions	Optional Interventions
Risk Control: Alcohol Use			
DEFINITION: Personal actions to prevent, eliminate, or reduce alcohol use that poses a threat to health	Health Education Substance Use Prevention	Coping Enhancement Decision-Making Support Health Screening Risk Identification Self-Awareness Enhancement Self-Modification Assistance Self-Responsibility Facilitation Support Group	Behavior Modification Counseling Grief Work Facilitation Mood Management Preconception Counseling Self-Esteem Enhancement Spiritual Growth Facilitation
Risk Control: Cancer			
DEFINITION: Personal actions to detect or reduce the threat of cancer	Health Education Health Screening	Risk Identification Risk Identification: Genetic Self-Modification Assistance Smoking Cessation Assistance Substance Use Prevention	Genetic Counseling Teaching: Individual
Risk Control: Cardiovascular Health			
DEFINITION: Personal actions to eliminate or reduce threats to cardiovascular health	Cardiac Precautions Health Education Health Screening	Exercise Promotion Medication Management Mutual Goal Setting Risk Identification Self-Modification Assistance Smoking Cessation Assistance Teaching: Prescribed Diet Teaching: Prescribed Medication Weight Reduction Assistance	Nutrition Management Teaching: Individual Vital Signs Monitoring

Outcome	Major Interventions	Suggested Interventions	Optional Interventions
Risk Control: Drug Use			
DEFINITION: Personal actions to prevent, eliminate, or reduce drug use that poses a threat to health	Health Education Substance Use Prevention	Coping Enhancement Decision-Making Support Health Screening Risk Identification Self-Awareness Enhancement Self-Modification Assistance Self-Responsibility Facilitation Support Group	Behavior Modification Counseling Grief Work Facilitation Mood Management Preconception Counseling Self-Esteem Enhancement
Risk Control: Hearing Impairment			
DEFINITION: Personal actions to prevent, eliminate, or reduce threats to hearing function	Environmental Risk Protection Risk Identification	Environmental Management: Worker Safety Fever Treatment Health Screening Medication Administration: Ear Medication Prescribing	Communication Enhancement: Hearing Deficit Ear Care Risk Identification: Genetic
Risk Control: Sexually Transmitted Diseases (STD)			
DEFINITION: Personal actions to prevent, eliminate, or reduce behaviors associated with sexually transmitted disease	Health Education Teaching: Safe Sex	Anticipatory Guidance Behavior Management: Sexual Health Screening Health System Guidance Infection Protection Self-Modification Assistance Self-Responsibility Facilitation Values Clarification	Assertiveness Training Behavior Modification Impulse Control Training

Continued

Outcome	Major Interventions	Suggested Interventions	Optional Interventions
Risk Control: Tobacco Use			
DEFINITION: Personal actions to prevent, eliminate, or reduce tobacco use	Environmental Risk Protection Smoking Cessation Assistance	Health Education Medication Prescribing Self-Modification Assistance	Environmental Management: Community Preconception Counseling
Risk Control: Unintended Pregnancy			
DEFINITION: Personal actions to prevent or reduce the possibility of unintended pregnancy	Family Planning: Contraception Self-Responsibility Facilitation	Health System Guidance Risk Identification Self-Esteem Enhancement Self-Modification Assistance Sexual Counseling Teaching: Safe Sex Teaching: Sexuality Values Clarification	Assertiveness Training Behavior Modification Counseling Emotional Support
Risk Control: Visual Impairment			
DEFINITION: Personal actions to prevent, eliminate, or reduce threats to visual function	Environmental Risk Protection Risk Identification	Contact Lens Care Health Education Health Screening Medication Administration: Eye Medication Prescribing Teaching: Disease Process	Communication Enhancement: Visual Deficit Eye Care Phototherapy: Neonate

NURSING DIAGNOSIS: Home Maintenance, Impaired

DEFINITION: Inability to independently maintain a safe growth-promoting immediate environment.

Outcome	Major Interventions	Suggested Interventions	Optional Interventions
Family Functioning			
DEFINITION: Capacity of the family system to meet the needs of its members during developmental transitions	Family Integrity Promotion Family Integrity Promotion: Childbearing Family	Family Mobilization Family Process Maintenance Family Support Parenting Promotion	Case Management Financial Resource Assistance Mutual Goal Setting Resiliency Promotion Role Enhancement
Family Physical Environment			
DEFINITION: Physical arrangements in the home that provide safety and stimulation to family members	Home Maintenance Assistance	Environmental Management: Home Preparation Environmental Management: Safety Family Support Referral Support System Enhancement	Caregiver Support Financial Resource Assistance Role Enhancement
Parenting Performance			
DEFINITION: Parental actions to provide a child a nurturing and constructive physical, emotional, and social environment	Home Maintenance Assistance Parenting Promotion	Abuse Protection Support: Child Environmental Management: Safety Family Support Parent Education: Childrearing Family Support System Enhancement Surveillance	Respite Care Security Enhancement Support Group Sustenance Support Telephone Consultation

Continued

Outcome	Major Interventions	Suggested Interventions	Optional Interventions
Parenting: Psychosocial Safety			
DEFINITION: Parental actions to protect a child from social contacts that might cause harm or injury	Parent Education: Adolescent Parent Education: Childrearing Family Risk Identification: Childbearing Family	Abuse Protection Support: Child Anticipatory Guidance Developmental Enhancement: Adolescent Developmental Enhancement: Child Family Integrity Promotion: Childbearing Family Surveillance: Safety	Abuse Protection Support: Religious Counseling Family Support Family Therapy Mutual Goal Setting Self-Modification Assistance Support Group Teaching: Individual
Role Performance			
DEFINITION: Congruence of an individual's role behavior with role expectations	Role Enhancement	Anticipatory Guidance Behavior Modification Caregiver Support Counseling Emotional Support Self-Awareness Enhancement Values Clarification	Decision-Making Support Family Therapy Health Education Mutual Goal Setting Respite Care Self-Esteem Enhancement Support Group Support System Enhancement Sustenance Support
Safe Home Environment			
DEFINITION: Physical arrangements to minimize environmental factors that might cause physical harm or injury in the home	Environmental Management: Safety	Environmental Management: Violence Prevention Fall Prevention Home Maintenance Assistance Risk Identification Teaching: Infant Safety Teaching: Toddler Safety	Environmental Management: Home Preparation Fire Setting Precautions Surveillance: Safety

NURSING DIAGNOSIS: Hopelessness

DEFINITION: Subjective state in which an individual sees limited or no alternatives or personal choices available and is unable to mobilize energy on own behalf.

Outcome	Major Interventions	Suggested Interventions	Optional Interventions
Depression Self-Control			
DEFINITION: Personal actions to minimize melancholy and maintain interest in life events	Mood Management Resiliency Promotion Self-Modification Assistance	Behavior Modification Coping Enhancement Emotional Support Energy Management Grief Work Facilitation Grief Work Facilitation: Perinatal Death Guilt Work Facilitation Hope Instillation Mutual Goal Setting Patient Contracting Self-Awareness Enhancement Therapy Group	Animal-Assisted Therapy Art Therapy Exercise Promotion Music Therapy Presence Recreation Therapy Socialization Enhancement Therapeutic Play
Depression Level			
DEFINITION: Severity of melancholic mood and loss of interest in life events	Hope Instillation Mood Management	Crisis Intervention Coping Enhancement Counseling Emotional Support Grief Work Facilitation Grief Work Facilitation: Perinatal Death Self-Esteem Enhancement Support Group Therapy Group	Activity Therapy Behavior Management: Self-Harm Cognitive Stimulation Electroconvulsive Therapy (ECT) Management Phototherapy: Mood/Sleep Regulation Recreation Therapy Resiliency Promotion Security Enhancement Spiritual Support Suicide Prevention

Continued

Outcome	Major Interventions	Suggested Interventions	Optional Interventions
Hope			
DEFINITION: Optimism that is personally satisfying and life-supporting	Hope Instillation Spiritual Growth Facilitation	Active Listening Coping Enhancement Complex Relationship Building Emotional Support Energy Management Reminiscence Therapy Resiliency Promotion Sleep Enhancement Spiritual Support Support Group Support System Enhancement Values Clarification	Counseling Family Mobilization Grief Work Facilitation Mutual Goal Setting Presence Socialization Enhancement Suicide Prevention Touch
Mood Equilibrium			
DEFINITION: Appropriate adjustment of prevailing emotional tone in response to circumstances	Mood Management	Anger Control Assistance Counseling Crisis Intervention Emotional Support Grief Work Facilitation Grief Work Facilitation: Perinatal Death Hope Instillation Presence Resiliency Promotion Spiritual Support Support Group Suicide Prevention Touch	Animal-Assisted Therapy Anxiety Reduction Exercise Promotion Music Therapy Pain Management Self-Care Assistance Sleep Enhancement Support System Enhancement Therapeutic Play Therapy Group

Outcome	Major Interventions	Suggested Interventions	Optional Interventions
Psychomotor Energy			
DEFINITION: Personal drive and energy to maintain activities of daily living, nutrition, and personal safety	Counseling Mood Management	Coping Enhancement Decision-Making Support Emotional Support Forgiveness Facilitation Grief Work Facilitation Guilt Work Facilitation Hope Instillation Self-Awareness Enhancement Self-Esteem Enhancement Therapy Group	Anger Control Assistance Animal-Assisted Therapy Body Image Enhancement Cognitive Restructuring Grief Work Facilitation: Perinatal Death Presence Resiliency Promotion
Quality of Life			
DEFINITION: Extent of positive perception of current life circumstances	Hope Instillation Values Clarification	Coping Enhancement Decision-Making Support Emotional Support Family Support Grief Work Facilitation Resiliency Promotion Role Enhancement Security Enhancement Self-Awareness Enhancement Socialization Enhancement Spiritual Support Support System Enhancement	Body Image Enhancement Guilt Work Facilitation Mood Management Reminiscence Therapy Support Group Sustenance Support

Continued

Outcome	Major Interventions	Suggested Interventions	Optional Interventions
Will to Live			
DEFINITION: Desire, determination, and effort to survive	Coping Enhancement Hope Instillation	Active Listening Counseling Emotional Support Grief Work Facilitation Self-Awareness Enhancement Self-Esteem Enhancement Spiritual Support Support Group Support System Enhancement Values Clarification	Animal-Assisted Therapy Behavior Management: Self-Harm Bibliotherapy Cognitive Restructuring Humor Music Therapy Reminiscence Therapy Self-Modification Assistance Socialization Enhancement Suicide Prevention

NURSING DIAGNOSIS: Hyperthermia

DEFINITION: Body temperature elevated above normal range.

Outcome	Major Interventions	Suggested Interventions	Optional Interventions

Thermoregulation
 	
DEFINITION:
Balance among heat production, heat gain, and heat loss
	Fever Treatment
	Malignant
	  Hyperthermia
	  Precautions
	Temperature
	  Regulation
		Bathing
		Environmental
		  Management
		Fluid Management
		Heat Exposure
		  Treatment
		Infection Control
		Medication
		  Administration
		Medication
		  Management
		Medication
		  Prescribing
		Temperature
		  Regulation:
		  Intraoperative
		Vital Signs
		  Monitoring
			Emergency Care
			Heat/Cold Application
			Infection Protection
			Shock Management
			Skin Surveillance

**Thermoregulation:
Newborn**
 	
DEFINITION:
Balance among heat production, heat gain, and heat loss during the first 28 days of life
	Fever Treatment
	Newborn Care
	Temperature
	  Regulation
		Bathing
		Environmental
		  Management
		Fluid Management
		Infection Control
		Newborn
		  Monitoring
		Vital Signs
		  Monitoring
			Heat Exposure
			  Treatment
			Infection Protection
			Parent Education: Infant
			Seizure Management
			Seizure Precautions
			Skin Surveillance

Continued

Outcome	Major Interventions	Suggested Interventions	Optional Interventions
Vital Signs			
DEFINITION: Extent to which temperature, pulse, respiration, and blood pressure are within normal range	Temperature Regulation Vital Signs Monitoring	Fever Treatment Heat Exposure Treatment Hemodynamic Regulation Shock Management Shock Prevention	Heat/Cold Application Medication Administration Medication Management Temperature Regulation: Intraoperative

NURSING DIAGNOSIS: Hypothermia

DEFINITION: Body temperature below normal range.

Outcome	Major Interventions	Suggested Interventions	Optional Interventions
Thermoregulation			
DEFINITION: Balance among heat production, heat gain, and heat loss	Hypothermia Treatment Temperature Regulation Temperature Regulation: Intraoperative Vital Signs Monitoring	Circulatory Precautions Environmental Management Hemodynamic Regulation Respiratory Monitoring Shock Management: Vasogenic Shock Prevention	Circulatory Care: Arterial Insufficiency Circulatory Care: Venous Insufficiency Electrolyte Monitoring Fluid/Electrolyte Management Fluid Management Heat/Cold Application Shock Management Shock Prevention
Thermoregulation: Newborn			
DEFINITION: Balance among heat production, heat gain, and heat loss during the first 28 days of life	Hypothermia Treatment Newborn Care Temperature Regulation Vital Signs Monitoring	Environmental Management Fluid Management Newborn Monitoring Respiratory Monitoring Technology Management	Acid-Base Management Heat/Cold Application Parent Education: Infant Shock Prevention
Vital Signs			
DEFINITION: Extent to which temperature, pulse, respiration, and blood pressure are within normal range	Hypothermia Treatment Vital Signs Monitoring	Circulatory Precautions Environmental Management Hemodynamic Regulation Respiratory Monitoring Shock Management Shock Prevention Temperature Regulation	Fluid Management Heat/Cold Application Skin Surveillance

NURSING DIAGNOSIS: Infant Behavior, Disorganized

DEFINITION: Disintegrated physiological and neurobehavioral responses to the environment.

Outcome	Major Interventions	Suggested Interventions	Optional Interventions
Child Development: 1 Month			
DEFINITION: Milestones of physical, cognitive, and psychosocial progression by 1 month of age	Developmental Care Neurologic Monitoring Newborn Care	Attachment Promotion Environmental Management: Attachment Process Environmental Management: Comfort Kangaroo Care Parent Education: Infant Presence Touch	Bottle Feeding Breastfeeding Assistance Nonnutritive Sucking Respiratory Monitoring Sleep Enhancement Teaching: Infant Safety
Child Development: 2 Months			
DEFINITION: Milestones of physical, cognitive, and psychosocial progression by 2 months of age	Infant Care	Attachment Promotion Environmental Management: Comfort Family Involvement Promotion Family Mobilization Kangaroo Care Nonnutritive Sucking Sleep Enhancement Touch	Energy Management Lactation Counseling Neurologic Monitoring Nutritional Monitoring Positioning Respiratory Monitoring Teaching: Infant Nutrition Teaching: Infant Safety

Outcome	Major Interventions	Suggested Interventions	Optional Interventions
Neurological Status DEFINITION: Ability of the peripheral and central nervous system to receive, process, and respond to internal and external stimuli	Developmental Care Neurologic Monitoring	Environmental Management Fluid Management Positioning Respiratory Monitoring Surveillance Temperature Regulation Vital Signs Monitoring	Laboratory Data Interpretation Medication Administration Medication Management Newborn Monitoring Sleep Enhancement
Preterm Infant Organization DEFINITION: Extrauterine integration of physiologic and behavioral function by the infant born 24 to 37 (term) weeks gestation	Developmental Care Environmental Management	Attachment Promotion Breastfeeding Assistance Environmental Management: Attachment Process Kangaroo Care Lactation Counseling Newborn Care Newborn Monitoring Nonnutritive Sucking Nutritional Monitoring Pain Management Respiratory Monitoring Sleep Enhancement Temperature Regulation	Bottle Feeding Cutaneous Stimulation Parent Education: Infant Phototherapy: Neonate Positioning Surveillance Sustenance Support Teaching: Infant Stimulation

Continued

Outcome	Major Interventions	Suggested Interventions	Optional Interventions
Sleep DEFINITION: Natural periodic suspension of consciousness during which the body is restored	Sleep Enhancement	Calming Technique Energy Management Environmental Management Environmental Management: Comfort Pain Management	Nonnutritive Sucking Presence
Thermoregulation: Newborn DEFINITION: Balance among heat production, heat gain, and heat loss during the first 28 days of life	Newborn Care Temperature Regulation	Environmental Management Fluid Management Newborn Monitoring Vital Signs Monitoring	Parent Education: Infant

NURSING DIAGNOSIS: Infant Behavior: Organized, Readiness for Enhanced

DEFINITION: A pattern of modulation of the physiologic and behavioral systems of functioning (i.e., autonomic, motor, state-organizational, self-regulatory, and attentional-interactional systems) in an infant that is satisfactory but that can be improved resulting in higher levels of integration in response to environmental stimuli.

Outcome	Major Interventions	Suggested Interventions	Optional Interventions
Child Development: 1 Month			
DEFINITION: Milestones of physical, cognitive, and psychosocial progression by 1 month of age	Developmental Care Newborn Care	Attachment Promotion Environmental Management: Attachment Process Kangaroo Care Parent Education: Infant Teaching: Infant Safety Teaching: Infant Stimulation Touch	Bottle Feeding Breastfeeding Assistance Caregiver Support Circumcision Care Nonnutritive Sucking
Child Development: 2 Months			
DEFINITION: Milestones of physical, cognitive, and psychosocial progression by 2 months of age	Infant Care	Attachment Promotion Environmental Management Environmental Management: Attachment Process Family Integrity Promotion: Childbearing Family Family Mobilization Kangaroo Care Nonnutritive Sucking Sleep Enhancement Touch	Lactation Counseling Newborn Care Newborn Monitoring Parent Education: Infant Surveillance

Continued

Outcome	Major Interventions	Suggested Interventions	Optional Interventions
Child Development: 4 Months			
DEFINITION: Milestones of physical, cognitive, and psychosocial progression by 4 months of age	Health Screening Infant Care	Bottle Feeding Family Integrity Promotion: Childbearing Family Infant Care Lactation Counseling Parent Education: Infant Sleep Enhancement Teaching: Infant Nutrition	Attachment Promotion Caregiver Support Environmental Management Health System Guidance Nonnutritive Sucking Support System Enhancement Surveillance
Newborn Adaptation			
DEFINITION: Adaptive response to the extrauterine environment by a physiologically mature newborn during the first 28 days	Developmental Care Newborn Care	Attachment Promotion Bottle Feeding Breastfeeding Assistance Environmental Management: Attachment Process Kangaroo Care Newborn Monitoring Nonnutritive Sucking Respiratory Monitoring Sleep Enhancement Teaching: Infant Stimulation Touch Vital Signs Monitoring	Laboratory Data Interpretation Lactation Counseling Pain Management Parent Education: Infant Phototherapy: Neonate

Outcome	Major Interventions	Suggested Interventions	Optional Interventions
Sleep			
DEFINITION: Natural periodic suspension of consciousness during which the body is restored	Sleep Enhancement	Calming Technique Energy Management Environmental Management Environmental Management: Comfort Music Therapy	Newborn Care Newborn Monitoring Vital Signs Monitoring

NURSING DIAGNOSIS: Infant Feeding Pattern, Ineffective

DEFINITION: Impaired ability to suck or coordinate the suck-swallow response.

Outcome	Major Interventions	Suggested Interventions	Optional Interventions
Breastfeeding Establishment: Infant			
DEFINITION: Infant attachment to and sucking from the mother's breast for nourishment during the first 3 weeks of breastfeeding	Breastfeeding Assistance Lactation Counseling	Calming Technique Environmental Management: Attachment Process Environmental Management: Comfort Infant Care Newborn Care Weight Management	Caregiver Support Nonnutritive Sucking Nutritional Monitoring Parent Education: Infant
Breastfeeding Maintenance			
DEFINITION: Continuation of breastfeeding for nourishment of an infant/toddler	Breastfeeding Assistance Lactation Counseling	Attachment Promotion Environmental Management Environmental Management: Comfort Infant Care Nutrition Management Weight Management	Caregiver Support Parent Education: Infant
Hydration			
DEFINITION: Adequate water in the intracellular and extracellular compartments of the body	Fluid Monitoring Infant Care	Bottle Feeding Breastfeeding Assistance Enteral Tube Feeding Fluid Management Weight Management	Intravenous (IV) Insertion Intravenous (IV) Therapy Lactation Counseling

Outcome	Major Interventions	Suggested Interventions	Optional Interventions
Nutritional Status: Food and Fluid Intake			
DEFINITION: Amount of food and fluid taken into the body over a 24-hour period	Bottle Feeding Breastfeeding Assistance Enteral Tube Feeding	Fluid Management Fluid Monitoring Lactation Counseling Nutrition Management Nutritional Monitoring Weight Management	Gastrointestinal Intubation Sustenance Support Teaching: Infant Nutrition Teaching: Infant Safety Teaching: Infant Stimulation
Swallowing Status			
DEFINITION: Safe passage of fluids and/or solids from the mouth to the stomach	Enteral Tube Feeding Nonnutritive Sucking	Aspiration Precautions Calming Technique Surveillance	Bottle Feeding Breastfeeding Assistance Nutrition Management Referral Swallowing Therapy

NURSING DIAGNOSIS: Intracranial Adaptive Capacity, Decreased

DEFINITION: Intracranial fluid dynamic mechanisms that normally compensate for increases in intracranial volumes are compromised, resulting in repeated disproportionate increases in intracranial pressure (ICP) in response to a variety of noxious and nonnoxious stimuli.

Outcome	Major Interventions	Suggested Interventions	Optional Interventions
Neurological Status			
DEFINITION: Ability of the peripheral and central nervous system to receive, process, and respond to internal and external stimuli	Cerebral Edema Management Cerebral Perfusion Promotion Intracranial Pressure (ICP) Monitoring Neurologic Monitoring	Fluid/Electrolyte Management Fluid Management Fluid Monitoring Laboratory Data Interpretation Medication Administration Medication Management Peripheral Sensation Management Positioning: Neurologic Surveillance Surveillance: Safety Tube Care: Ventriculostomy/ Lumbar Drain Vital Signs Monitoring	Acid-Base Management Acid-Base Monitoring Airway Management Anxiety Reduction Code Management Emergency Care Intravenous (IV) Insertion Intravenous (IV) Therapy Positioning Respiratory Monitoring Seizure Management Seizure Precautions

Outcome	Major Interventions	Suggested Interventions	Optional Interventions
Neurological Status: Consciousness			
DEFINITION: Arousal, orientation, and attention to the environment	Cerebral Edema Management Cerebral Perfusion Promotion Neurologic Monitoring	Airway Management Aspiration Precautions Emergency Care Intracranial Pressure (ICP) Monitoring Intravenous (IV) Insertion Intravenous (IV) Therapy Laboratory Data Interpretation Medication Administration Medication Management Respiratory Monitoring Surveillance Vital Signs Monitoring	Anxiety Reduction Environmental Management: Safety Medication Administration: Ventricular Reservoir Patient Rights Protection Presence Seizure Precautions Skin Surveillance Touch
Seizure Control			
DEFINITION: Personal actions to reduce or minimize the occurrence of seizure episodes	Cerebral Edema Management Seizure Management Seizure Precautions Surveillance	Airway Management Aspiration Precautions Intracranial Pressure (ICP) Monitoring Medication Administration Neurologic Monitoring	Emergency Care Environmental Management: Safety

Continued

Outcome	Major Interventions	Suggested Interventions	Optional Interventions
Tissue Perfusion: Cerebral			
DEFINITION: Adequacy of blood flow through the cerebral vasculature to maintain brain function	Cerebral Edema Management Cerebral Perfusion Promotion Intracranial Pressure (ICP) Monitoring	Fluid Management Neurologic Monitoring Positioning: Neurologic Subarachnoid Hemorrhage Precautions Vital Signs Monitoring	Airway Management Respiratory Monitoring Seizure Management Seizure Precautions

NURSING DIAGNOSIS: Knowledge, Deficient (Specify)

DEFINITION: Absence or deficiency of cognitive information related to a specific topic.

Outcome	Major Interventions	Suggested Interventions	Optional Interventions
Knowledge: Body Mechanics			
DEFINITION: Extent of understanding conveyed about proper body alignment, balance and coordinated movement	Body Mechanics Promotion Teaching: Prescribed Activity/Exercise	Health Education Learning Facilitation Learning Readiness Enhancement Risk Identification Teaching: Individual	Exercise Promotion: Strength Training Exercise Promotion: Stretching Exercise Therapy: Ambulation Exercise Therapy: Balance Exercise Therapy: Joint Mobility Exercise Therapy: Muscle Control
Knowledge: Breastfeeding			
DEFINITION: Extent of understanding conveyed about lactation and nourishment of an infant through breastfeeding	Breastfeeding Assistance Lactation Counseling	Childbirth Preparation Learning Facilitation Learning Readiness Enhancement Teaching: Infant Nutrition	Infant Care Lactation Suppression Nonnutritive Sucking Parent Education: Infant
Knowledge: Cardiac Disease Management			
DEFINITION: Extent of understanding conveyed about heart disease and the prevention of complications	Teaching: Disease Process	Cardiac Care Learning Facilitation Learning Readiness Enhancement Teaching: Prescribed Activity/Exercise Teaching: Prescribed Diet Teaching: Prescribed Medication	Anxiety Reduction Behavior Modification Teaching: Individual Teaching: Procedure/ Treatment

Continued

K

Outcome	Major Interventions	Suggested Interventions	Optional Interventions
Knowledge: Child Physical Safety			
DEFINITION: Extent of understanding conveyed about safely caring for a child from 1 year through 17 years of age	Teaching: Infant Safety Teaching: Toddler Safety	Health Education Learning Facilitation Learning Readiness Enhancement Parent Education: Infant Risk Identification Surveillance: Safety Teaching: Individual	Counseling Parenting Promotion Risk Identification: Childbearing Family Teaching: Group Vehicle Safety Promotion
Knowledge: Conception Prevention			
DEFINITION: Extent of understanding conveyed about prevention of unintended pregnancy	Family Planning: Contraception Teaching: Safe Sex	Health Education Parent Education: Adolescent Parenting Promotion Learning Facilitation Learning Readiness Enhancement Self-Responsibility Facilitation Teaching: Individual	Behavior Management: Sexual Behavior Modification Family Planning: Unplanned Pregnancy Impulse Control Training Pregnancy Termination Care
Knowledge: Diabetes Management			
DEFINITION: Extent of understanding conveyed about diabetes mellitus and the prevention of complications	Teaching: Disease Process Teaching: Prescribed Diet Teaching: Prescribed Medication	Hyperglycemia Management Hypoglycemia Management Learning Facilitation Learning Readiness Enhancement Medication Administration: Subcutaneous Teaching: Foot Care Teaching: Prescribed Activity/Exercise Teaching: Psychomotor Skill	Behavior Modification Health Education Medication Management Nutrition Management Referral

Outcome	Major Interventions	Suggested Interventions	Optional Interventions
Knowledge: Diet			
DEFINITION: Extent of understanding conveyed about recommended diet	Teaching: Infant Nutrition Teaching: Prescribed Diet Teaching: Toddler Nutrition	Breastfeeding Assistance Health Education Lactation Counseling Learning Facilitation Learning Readiness Enhancement Nutritional Counseling Preconception Counseling Teaching: Individual	Behavior Management Chemotherapy Management Eating Disorders Management Nutrition Management Prenatal Care Self-Modification Assistance Teaching: Group Weight Management
Knowledge: Disease Process			
DEFINITION: Extent of understanding conveyed about a specific disease process	Teaching: Disease Process	Health System Guidance Learning Facilitation Learning Readiness Enhancement Teaching: Individual	Admission Care Allergy Management Anxiety Reduction Asthma Management Discharge Planning Risk Identification Teaching: Group
Knowledge: Energy Conservation			
DEFINITION: Extent of understanding conveyed about energy conservation techniques	Teaching: Prescribed Activity/Exercise	Health Education Learning Facilitation Learning Readiness Enhancement Teaching: Disease Process Teaching: Individual	Body Mechanics Promotion Energy Management Exercise Promotion Progressive Muscle Relaxation Recreation Therapy Simple Relaxation Therapy Teaching: Group

Continued

K

Outcome	Major Interventions	Suggested Interventions	Optional Interventions
Knowledge: Fall Prevention			
DEFINITION: Extent of understanding conveyed about prevention of falls	Fall Prevention Teaching: Individual	Exercise Promotion: Strength Training Exercise Promotion: Stretching Exercise Therapy: Ambulation Exercise Therapy: Balance Learning Facilitation Learning Readiness Enhancement Teaching: Prescribed Activity/Exercise Teaching: Toddler Safety	Surveillance: Safety
Knowledge: Fertility Promotion			
DEFINITION: Extent of understanding conveyed about fertility testing and the conditions that affect conception	Family Planning: Infertility Fertility Preservation Reproductive Technology Management	Learning Facilitation Learning Readiness Enhancement Patient Rights Protection Preconception Counseling Teaching: Procedure/ Treatment	Counseling Decision-Making Support Genetic Counseling Specimen Management

Outcome	Major Interventions	Suggested Interventions	Optional Interventions
Knowledge: Health Behavior			
DEFINITION: Extent of understanding conveyed about the promotion and protection of health	Health Education Teaching: Individual	Active Listening Anticipatory Guidance Breast Examination Health System Guidance Learning Facilitation Learning Readiness Enhancement Parent Education: Adolescent Parent Education: Childrearing Family Parent Education: Infant Teaching: Group Teaching: Safe Sex Values Clarification	Behavior Modification Genetic Counseling Health Screening Infection Protection Oral Health Promotion Preconception Counseling Risk Identification Substance Use Prevention Vehicle Safety Promotion
Knowledge: Health Promotion			
DEFINITION: Extent of understanding conveyed about information needed to obtain and maintain optimal health	Health Education Teaching: Individual	Anticipatory Guidance Learning Facilitation Learning Readiness Enhancement Teaching: Foot Care Teaching: Prescribed Activity/Exercise Teaching: Prescribed Diet Teaching: Prescribed Medication Teaching: Safe Sex Teaching: Sexuality	Allergy Management Asthma Management Immunization/ Vaccination Management Nutrition Management Weight Management

Continued

Outcome	Major Interventions	Suggested Interventions	Optional Interventions
Knowledge: Health Resources			
DEFINITION: Extent of understanding conveyed about relevant health care resources	Health System Guidance Teaching: Individual	Discharge Planning Health Education Learning Facilitation Learning Readiness Enhancement Support System Enhancement	Health Care Information Exchange Teaching: Group Telephone Consultation
Knowledge: Illness Care			
DEFINITION: Extent of understanding conveyed about illness-related information needed to achieve and maintain optimal health	Teaching: Individual Teaching: Procedure/ Treatment	Learning Facilitation Learning Readiness Enhancement Preparatory Sensory Information Teaching: Disease Process Teaching: Preoperative Teaching: Prescribed Activity/Exercise Teaching: Prescribed Diet Teaching: Prescribed Medication	Energy Management Health System Guidance Pain Management

Outcome	Major Interventions	Suggested Interventions	Optional Interventions
Knowledge: Infant Care			
DEFINITION: Extent of understanding conveyed about caring for a baby from birth to 1st birthday	Parent Education: Infant	Breastfeeding Assistance Lactation Counseling Learning Facilitation Learning Readiness Enhancement Teaching: Individual Teaching: Infant Nutrition Teaching: Infant Safety Teaching: Infant Stimulation	Circumcision Care Infant Care Newborn Care Parenting Promotion
Knowledge: Infection Control			
DEFINITION: Extent of understanding conveyed about prevention and control of infection	Infection Protection Risk Identification Teaching: Safe Sex	Health Education Incision Site Care Infection Control Learning Facilitation Learning Readiness Enhancement Teaching: Disease Process Teaching: Individual Teaching: Procedure/ Treatment Teaching: Psychomotor Skill	Home Maintenance Assistance Immunization/ Vaccination Management Medication Management Teaching: Group Teaching: Preoperative Teaching: Prescribed Medication Urinary Elimination Management Wound Care

Continued

Outcome	Major Interventions	Suggested Interventions	Optional Interventions
Knowledge: Labor and Delivery			
DEFINITION: Extent of understanding conveyed about labor and vaginal delivery	Childbirth Preparation	Anticipatory Guidance Learning Facilitation Learning Readiness Enhancement Prenatal Care Teaching: Individual	Intrapartal Care Labor Induction Labor Suppression Teaching: Group
Knowledge: Medication			
DEFINITION: Extent of understanding conveyed about the safe use of medication	Teaching: Prescribed Medication	Allergy Management Analgesic Administration Asthma Management Chemotherapy Management Learning Facilitation Learning Readiness Enhancement Medication Management Patient-Controlled Analgesia (PCA) Assistance Teaching: Disease Process Teaching: Individual	Constipation/Impaction Management Hyperglycemia Management Hypoglycemia Management Immunization/ Vaccination Management Pain Management Preconception Counseling Prenatal Care Teaching: Group
Knowledge: Ostomy Care			
DEFINITION: Extent of understanding conveyed about maintenance of an ostomy for elimination	Ostomy Care Teaching: Individual	Learning Facilitation Learning Readiness Enhancement Skin Care: Topical Treatments Skin Surveillance Teaching: Procedure/ Treatment Teaching: Psychomotor Skill	Infection Protection Teaching: Prescribed Diet Wound Care

Outcome	Major Interventions	Suggested Interventions	Optional Interventions
Knowledge: Parenting			
DEFINITION: Extent of understanding conveyed about provision of a nurturing and constructive environment for a child from 1 year through 17 years of age	Parent Education: Adolescent Parent Education: Childrearing Family Parent Education: Infant	Anticipatory Guidance Learning Facilitation Learning Readiness Enhancement Parenting Promotion Teaching: Infant Nutrition Teaching: Infant Safety Teaching: Infant Stimulation Teaching: Toddler Nutrition Teaching: Toddler Safety Teaching: Toilet Training	Attachment Promotion Bowel Incontinence Care: Encopresis Developmental Enhancement: Adolescent Developmental Enhancement: Child Teaching: Individual
Knowledge: Personal Safety			
DEFINITION: Extent of understanding conveyed about prevention of unintentional injuries	Health Education Teaching: Infant Safety Teaching: Toddler Safety	Counseling Learning Facilitation Learning Readiness Enhancement Patient Rights Protection Risk Identification Teaching: Individual	Abuse Protection Support Abuse Protection Support: Child Abuse Protection Support: Domestic Partner Abuse Protection Support: Elder Fall Prevention Infection Protection Substance Use Prevention Teaching: Psychomotor Skill Vehicle Safety Promotion

Continued

Outcome	Major Interventions	Suggested Interventions	Optional Interventions
Knowledge: Postpartum Maternal Health			
DEFINITION: Extent of understanding conveyed about maternal health following delivery	Lactation Counseling Teaching: Prescribed Activity/Exercise	Health Education Learning Facilitation Learning Readiness Enhancement Nutritional Counseling Teaching: Individual Weight Reduction Assistance	Cesarean Section Care Health System Guidance Postpartal Care
Knowledge: Preconception Maternal Health			
DEFINITION: Extent of understanding conveyed about maternal health prior to conception to insure a healthy pregnancy	Health Education Preconception Counseling	Counseling Genetic Counseling Learning Facilitation Learning Readiness Enhancement Teaching: Individual	Behavior Modification Sexual Counseling Substance Use Prevention
Knowledge: Pregnancy			
DEFINITION: Extent of understanding conveyed about promotion of a healthy pregnancy and prevention of complications	Childbirth Preparation	Anticipatory Guidance Health Education Learning Facilitation Learning Readiness Enhancement Teaching: Individual Teaching: Prescribed Diet Teaching: Prescribed Medication	Health System Guidance High-Risk Pregnancy Care Prenatal Care

Outcome	Major Interventions	Suggested Interventions	Optional Interventions
Knowledge: Prescribed Activity			
DEFINITION: Extent of understanding conveyed about prescribed activity and exercise	Teaching: Prescribed Activity/Exercise	Energy Management Exercise Promotion Learning Facilitation Learning Readiness Enhancement Patient Contracting Teaching: Individual	Activity Therapy Behavior Modification Recreation Therapy Self-Modification Assistance Teaching: Group Therapeutic Play
Knowledge: Sexual Functioning			
DEFINITION: Extent of understanding conveyed about sexual development and responsible sexual practices	Teaching: Safe Sex Teaching: Sexuality	Behavior Management: Sexual Family Planning: Contraception Learning Facilitation Learning Readiness Enhancement Sexual Counseling Teaching: Individual	Genetic Counseling Patient Rights Protection Self-Awareness Enhancement
Knowledge: Substance Use Control			
DEFINITION: Extent of understanding conveyed about controlling the use of drugs, tobacco, or alcohol	Health Education Substance Use Prevention	Behavior Management Learning Facilitation Learning Readiness Enhancement Medication Management Teaching: Group Teaching: Individual Teaching: Prescribed Medication	Analgesic Administration Health System Guidance Mutual Goal Setting Patient Contracting Preconception Counseling Smoking Cessation Assistance Substance Use Treatment

Continued

Outcome	Major Interventions	Suggested Interventions	Optional Interventions
Knowledge: Treatment Procedure(s)			
DEFINITION: Extent of understanding conveyed about procedure(s) required as part of a treatment regimen	Preparatory Sensory Information Teaching: Procedure/ Treatment Teaching: Psychomotor Skill	Anticipatory Guidance Learning Facilitation Learning Readiness Enhancement Patient Rights Protection Teaching: Disease Process Teaching: Individual	Anxiety Reduction Culture Brokerage Decision-Making Support Examination Assistance Labor Induction
Knowledge: Treatment Regimen			
DEFINITION: Extent of understanding conveyed about a specific treatment regimen	Teaching: Disease Process Teaching: Preoperative Teaching: Procedure/ Treatment	Allergy Management Anticipatory Guidance Asthma Management Chemotherapy Management Learning Facilitation Learning Readiness Enhancement Medication Management Nutrition Management Radiation Therapy Management Teaching: Individual Teaching: Prescribed Activity/Exercise Teaching: Prescribed Diet Teaching: Prescribed Medication	Health System Guidance Labor Induction Prenatal Care Prosthesis Care Teaching: Group Weight Gain Assistance Weight Management Weight Reduction Assistance

NURSING DIAGNOSIS: Knowledge (Specify), Readiness for Enhanced*

DEFINITION: The presence or acquisition of cognitive information related to a specific topic is sufficient for meeting health-related goals and can be strengthened.

Outcome	Major Interventions	Suggested Interventions	Optional Interventions
Knowledge: Health Behavior DEFINITION: Extent of understanding conveyed about the promotion and protection of health	Health Education Learning Facilitation Learning Readiness Enhancement	Anticipatory Guidance Energy Management Family Planning: Contraception Health System Guidance Nutrition Management Substance Use Prevention Teaching: Safe Sex	Health Screening Oral Health Promotion Preconception Counseling Self-Modification Assistance Self-Responsibility Facilitation Sexual Counseling Smoking Cessation Assistance Sports-Injury Prevention: Youth Vehicle Safety Promotion

Continued

*See areas of specific knowledge under Knowledge, Deficient.

Outcome	Major Interventions	Suggested Interventions	Optional Interventions
Knowledge: Health Promotion			
DEFINITION: Extent of understanding conveyed about information needed to obtain and maintain optimal health	Health Education Learning Facilitation Learning Readiness Enhancement	Coping Enhancement Immunization/ Vaccination Management Infection Protection Substance Use Prevention Teaching: Individual Teaching: Prescribed Activity/Exercise Teaching: Prescribed Diet Teaching: Prescribed Medication Teaching: Procedure/ Treatment Teaching: Safe Sex	Breast Examination Smoking Cessation Assistance Weight Management
Knowledge: Health Resources			
DEFINITION: Extent of understanding conveyed about relevant health care resources	Health System Guidance Learning Facilitation Learning Readiness Enhancement	Case Management Culture Brokerage Discharge Planning Health Education Teaching: Individual	Financial Resource Assistance Teaching: Group Telephone Consultation

NURSING DIAGNOSIS: Latex Allergy Response

DEFINITION: An allergic response to natural latex rubber products.

Outcome	Major Interventions	Suggested Interventions	Optional Interventions
Allergic Response: Localized			
DEFINITION: Severity of localized hypersensitive immune response to a specific environmental (exogenous) antigen	Allergy Management Latex Precautions	Environmental Management Medication Administration Medication Administration: Nasal Medication Administration: Skin Risk Identification Skin Care: Topical Treatments Skin Surveillance Teaching: Individual	Pruritus Management Respiratory Monitoring
Allergic Response: Systemic			
DEFINITION: Severity of systemic hypersensitive immune response to a specific environmental (exogenous) antigen	Airway Management Anaphylaxis Management Emergency Care Respiratory Monitoring	Airway Suctioning Fluid Management Intravenous (IV) Insertion Intravenous (IV) Therapy Latex Precautions Medication Administration Medication Administration: Intravenous (IV) Medication Management Oxygen Therapy Risk Identification Shock Prevention	Airway Insertion and Stabilization Artificial Airway Management Code Management Eye Care

Continued

Outcome	Major Interventions	Suggested Interventions	Optional Interventions
Tissue Integrity: Skin & Mucous Membranes			
DEFINITION: Structural intactness and normal physiological function of skin and mucous membranes	Latex Precautions Skin Surveillance	Medication Administration Medication Administration: Skin Medication Management Skin Care: Topical Treatments Teaching: Individual	Fluid Management Pruritus Management Wound Care

NURSING DIAGNOSIS: Lifestyle, Sedentary

DEFINITION: Reports of a habit of life that is characterized by a low physical activity level.

Outcome	Major Interventions	Suggested Interventions	Optional Interventions
Activity Tolerance			
DEFINITION: Physiologic response to energy-consuming movements with daily activities	Activity Therapy Exercise Promotion	Behavior Modification Energy Management Exercise Promotion: Strength Training Mutual Goal Setting Self-Modification Assistance Teaching: Prescribed Activity/Exercise	Emotional Support Recreation Therapy Smoking Cessation Assistance Support Group Weight Management
Endurance			
DEFINITION: Capacity to sustain activity	Exercise Promotion Exercise Promotion: Strength Training	Activity Therapy Exercise Promotion: Stretching Exercise Therapy: Ambulation Mutual Goal Setting Teaching: Prescribed Activity/Exercise	Body Mechanics Promotion Nutrition Management Sleep Enhancement Smoking Cessation Assistance Weight Management

Continued

Outcome	Major Interventions	Suggested Interventions	Optional Interventions
Physical Fitness			
DEFINITION: Performance of physical activities with vigor	Activity Therapy Teaching: Prescribed Activity/Exercise	Behavior Modification Body Mechanics Promotion Exercise Promotion Nutrition Management Recreation Therapy Smoking Cessation Assistance Weight Management	Energy Management Self-Modification Assistance Sleep Enhancement

NURSING DIAGNOSIS: Memory, Impaired

DEFINITION: Inability to remember or recall bits of information or behavioral skills. May be attributed to pathophysiological or situational causes that are either temporary or permanent.

Outcome	Major Interventions	Suggested Interventions	Optional Interventions
Cognition			
DEFINITION: Ability to execute complex mental processes	Cognitive Stimulation Dementia Management Memory Training	Active Listening Anxiety Reduction Cerebral Perfusion Promotion Environmental Management Reality Orientation Reminiscence Therapy	Animal-Assisted Therapy Coping Enhancement Patient Rights Protection Recreation Therapy Security Enhancement
Cognitive Orientation			
DEFINITION: Ability to identify person, place, and time accurately	Delirium Management Dementia Management Reality Orientation	Cognitive Stimulation Electrolyte Monitoring Environmental Management Environmental Management: Safety Medication Management Memory Training Surveillance: Safety	Animal-Assisted Therapy Area Restriction Calming Technique Milieu Therapy Neurologic Monitoring Patient Rights Protection Reminiscence Therapy Substance Use Treatment Surveillance Visitation Facilitation
Concentration			
DEFINITION: Ability to focus on a specific stimulus	Anxiety Reduction Cognitive Stimulation	Cerebral Perfusion Promotion Dementia Management Environmental Management Learning Facilitation Medication Management	Communication Enhancement: Hearing Deficit Communication Enhancement: Visual Deficit Reminiscence Therapy

Continued

M

Outcome	Major Interventions	Suggested Interventions	Optional Interventions
Memory DEFINITION: Ability to cognitively retrieve and report previously stored information	Dementia Management Memory Training	Active Listening Anxiety Reduction Cognitive Stimulation Medication Management Milieu Therapy Reminiscence Therapy	Coping Enhancement Emotional Support Family Support Oxygen Therapy Patient Rights Protection Reality Orientation
Neurological Status DEFINITION: Ability of the peripheral and central nervous system to receive, process, and respond to internal and external stimuli	Cerebral Perfusion Promotion Neurologic Monitoring	Electrolyte Management Electrolyte Monitoring Fluid/Electrolyte Management Fluid Management Fluid Monitoring Medication Administration Medication Management Substance Use Treatment Surveillance	Oxygen Therapy Respiratory Monitoring Vital Signs Monitoring

NURSING DIAGNOSIS: Mobility: Bed, Impaired

DEFINITION: Limitation of independent movement from one bed position to another.

Outcome	Major Interventions	Suggested Interventions	Optional Interventions
Body Positioning: Self-Initiated			
DEFINITION: Ability to change own body position independently with or without assistive device	Exercise Promotion: Strength Training Self-Care Assistance	Body Mechanics Promotion Exercise Promotion: Stretching Exercise Therapy: Joint Mobility Exercise Therapy: Muscle Control Positioning Teaching: Prescribed Activity/Exercise	Energy Management Fall Prevention Self-Care Assistance: Transfer Traction/Immobilization Care
Body Mechanics Performance			
DEFINITION: Personal actions to maintain proper body alignment and to prevent muscular skeletal strain	Body Mechanics Promotion	Exercise Promotion: Strength Training Exercise Promotion: Stretching Exercise Therapy: Joint Mobility Exercise Therapy: Muscle Control Self-Care Assistance	Pain Management Self-Care Assistance: Feeding Self-Care Assistance: Toileting Self-Care Assistance: Transfer
Coordinated Movement			
DEFINITION: Ability of muscles to work together voluntarily for purposeful movement	Exercise Promotion: Strength Training Exercise Therapy: Muscle Control	Body Mechanics Promotion Exercise Promotion: Stretching Exercise Therapy: Joint Mobility Teaching: Prescribed Activity/Exercise	Pain Management Progressive Muscle Relaxation Simple Massage Simple Relaxation Therapy

Continued

M

Outcome	Major Interventions	Suggested Interventions	Optional Interventions
Immobility Consequences: Physiological DEFINITION: Severity of compromise in physiological functioning due to impaired physical mobility	Bed Rest Care Positioning	Embolus Precautions Exercise Promotion Exercise Promotion: Strength Training Exercise Promotion: Stretching Exercise Therapy: Joint Mobility Exercise Therapy: Muscle Control	Positioning: Neurologic Pressure Management Simple Massage Teaching: Prescribed Activity/Exercise
Joint Movement: (Specify Joint) DEFINITION: Active range of motion of _____ (specify joint) with self-initiated movement	Exercise Promotion: Strength Training Exercise Therapy: Joint Mobility	Energy Management Exercise Promotion: Stretching Exercise Therapy: Muscle Control	Heat/Cold Application Pain Management Traction/Immobilization Care
Joint Movement: Passive DEFINITION: Joint movement with assistance	Exercise Therapy: Joint Mobility	Exercise Promotion: Stretching Exercise Therapy: Muscle Control Pain Management	Heat/Cold Application Traction/Immobilization Care

Outcome	Major Interventions	Suggested Interventions	Optional Interventions
Mobility			
DEFINITION: Ability to move purposefully in own environment independently with or without assistive device	Exercise Promotion: Strength Training Exercise Therapy: Joint Mobility Exercise Therapy: Muscle Control	Bed Rest Care Body Mechanics Promotion Exercise Promotion Exercise Promotion: Stretching Teaching: Prescribed Activity/Exercise	Medication Management Pain Management Positioning Self-Care Assistance Self-Care Assistance: Bathing/Hygiene Self-Care Assistance: Dressing/Grooming Self-Care Assistance: Toileting Self-Care Assistance: Transfer Sleep Enhancement

M

M

NURSING DIAGNOSIS: Mobility: Physical, Impaired

DEFINITION: Limitation in independent, purposeful physical movement of the body or of one or more extremities.

Outcome	Major Interventions	Suggested Interventions	Optional Interventions
Ambulation DEFINITION: Ability to walk from place to place independently with or without assistive device	Exercise Promotion: Strength Training Exercise Therapy: Ambulation	Body Mechanics Promotion Energy Management Exercise Promotion Exercise Promotion: Stretching Exercise Therapy: Balance Exercise Therapy: Joint Mobility Exercise Therapy: Muscle Control Teaching: Prescribed Activity/Exercise	Activity Therapy Environmental Management: Safety Fall Prevention Pain Management Surveillance: Safety Weight Management Weight Reduction Assistance
Ambulation: Wheelchair DEFINITION: Ability to move from place to place in a wheelchair	Exercise Promotion: Strength Training Positioning: Wheelchair	Body Mechanics Promotion Energy Management Environmental Management: Safety Exercise Therapy: Balance Exercise Therapy: Joint Mobility Exercise Therapy: Muscle Control Fall Prevention Self-Care Assistance Teaching: Prescribed Activity/Exercise	Environmental Management Exercise Promotion Pain Management Self-Care Assistance: Transfer Surveillance: Safety Weight Management Weight Reduction Assistance

Outcome	Major Interventions	Suggested Interventions	Optional Interventions
Balance DEFINITION: Ability to maintain body equilibrium	Exercise Promotion: Strength Training Exercise Therapy: Balance	Exercise Promotion Exercise Therapy: Joint Mobility Exercise Therapy: Muscle Control Fall Prevention	Activity Therapy Body Mechanics Promotion Energy Management Environmental Management: Safety Pain Management Weight Management
Body Mechanics Performance DEFINITION: Personal actions to maintain proper body alignment and to prevent muscular skeletal strain	Body Mechanics Promotion Exercise Therapy: Ambulation	Exercise Promotion: Strength Training Exercise Promotion: Stretching Exercise Therapy: Balance Exercise Therapy: Joint Mobility Exercise Therapy: Muscle Control Teaching: Individual	Pain Management Self-Care Assistance Self-Care Assistance: IADL Self-Care Assistance: Toileting Self-Care Assistance: Transfer
Coordinated Movement DEFINITION: Ability of muscles to work together voluntarily for purposeful movement	Exercise Promotion: Strength Training Exercise Therapy: Muscle Control	Body Mechanics Promotion Exercise Promotion: Stretching Exercise Therapy: Ambulation Exercise Therapy: Balance Exercise Therapy: Joint Mobility	Energy Management Pain Management Teaching: Prescribed Activity/Exercise

Continued

Outcome	Major Interventions	Suggested Interventions	Optional Interventions
Joint Movement: (Specify Joint)			
DEFINITION: Active range of motion of _____ (specify joint) with self-initiated movement	Exercise Therapy: Joint Mobility	Energy Management Exercise Promotion: Strength Training Exercise Promotion: Stretching Exercise Therapy: Muscle Control	Analgesic Administration Body Mechanics Promotion Exercise Promotion Exercise Therapy: Ambulation Exercise Therapy: Balance Pain Management Teaching: Prescribed Activity/Exercise
Mobility			
DEFINITION: Ability to move purposefully in own environment independently with or without assistive device	Exercise Therapy: Ambulation Exercise Therapy: Balance Exercise Therapy: Joint Mobility Exercise Therapy: Muscle Control	Body Mechanics Promotion Energy Management Exercise Promotion Exercise Promotion: Strength Training Exercise Promotion: Stretching Fall Prevention Pain Management Positioning Surveillance: Safety Teaching: Prescribed Activity/Exercise Traction/ Immobilization Care	Activity Therapy Cast Care: Maintenance Cast Care: Wet Circulatory Precautions Neurologic Monitoring Pain Management Peripheral Sensation Management Positioning: Intraoperative Positioning: Neurologic Positioning: Wheelchair Pressure Management Skin Surveillance Weight Management

Outcome	Major Interventions	Suggested Interventions	Optional Interventions
Skeletal Function			
DEFINITION: Ability of the bones to support the body and facilitate movement	Body Mechanics Promotion Exercise Therapy: Ambulation	Exercise Promotion Exercise Promotion: Strength Training Exercise Promotion: Stretching Exercise Therapy: Balance Exercise Therapy: Joint Mobility Exercise Therapy: Muscle Control	Energy Management Medication Administration: Intraosseous Positioning Self-Care Assistance: Transfer Traction/Immobilization Care Weight Management
Transfer Performance			
DEFINITION: Ability to change body location independently with or without assistive device	Exercise Promotion: Strength Training Exercise Therapy: Muscle Control Self-Care Assistance: Transfer	Body Mechanics Promotion Energy Management Exercise Therapy: Balance Exercise Therapy: Joint Mobility Fall Prevention Positioning Positioning: Wheelchair Teaching: Psychomotor Skill	Anxiety Reduction Environmental Management: Safety Exercise Promotion Exercise Promotion: Stretching Pain Management Self-Care Assistance Surveillance: Safety Teaching: Prescribed Activity/Exercise

M

M

NURSING DIAGNOSIS: Mobility: Wheelchair, Impaired

DEFINITION: Limitation of independent operation of wheelchair within environment.

Outcome	Major Interventions	Suggested Interventions	Optional Interventions
Ambulation: Wheelchair			
DEFINITION: Ability to move from place to place in a wheelchair	Exercise Promotion: Strength Training Positioning: Wheelchair	Body Mechanics Promotion Energy Management Environmental Management: Safety Exercise Promotion Exercise Promotion: Stretching Exercise Therapy: Balance Exercise Therapy: Muscle Control Fall Prevention Self-Care Assistance: Transfer Teaching: Prescribed Activity/Exercise	Medication Management Pain Management Positioning: Neurologic Weight Management
Balance			
DEFINITION: Ability to maintain body equilibrium	Exercise Promotion: Strength Training Exercise Therapy: Balance	Energy Management Exercise Therapy: Ambulation Exercise Therapy: Joint Mobility Exercise Therapy: Muscle Control Fall Prevention Positioning: Wheelchair	Environmental Management: Safety Exercise Promotion Weight Management

Outcome	Major Interventions	Suggested Interventions	Optional Interventions
Coordinated Movement DEFINITION: Ability of muscles to work together voluntarily for purposeful movement	Exercise Promotion: Strength Training Exercise Therapy: Muscle Control	Body Mechanics Promotion Exercise Promotion: Stretching Exercise Therapy: Joint Mobility Positioning: Wheelchair Teaching: Prescribed Activity/Exercise	Energy Management Pain Management Weight Management
Mobility DEFINITION: Ability to move purposefully in own environment independently with or without assistive device	Exercise Promotion: Strength Training Positioning: Wheelchair	Body Mechanics Promotion Energy Management Exercise Promotion: Stretching Exercise Therapy: Balance Exercise Therapy: Muscle Control Fall Prevention	Environmental Management: Safety Exercise Promotion Mutual Goal Setting Pain Management Positioning Teaching: Prescribed Activity/Exercise
Transfer Performance DEFINITION: Ability to change body location independently with or without assistive device	Positioning: Wheelchair Self-Care Assistance: Transfer	Body Mechanics Promotion Exercise Promotion: Strength Training Exercise Promotion: Stretching Exercise Therapy: Joint Mobility Exercise Therapy: Muscle Control Teaching: Prescribed Activity/Exercise	Energy Management Nutrition Management Pain Management Weight Management

M

NURSING DIAGNOSIS: Nausea

DEFINITION: A subjective unpleasant, wave-like sensation in the back of the throat, epigastrium, or abdomen, that may lead to the urge or need to vomit.

Outcome	Major Interventions	Suggested Interventions	Optional Interventions
Appetite			
DEFINITION: Desire to eat when ill or receiving treatment	Nausea Management Nutritional Monitoring	Diet Staging Fluid Monitoring Medication Management Oral Health Maintenance Vomiting Management	Calming Technique Pain Management Self-Care Assistance: Feeding
Comfort Level			
DEFINITION: Extent of positive perception of physical and psychological ease	Medication Management Nausea Management	Calming Technique Medication Administration Medication Prescribing Pain Management Simple Relaxation Therapy Vomiting Management	Acupressure Environmental Management: Comfort
Hydration			
DEFINITION: Adequate water in the intracellular and extracellular compartments of the body	Fluid/Electrolyte Management	Electrolyte Management Electrolyte Monitoring Fluid Management Fluid Monitoring Fluid Resuscitation Intravenous (IV) Insertion Intravenous (IV) Therapy Vomiting Management	Temperature Regulation Venous Access Device (VAD) Maintenance

Outcome	Major Interventions	Suggested Interventions	Optional Interventions
Nausea & Vomiting Control			
DEFINITION: Personal actions to control nausea, retching, and vomiting symptoms	Medication Management Nausea Management Vomiting Management	Aspiration Precautions Diet Staging Oral Health Maintenance Pain Management Simple Relaxation Therapy	Distraction Oral Health Promotion Self-Hypnosis Facilitation
Nausea & Vomiting: Disruptive Effect			
DEFINITION: Severity of observed or reported disruptive effects of nausea, retching, and vomiting on daily functioning	Nausea Management Vomiting Management	Electrolyte Monitoring Fluid/Electrolyte Monitoring Fluid Management Fluid Monitoring Medication Administration Medication Management Nutritional Counseling Simple Relaxation Therapy Sleep Enhancement	Chemotherapy Management Emotional Support Intravenous (IV) Insertion Intravenous (IV) Therapy Mood Management Pain Management Total Parenteral Nutrition (TPN) Administration

Continued

Outcome	Major Interventions	Suggested Interventions	Optional Interventions
Nausea & Vomiting Severity			
DEFINITION: Severity of nausea, retching, and vomiting symptoms	Nausea Management Vomiting Management	Aspiration Precautions Fluid/Electrolyte Management Fluid Management Fluid Monitoring Intravenous (IV) Insertion Intravenous (IV) Therapy Medication Administration Medication Management	Calming Technique Oral Health Maintenance Peripherally Inserted Central (PIC) Catheter Care Temperature Regulation Venous Access Device (VAD) Maintenance
Nutritional Status: Food & Fluid Intake			
DEFINITION: Amount of food and fluid taken into the body over a 24-hour period	Fluid Monitoring Nutritional Monitoring	Diet Staging Fluid Management Nausea Management Nutrition Management Vomiting Management	Intravenous (IV) Insertion Intravenous (IV) Therapy

NURSING DIAGNOSIS: Noncompliance

DEFINITION: Behavior of person and/or caregiver that fails to coincide with a health-promoting or therapeutic plan agreed on by the person (and/or family and/or community) and health care professional. In the presence of an agreed-on, health-promoting or therapeutic plan, person's or caregiver's behavior is fully or partially nonadherent and may lead to clinically ineffective or partially ineffective outcomes.

Outcome	Major Interventions	Suggested Interventions	Optional Interventions
Adherence Behavior DEFINITION: Self-initiated actions to promote wellness, recovery, and rehabilitation	Health Education Self-Modification Assistance Self-Responsibility Facilitation	Behavior Modification Coping Enhancement Counseling Decision-Making Support Health System Guidance Support System Enhancement Telephone Consultation Values Clarification	Prenatal Care Risk Identification Smoking Cessation Assistance Substance Use Prevention Teaching: Individual

Continued

Outcome	Major Interventions	Suggested Interventions	Optional Interventions
Caregiver Performance: Direct Care			
DEFINITION: Provision by family care provider of appropriate personal and health care for a family member	Caregiver Support Learning Facilitation	Anticipatory Guidance Coping Enhancement Discharge Planning Teaching: Disease Process Teaching: Prescribed Activity/Exercise Teaching: Prescribed Diet Teaching: Prescribed Medication Teaching: Procedure/ Treatment Teaching: Psychomotor Skill	Family Involvement Promotion Home Maintenance Assistance Referral Respite Care Support System Enhancement
Caregiver Performance: Indirect Care			
DEFINITION: Arrangement and oversight by family care provider of appropriate care for a family member	Caregiver Support Health System Guidance	Coping Enhancement Culture Brokerage Decision-Making Support Financial Resource Assistance Support System Enhancement	Case Management Family Involvement Promotion Home Maintenance Assistance Insurance Authorization Patient Rights Protection Referral

Outcome	Major Interventions	Suggested Interventions	Optional Interventions
Compliance Behavior DEFINITION: Personal actions to promote wellness, recovery, and rehabilitation based on professional advice	Health System Guidance Mutual Goal Setting Patient Contracting	Behavior Modification Counseling Culture Brokerage Decision-Making Support Financial Resource Assistance Learning Facilitation Learning Readiness Enhancement Patient Rights Protection Self-Modification Assistance Self-Responsibility Facilitation Support System Enhancement Teaching: Disease Process Teaching: Individual Teaching: Prescribed Activity/Exercise Teaching: Prescribed Diet Teaching: Prescribed Medication Teaching: Procedure/ Treatment Teaching: Psychomotor Skill Telephone Consultation Values Clarification	Case Management Discharge Planning Elopement Precautions Family Involvement Promotion Parent Education: Adolescent Referral Smoking Cessation Assistance Substance Use Prevention Support Group Surveillance Teaching: Infant Nutrition Teaching: Infant Safety Teaching: Safe Sex Teaching: Toddler Nutrition Teaching: Toddler Safety Truth Telling

Continued

Outcome	Major Interventions	Suggested Interventions	Optional Interventions
Motivation			
DEFINITION: Inner urge that moves or prompts an individual to positive action(s)	Self-Modification Assistance Self-Responsibility Facilitation	Coping Enhancement Counseling Decision-Making Support Mutual Goal Setting Role Enhancement Teaching: Individual Values Clarification	Family Involvement Promotion Hope Instillation Support Group

Outcome	Major Interventions	Suggested Interventions	Optional Interventions
Treatment Behavior: Illness or Injury DEFINITION: Personal actions to palliate or eliminate pathology	Self-Responsibility Facilitation Teaching: Disease Process Teaching: Individual	Behavior Modification Coping Enhancement Counseling Health Education Health System Guidance Learning Facilitation Learning Readiness Enhancement Mutual Goal Setting Patient Contracting Self-Modification Assistance Support System Enhancement Surveillance Teaching: Prescribed Activity/Exercise Teaching: Prescribed Diet Teaching: Prescribed Medication Teaching: Procedure/ Treatment Teaching: Psychomotor Skill Telephone Consultation Values Clarification	Allergy Management Asthma Management Chemotherapy Management Family Involvement Promotion Home Maintenance Assistance Radiation Therapy Management Referral Self-Care Assistance Smoking Cessation Assistance Substance Use Treatment Support Group Weight Gain Assistance Weight Reduction Assistance

N

NURSING DIAGNOSIS: Nutrition: Imbalanced, Less than Body Requirements

DEFINITION: Intake of nutrients insufficient to meet metabolic needs.

Outcome	Major Interventions	Suggested Interventions	Optional Interventions
Appetite			
DEFINITION: Desire to eat when ill or receiving treatment	Nutrition Therapy Nutritional Monitoring	Diet Staging Eating Disorders Management Environmental Management Fluid Management Nutrition Management Oral Health Maintenance	Fluid/Electrolyte Management Oral Health Promotion Weight Gain Assistance Weight Management
Breastfeeding Establishment: Infant			
DEFINITION: Infant attachment to and sucking from the mother's breast for nourishment during the first 3 weeks of breastfeeding	Breastfeeding Assistance Lactation Counseling	Calming Technique Environmental Management: Attachment Process Newborn Care Newborn Monitoring Weight Gain Assistance	Caregiver Support Fluid Management Parent Education: Infant

Outcome	Major Interventions	Suggested Interventions	Optional Interventions
Nutritional Status DEFINITION: Extent to which nutrients are available to meet metabolic needs	Eating Disorders Management Nutrition Management Weight Gain Assistance	Diet Staging Fluid/Electrolyte Management Nutrition Therapy Nutritional Counseling Nutritional Monitoring Teaching: Prescribed Diet Vital Signs Monitoring Weight Management	Energy Management Enteral Tube Feeding Gastrointestinal Intubation Self-Care Assistance: Feeding Sustenance Support Total Parenteral Nutrition (TPN) Administration

Continued

Outcome	Major Interventions	Suggested Interventions	Optional Interventions
Nutritional Status: Biochemical Measures			
DEFINITION: Body fluid components and chemical indices of nutritional status	Electrolyte Management Electrolyte Monitoring Fluid/Electrolyte Management	Acid-Base Management Eating Disorders Management Electrolyte Management: Hypocalcemia Electrolyte Management: Hyponatremia Hyperglycemia Management Hypervolemia Management Hypoglycemia Management Hypovolemia Management Nutrition Management Nutrition Therapy Nutritional Counseling Weight Gain Assistance	Enteral Tube Feeding Teaching: Prescribed Diet Total Parenteral Nutrition (TPN) Administration

Outcome	Major Interventions	Suggested Interventions	Optional Interventions
Nutritional Status: Food & Fluid Intake			
DEFINITION: Amount of food and fluid taken into the body over a 24-hour period	Fluid Monitoring Nutritional Monitoring	Enteral Tube Feeding Feeding Fluid Management Nutrition Management Nutrition Therapy Self-Care Assistance: Feeding Swallowing Therapy	Bottle Feeding Hypoglycemia Management Intravenous (IV) Therapy Sustenance Support Teaching: Prescribed Diet Total Parenteral Nutrition (TPN) Administration Weight Gain Assistance Weight Management
Nutritional Status: Nutrient Intake			
DEFINITION: Adequacy of usual pattern of nutrient intake	Nutrition Management Nutritional Monitoring	Enteral Tube Feeding Medication Management Nutrition Therapy Nutritional Counseling Teaching: Prescribed Diet Total Parenteral Nutrition (TPN) Administration	Bottle Feeding Feeding Laboratory Data Interpretation Self-Care Assistance: Feeding Sustenance Support Swallowing Therapy Swallowing Therapy Weight Gain Assistance Weight Management

Continued

Outcome	Major Interventions	Suggested Interventions	Optional Interventions
Self-Care: Eating			
DEFINITION: Ability to prepare and ingest food and fluid independently with or without assistive device	Self-Care Assistance: Feeding	Dementia Management Environmental Management Feeding Nutrition Management Nutritional Monitoring Teaching: Prescribed Diet	Nutrition Therapy Nutritional Counseling Oral Health Maintenance Swallowing Therapy
Weight: Body Mass			
DEFINITION: Extent to which body weight, muscle, and fat are congruent to height, frame, gender, and age	Eating Disorders Management Weight Gain Assistance	Nutrition Management Nutrition Therapy Nutritional Counseling Nutritional Monitoring Weight Management	Behavior Modification Exercise Promotion Mutual Goal Setting Patient Contracting Teaching: Individual

NURSING DIAGNOSIS: Nutrition: Imbalanced, More than Body Requirements

DEFINITION: Intake of nutrients that exceeds metabolic needs.

Outcome	Major Interventions	Suggested Interventions	Optional Interventions
Nutritional Status			
DEFINITION: Extent to which nutrients are available to meet metabolic needs	Nutrition Management Weight Reduction Assistance	Fluid Management Nutritional Counseling Nutritional Monitoring Weight Management	Fluid Management Teaching: Prescribed Diet
Nutritional Status: Food & Fluid Intake			
DEFINITION: Amount of food and fluid taken into the body over a 24-hour period	Behavior Modification Nutritional Counseling	Behavior Management Fluid Monitoring Nutrition Management Nutritional Monitoring Teaching: Prescribed Diet Weight Reduction Assistance	Eating Disorders Management Mutual Goal Setting Self-Responsibility Facilitation Weight Management
Nutritional Status: Nutrient Intake			
DEFINITION: Adequacy of usual pattern of nutrient intake	Nutrition Management Nutritional Monitoring	Eating Disorders Management Nutritional Counseling Teaching: Prescribed Diet Weight Management Weight Reduction Assistance	Behavior Modification Bottle Feeding Fluid Management Hyperglycemia Management

Continued

Outcome	Major Interventions	Suggested Interventions	Optional Interventions
Weight Control			
DEFINITION: Personal actions to achieve and maintain optimum body weight	Behavior Modification Weight Reduction Assistance	Behavior Management Exercise Promotion Mutual Goal Setting Nutrition Management Nutritional Counseling Nutritional Monitoring Patient Contracting Self-Responsibility Facilitation Teaching: Prescribed Diet	Anxiety Reduction Coping Enhancement Exercise Therapy: Ambulation Limit Setting Referral

NURSING DIAGNOSIS: Nutrition, Readiness for Enhanced

DEFINITION: A pattern of nutrient intake that is sufficient for meeting metabolic needs and can be strengthened.

Outcome	Major Interventions	Suggested Interventions	Optional Interventions
Knowledge: Diet			
DEFINITION: Extent of understanding conveyed about recommended diet	Teaching: Individual Teaching: Prescribed Diet	Learning Facilitation Learning Readiness Enhancement Nutritional Counseling	Health Education Parent Education: Childrearing Family Prenatal Care Teaching: Group
Nutritional Status			
DEFINITION: Extent to which nutrients are available to meet metabolic needs	Nutrition Management Nutritional Counseling	Nutritional Monitoring Prenatal Care Teaching: Prescribed Diet Weight Management	Weight Gain Assistance Weight Reduction Assistance
Nutritional Status: Nutrient Intake			
DEFINITION: Adequacy of usual pattern of nutrient intake	Nutrition Management Nutritional Counseling	Nutritional Monitoring Teaching: Prescribed Diet Weight Management	Medication Management Self-Care Assistance: Feeding Weight Gain Assistance Weight Reduction Assistance

NURSING DIAGNOSIS: Oral Mucous Membrane, Impaired

DEFINITION: Disruption of the lips and soft tissue of the oral cavity.

Outcome	Major Interventions	Suggested Interventions	Optional Interventions
Oral Hygiene			
DEFINITION: Condition of the mouth, teeth, gums, and tongue	Oral Health Restoration	Chemotherapy Management Fluid/Electrolyte Management Fluid Management Nutrition Management Oral Health Maintenance Oral Health Promotion	Airway Suctioning Artificial Airway Management Dying Care Pain Management
Tissue Integrity: Skin & Mucous Membranes			
DEFINITION: Structural intactness and normal physiological function of skin and mucous membranes	Oral Health Restoration	Chemotherapy Management Infection Protection Medication Administration: Skin Medication Management Nutrition Management Oral Health Maintenance Radiation Therapy Management	Fluid Management Wound Care Wound Irrigation

NURSING DIAGNOSIS: Pain, Acute

DEFINITION: Unpleasant sensory and emotional experience arising from actual or potential tissue damage or described in terms of such damage (International Association for the Study of Pain); sudden or slow onset of any intensity from mild to severe with an anticipated or predictable end and a duration of less than 6 months.

Outcome	Major Interventions	Suggested Interventions	Optional Interventions
Comfort Level			
DEFINITION: Extent of positive perception of physical and psychological ease	Medication Management Pain Management	Acupressure Analgesic Administration Biofeedback Coping Enhancement Emotional Support Environmental Management: Comfort Humor Medication Administration Medication Administration: Intramuscular (IM) Medication Administration: Intravenous (IV) Medication Administration: Oral Medication Prescribing Meditation Facilitation Positioning Presence Sedation Management Simple Guided Imagery Simple Massage Simple Relaxation Therapy	Animal-Assisted Therapy Anxiety Reduction Autogenic Training Bathing Bowel Management Calming Technique Cutaneous Stimulation Distraction Dying Care Energy Management Exercise Promotion Flatulence Reduction Heat/Cold Application Hope Instillation Hypnosis Lactation Suppression Music Therapy Oxygen Therapy Progressive Muscle Relaxation Security Enhancement Sleep Enhancement Splinting Therapeutic Touch

Continued

Outcome	Major Interventions	Suggested Interventions	Optional Interventions
Pain Control			
DEFINITION: Personal actions to control pain	Medication Management Pain Management Patient-Controlled Analgesia (PCA) Assistance	Biofeedback Health Screening Medication Prescribing Mutual Goal Setting Patient Contracting Preparatory Sensory Information Self-Hypnosis Facilitation Self-Modification Assistance Self-Responsibility Facilitation Simple Guided Imagery Simple Relaxation Therapy Sleep Enhancement Teaching: Disease Process Teaching: Individual Teaching: Prescribed Medication Teaching: Procedure/ Treatment Telephone Consultation	Autogenic Training Coping Enhancement Distraction Environmental Management: Comfort Family Support Heat/Cold Application Rectal Prolapse Management Splinting Support System Enhancement Surveillance

Outcome	Major Interventions	Suggested Interventions	Optional Interventions
Pain Level			
DEFINITION: Severity of observed or reported pain	Analgesic Administration Pain Management Sedation Management	Acupressure Analgesic Administration: Intraspinal Anesthesia Administration Anxiety Reduction Cutaneous Stimulation Environmental Management: Comfort Flatulence Reduction Heat/Cold Application Medication Administration Medication Administration: Intramuscular (IM) Medication Administration: Intravenous (IV) Medication Administration: Oral Medication Management Medication Prescribing Positioning Simple Guided Imagery Splinting Surveillance Transcutaneous Electrical Nerve Stimulation (TENS)	Biofeedback Distraction Hypnosis Music Therapy Presence Progressive Muscle Relaxation Simple Massage Simple Relaxation Therapy Therapeutic Touch Touch Vital Signs Monitoring

P

NURSING DIAGNOSIS: Pain, Chronic

DEFINITION: Unpleasant sensory and emotional experience arising from actual or potential tissue damage or described in terms of such damage (International Association for the Study of Pain); sudden or slow onset of any intensity from mild to severe, constant or recurring without an anticipated or predictable end and a duration of greater than 6 months.

Outcome	Major Interventions	Suggested Interventions	Optional Interventions
Comfort Level			
DEFINITION: Extent of positive perception of physical and psychological ease	Medication Management Pain Management	Acupressure Environmental Management: Comfort Medication Administration Medication Prescribing Positioning Simple Massage Simple Relaxation Therapy Sleep Enhancement	Autogenic Training Biofeedback Cutaneous Stimulation Distraction Dying Care Heat/Cold Application Hypnosis Meditation Facilitation Progressive Muscle Relaxation Therapeutic Touch
Depression Level			
DEFINITION: Severity of melancholic mood and loss of interest in life events	Mood Management Pain Management	Counseling Emotional Support Hope Instillation Medication Administration Medication Management Sleep Enhancement	Animal-Assisted Therapy Art Therapy Biofeedback Environmental Management: Comfort Humor Music Therapy Presence Touch

Outcome	Major Interventions	Suggested Interventions	Optional Interventions
Depression Self-Control			
DEFINITION: Personal actions to minimize melancholy and maintain interest in life events	Mood Management Pain Management Patient Contracting	Behavior Management Behavior Management: Self-Harm Coping Enhancement Exercise Promotion Medication Management Sleep Enhancement Teaching: Prescribed Medication	Animal-Assisted Therapy Art Therapy Hope Instillation Humor Spiritual Support
Pain: Adverse Psychological Response			
DEFINITION: Severity of observed or reported adverse cognitive and emotional responses to physical pain	Cognitive Restructuring Mood Management	Active Listening Analgesic Administration Behavior Management Coping Enhancement Emotional Support Hope Instillation Medication Administration Sleep Enhancement Spiritual Support Support System Enhancement Transcutaneous Electrical Nerve Stimulation (TENS)	Anger Control Assistance Animal-Assisted Therapy Art Therapy Humor Music Therapy Presence Simple Guided Imagery Touch

Continued

P

Outcome	Major Interventions	Suggested Interventions	Optional Interventions
Pain Control			
DEFINITION: Personal actions to control pain	Medication Management Pain Management Self-Responsibility Facilitation	Behavior Modification Biofeedback Heat/Cold Application Mutual Goal Setting Patient Contracting Self-Hypnosis Facilitation Self-Modification Assistance Simple Guided Imagery Simple Relaxation Therapy Splinting Teaching: Individual Teaching: Prescribed Medication Teaching: Procedure/Treatment Transcutaneous Electrical Nerve Stimulation (TENS)	Autogenic Training Environmental Management: Comfort Exercise Promotion: Stretching Exercise Therapy: Ambulation Exercise Therapy: Joint Mobility Exercise Therapy: Muscle Control Family Involvement Promotion Support System Enhancement Surveillance Telephone Consultation

Outcome	Major Interventions	Suggested Interventions	Optional Interventions
Pain: Disruptive Effects			
DEFINITION: Severity of observed or reported disruptive effects of chronic pain on daily functioning	Behavior Modification Coping Enhancement	Analgesic Administration Emotional Support Energy Management Hope Instillation Medication Administration Medication Management Medication Prescribing Mood Management Nutrition Management Pain Management Self-Care Assistance Simple Relaxation Therapy Sleep Enhancement	Acupressure Anxiety Reduction Autogenic Training Biofeedback Body Mechanics Promotion Cutaneous Stimulation Distraction Environmental Management: Comfort Heat/Cold Application Hypnosis Meditation Facilitation Progressive Muscle Relaxation Role Enhancement Simple Guided Imagery Simple Massage Therapeutic Touch Transcutaneous Electrical Nerve Stimulation (TENS)

Continued

Outcome	Major Interventions	Suggested Interventions	Optional Interventions
Pain Level DEFINITION: Severity of observed or reported pain	Pain Management Patient-Controlled Analgesia (PCA) Assistance	Acupressure Analgesic Administration Analgesic Administration: Intraspinal Distraction Environmental Management: Comfort Medication Administration Medication Management Medication Prescribing Positioning Presence Simple Massage Splinting Surveillance Touch Transcutaneous Electrical Nerve Stimulation (TENS) Vital Signs Monitoring	Biofeedback Cutaneous Stimulation Heat/Cold Application Hypnosis Progressive Muscle Relaxation Self-Hypnosis Facilitation Simple Guided Imagery Simple Relaxation Therapy Therapeutic Touch

NURSING DIAGNOSIS: Parental Role Conflict

DEFINITION: Parent experience of role confusion and conflict in response to crisis.

Outcome	Major Interventions	Suggested Interventions	Optional Interventions
Caregiver Adaptation to Patient Institutionalization			
DEFINITION: Adaptive response of family caregiver when the care recipient is moved to an institution	Caregiver Support Decision-Making Support	Active Listening Anticipatory Guidance Anxiety Reduction Coping Enhancement Emotional Support Family Involvement Promotion Family Process Maintenance Family Support Guilt Work Facilitation Health System Guidance Role Enhancement Support System Enhancement	Counseling Culture Brokerage Family Presence Facilitation Family Therapy Support Group Values Clarification Visitation Facilitation

Continued

Outcome	Major Interventions	Suggested Interventions	Optional Interventions
Caregiver Home Care Readiness			
DEFINITION: Extent of preparedness of a caregiver to assume responsibility for the health care of a family member in the home	Caregiver Support Family Involvement Promotion Role Enhancement	Anticipatory Guidance Anxiety Reduction Coping Enhancement Decision-Making Support Discharge Planning Family Mobilization Family Process Maintenance Family Support Normalization Promotion	Childbirth Preparation Health System Guidance Home Maintenance Assistance Risk Identification Security Enhancement Support System Enhancement Teaching: Individual
Caregiver Lifestyle Disruption			
DEFINITION: Severity of disturbances in the lifestyle of a family member due to caregiving	Caregiver Support Role Enhancement	Assertiveness Training Coping Enhancement Emotional Support Health System Guidance Respite Care Support Group Support System Enhancement	Anticipatory Guidance Family Integrity Promotion Family Involvement Promotion Insurance Authorization

Outcome	Major Interventions	Suggested Interventions	Optional Interventions
Coping			
DEFINITION: Personal actions to manage stressors that tax an individual's resources	Coping Enhancement Counseling Crisis Intervention	Anxiety Reduction Caregiver Support Decision-Making Support Emotional Support Family Support Family Therapy Grief Work Facilitation: Perinatal Death Respite Care Self-Esteem Enhancement Socialization Enhancement Spiritual Support Support Group Values Clarification	Normalization Promotion Parent Education: Adolescent Parent Education: Childrearing Family Parent Education: Infant Parenting Promotion Sibling Support Support System Enhancement Therapy Group Trauma Therapy: Child
Family Functioning			
DEFINITION: Capacity of the family system to meet the needs of its members during developmental transitions	Crisis Intervention Family Process Maintenance	Childbirth Preparation Counseling Decision-Making Support Family Integrity Promotion Family Integrity Promotion: Childbearing Family Family Involvement Promotion Family Support Family Therapy Parenting Promotion	Abuse Protection Support: Child Consultation High-Risk Pregnancy Care Socialization Enhancement

Continued

Outcome	Major Interventions	Suggested Interventions	Optional Interventions
Family Social Climate DEFINITION: Supportive milieu as characterized by family member relationships and goals	Family Process Maintenance Parenting Promotion	Counseling Family Integrity Promotion Family Integrity Promotion: Childbearing Family Socialization Enhancement	Abuse Protection Support: Child Caregiver Support Family Therapy Support System Enhancement
Parenting Performance DEFINITION: Parental actions to provide a child a nurturing and constructive physical, emotional, and social environment	Crisis Intervention Family Process Maintenance Parenting Promotion	Abuse Protection Support: Child Coping Enhancement Counseling Environmental Management: Attachment Process Family Integrity Promotion: Childbearing Family Family Support Normalization Promotion Role Enhancement Sibling Support Support System Enhancement	Breastfeeding Assistance Childbirth Preparation Emotional Support Family Integrity Promotion Family Therapy Health System Guidance Home Maintenance Assistance Self-Esteem Enhancement Socialization Enhancement Support Group

Outcome	Major Interventions	Suggested Interventions	Optional Interventions
Psychosocial Adjustment: Life Change			
DEFINITION: Adaptive psychosocial response of an individual to a significant life change	Anticipatory Guidance Coping Enhancement	Childbirth Preparation Counseling Decision-Making Support Family Support Parent Education: Adolescent Parent Education: Childrearing Family Parenting Promotion Role Enhancement Spiritual Support	Family Integrity Promotion Family Integrity Promotion: Childbearing Family Family Mobilization Family Process Maintenance Sustenance Support
Role Performance			
DEFINITION: Congruence of an individual's role behavior with role expectations	Parenting Promotion Role Enhancement	Behavior Modification Caregiver Support Counseling Emotional Support Self-Awareness Enhancement Values Clarification	Attachment Promotion Childbirth Preparation Decision-Making Support Family Integrity Promotion Family Therapy Self-Esteem Enhancement Support Group Support System Enhancement

NURSING DIAGNOSIS: Parenting, Impaired

DEFINITION: Inability of the primary caretaker to create, maintain, or regain an environment that promotes the optimum growth and development of the child.

Outcome	Major Interventions	Suggested Interventions	Optional Interventions
Child Development: 1 Month DEFINITION: Milestones of physical, cognitive, and psychosocial progression by 1 month of age	Attachment Promotion Newborn Care	Anticipatory Guidance Bottle Feeding Breastfeeding Assistance Environmental Management: Attachment Process Family Integrity Promotion: Childbearing Family Family Involvement Promotion Parent Education: Infant Teaching: Infant Safety Teaching: Infant Stimulation	Anxiety Reduction Coping Enhancement Family Support Home Maintenance Assistance Lactation Counseling

Outcome	Major Interventions	Suggested Interventions	Optional Interventions
Child Development: 2 Months			
DEFINITION: Milestones of physical, cognitive, and psychosocial progression by 2 months of age	Family Integrity Promotion: Childbearing Family Parent Education: Infant Parenting Promotion	Anticipatory Guidance Attachment Promotion Bottle Feeding Breastfeeding Assistance Family Involvement Promotion Family Process Maintenance Family Support Infant Care Lactation Counseling Role Enhancement Teaching: Infant Nutrition Teaching: Infant Safety	Abuse Protection Support: Child Behavior Modification Caregiver Support Environmental Management: Attachment Process Health System Guidance Home Maintenance Assistance Newborn Care Respite Care Sibling Support Support System Enhancement Surveillance

Continued

Outcome	Major Interventions	Suggested Interventions	Optional Interventions
Child Development: 4 Months			
DEFINITION: Milestones of physical, cognitive, and psychosocial progression by 4 months of age	Family Integrity Promotion: Childbearing Family Parent Education: Infant Parenting Promotion	Anticipatory Guidance Bottle Feeding Family Involvement Promotion Family Process Maintenance Family Support Infant Care Lactation Counseling Role Enhancement Security Enhancement Teaching: Infant Nutrition Teaching: Infant Safety	Abuse Protection Support: Child Attachment Promotion Behavior Modification Caregiver Support Environmental Management: Safety Family Mobilization Health System Guidance Respite Care Sibling Support Support System Enhancement Surveillance Sustenance Support
Child Development: 6 Months			
DEFINITION: Milestones of physical, cognitive, and psychosocial progression by 6 months of age	Family Integrity Promotion: Childbearing Family Parenting Promotion	Anticipatory Guidance Bottle Feeding Family Involvement Promotion Family Process Maintenance Family Support Infant Care Lactation Counseling Parent Education: Infant Role Enhancement Security Enhancement Teaching: Infant Nutrition Teaching: Infant Safety	Abuse Protection Support: Child Attachment Promotion Caregiver Support Environmental Management: Safety Health System Guidance Respite Care Sibling Support Support System Enhancement Surveillance Sustenance Support

Outcome	Major Interventions	Suggested Interventions	Optional Interventions
Child Development: 12 Months			
DEFINITION: Milestones of physical, cognitive, and psychosocial progression by 12 months of age	Family Integrity Promotion: Childbearing Family Parenting Promotion	Anticipatory Guidance Bottle Feeding Developmental Enhancement: Child Family Involvement Promotion Family Process Maintenance Family Support Infant Care Lactation Counseling Parent Education: Infant Parent Education: Childrearing Family Role Enhancement Security Enhancement Socialization Enhancement Teaching: Toddler Nutrition Teaching: Toddler Safety Teaching: Toilet Training	Abuse Protection Support: Child Attachment Promotion Caregiver Support Environmental Management: Safety Health System Guidance Nutrition Management Respite Care Sibling Support Support System Enhancement Surveillance Sustenance Support Therapeutic Play

Continued

Outcome	Major Interventions	Suggested Interventions	Optional Interventions
Child Development: 2 Years DEFINITION: Milestones of physical, cognitive, and psychosocial progression by 2 years of age	Developmental Enhancement: Child Environmental Management: Safety Parenting Promotion	Anticipatory Guidance Family Integrity Promotion Family Involvement Promotion Parent Education: Childrearing Family Role Enhancement Security Enhancement Socialization Enhancement Teaching: Toddler Nutrition Teaching: Toddler Safety Teaching: Toilet Training	Abuse Protection Support: Child Bowel Training Counseling Family Process Maintenance Family Support Family Therapy Health System Guidance Sibling Support Support System Enhancement Surveillance Sustenance Support Urinary Habit Training

Outcome	Major Interventions	Suggested Interventions	Optional Interventions
Child Development: 3 Years			
DEFINITION: Milestones of physical, cognitive, and psychosocial progression by 3 years of age	Developmental Enhancement: Child Environmental Management: Safety Parenting Promotion	Anticipatory Guidance Bowel Management Family Integrity Promotion Family Involvement Promotion Parent Education: Childrearing Family Role Enhancement Security Enhancement Socialization Enhancement Support System Enhancement Urinary Habit Training	Abuse Protection Support: Child Behavior Management: Overactivity/ Inattention Counseling Family Process Maintenance Family Support Family Therapy Health System Guidance Sibling Support Sleep Enhancement Surveillance Sustenance Support Urinary Incontinence Care: Enuresis
Child Development: 4 Years			
DEFINITION: Milestones of physical, cognitive, and psychosocial progression by 4 years of age	Developmental Enhancement: Child Parenting Promotion	Anticipatory Guidance Environmental Management: Safety Family Integrity Promotion Family Involvement Promotion Parent Education: Childrearing Family Security Enhancement Socialization Enhancement Support System Enhancement	Abuse Protection Support: Child Behavior Management: Overactivity/ Inattention Counseling Family Process Maintenance Family Support Family Therapy Health System Guidance Sibling Support Sustenance Support Urinary Habit Training Urinary Incontinence Care: Enuresis

Continued

Outcome	Major Interventions	Suggested Interventions	Optional Interventions
Child Development: 5 Years			
DEFINITION: Milestones of physical, cognitive, and psychosocial progression by 5 years of age	Developmental Enhancement: Child Parent Education: Childrearing Family Parenting Promotion	Anticipatory Guidance Environmental Management: Safety Family Integrity Promotion Family Involvement Promotion Security Enhancement Socialization Enhancement Support System Enhancement	Abuse Protection Support: Child Behavior Management: Overactivity/ Inattention Counseling Family Process Maintenance Family Support Family Therapy Health System Guidance Sibling Support Sustenance Support Urinary Incontinence Care: Enuresis
Child Development: Middle Childhood			
DEFINITION: Milestones of physical, cognitive, and psychosocial progression from 6 years through 11 years of age	Developmental Enhancement: Child Parent Education: Childrearing Family Parenting Promotion	Anticipatory Guidance Family Integrity Promotion Family Involvement Promotion Mutual Goal Setting Spiritual Support Substance Use Prevention Teaching: Individual Values Clarification	Abuse Protection Support: Child Counseling Family Process Maintenance Family Support Family Therapy Health System Guidance Sibling Support Sports-Injury Prevention: Youth Sustenance Support

Outcome	Major Interventions	Suggested Interventions	Optional Interventions
Child Development: Adolescence			
DEFINITION: Milestones of physical, cognitive, and psychosocial progression from 12 years through 17 years of age	Developmental Enhancement: Adolescent Parenting Promotion	Anticipatory Guidance Family Integrity Promotion Family Involvement Promotion Health System Guidance Mutual Goal Setting Parent Education: Adolescent Role Enhancement Spiritual Support Substance Use Prevention Teaching: Individual Values Clarification	Abuse Protection Support Counseling Family Process Maintenance Family Support Family Therapy Sibling Support Sports-Injury Prevention: Youth Support System Enhancement Sustenance Support
Family Coping			
DEFINITION: Family actions to manage stressors that tax family resources	Coping Enhancement Family Process Maintenance Family Support	Caregiver Support Counseling Family Integrity Promotion Family Therapy Grief Work Facilitation Guilt Work Facilitation Normalization Promotion Parenting Promotion	Abuse Protection Support: Child Family Involvement Promotion Financial Resource Assistance Home Maintenance Assistance Respite Care

Continued

Outcome	Major Interventions	Suggested Interventions	Optional Interventions
Family Functioning			
DEFINITION: Capacity of the family system to meet the needs of its members during developmental transitions	Developmental Enhancement: Adolescent Developmental Enhancement: Child Family Process Maintenance	Family Integrity Promotion Family Involvement Promotion Family Support Family Therapy Parent Education: Childrearing Family Parenting Promotion	Childbirth Preparation Sibling Support
Family Social Climate			
DEFINITION: Supportive milieu as characterized by family member relationships and goals	Family Integrity Promotion Family Integrity Promotion: Childbearing Family	Abuse Protection Support: Child Attachment Promotion Family Support Family Process Maintenance Parenting Promotion	Coping Enhancement Family Involvement Promotion Family Therapy Resiliency Promotion
Parent-Infant Attachment			
DEFINITION: Parent and infant behaviors that demonstrate an enduring affectionate bond	Attachment Promotion Environmental Management: Attachment Process Kangaroo Care	Breastfeeding Assistance Family Integrity Promotion Infant Care Intrapartal Care Lactation Counseling Parent Education: Infant Risk Identification: Childbearing Family	Anticipatory Guidance Coping Enhancement Emotional Support Role Enhancement

Outcome	Major Interventions	Suggested Interventions	Optional Interventions
Parenting Performance DEFINITION: Parental actions to provide a child a nurturing and constructive physical, emotional, and social environment	Abuse Protection Support: Child Developmental Enhancement: Child Parenting Promotion	Anticipatory Guidance Anxiety Reduction Caregiver Support Coping Enhancement Counseling Developmental Enhancement: Adolescent Family Integrity Promotion Family Involvement Promotion Family Support Normalization Promotion Parent Education: Adolescent Parent Education: Childrearing Family Respite Care Role Enhancement Support System Enhancement Surveillance Values Clarification	Breastfeeding Assistance Emotional Support Family Integrity Promotion Family Process Maintenance Family Therapy Health System Guidance Home Maintenance Assistance Parent Education: Infant Prenatal Care Security Enhancement Self-Esteem Enhancement Socialization Enhancement Support Group Telephone Consultation

Continued

Outcome	Major Interventions	Suggested Interventions	Optional Interventions
Parenting: Psychosocial Safety			
DEFINITION: Parental actions to protect a child from social contacts that might cause harm or injury	Abuse Protection Support: Child Parent Education: Adolescent Parent Education: Childrearing Family Risk Identification: Childbearing Family	Anticipatory Guidance Developmental Enhancement: Child Family Integrity Promotion Family Integrity Promotion: Childbearing Family Health Screening Risk Identification Socialization Enhancement Surveillance: Safety	Counseling Emotional Support Family Support Family Therapy Mutual Goal Setting Parent Education: Infant Self-Esteem Enhancement Self-Modification Assistance Self-Responsibility Facilitation Substance Use Prevention Support Group Teaching: Individual Trauma Therapy: Child
Role Performance			
DEFINITION: Congruence of an individual's role behavior with role expectations	Parent Education: Adolescent Parent Education: Childrearing Family Parent Education: Infant Role Enhancement	Anticipatory Guidance Behavior Modification Caregiver Support Counseling Decision-Making Support Emotional Support Self-Awareness Enhancement Values Clarification	Attachment Promotion Childbirth Preparation Family Integrity Promotion Family Therapy Health Education Self-Esteem Enhancement Support Group Support System Enhancement

Outcome	Major Interventions	Suggested Interventions	Optional Interventions
Safe Home Environment DEFINITION: Physical arrangements to minimize environmental factors that might cause physical harm or injury in the home	Environmental Management: Safety Surveillance: Safety	Environmental Management: Violence Prevention Home Maintenance Assistance Risk Identification Teaching: Infant Safety Teaching: Toddler Safety	Patient Contracting Parent Education: Childrearing Family Parent Education: Infant Vehicle Safety Promotion
Social Support DEFINITION: Perceived availability and actual provision of reliable assistance from others	Family Involvement Promotion Support Group Support System Enhancement	Caregiver Support Emotional Support Family Support Referral Telephone Consultation	Coping Enhancement Financial Resource Assistance Spiritual Support Sustenance Support Therapy Group

NURSING DIAGNOSIS: Parenting, Readiness for Enhanced

DEFINITION: A pattern of providing an environment for children or other dependent person(s) that is sufficient to nurture growth and development and can be strengthened.

Outcome	Major Interventions	Suggested Interventions	Optional Interventions
Family Functioning			
DEFINITION: Capacity of the family system to meet the needs of its members during developmental transitions	Developmental Enhancement: Adolescent Developmental Enhancement: Child Family Integrity Promotion	Family Integrity Promotion: Childbearing Family Family Support Parent Education: Childrearing Family	Parent Education: Adolescent Parenting Promotion Support System Enhancement
Knowledge: Child Physical Safety			
DEFINITION: Extent of understanding conveyed about safely caring for a child from 1 year through 17 years of age	Teaching: Infant Safety Teaching: Toddler Safety	Developmental Enhancement: Child Learning Readiness Enhancement Parent Education: Childrearing Family	Environmental Management: Safety Sports-Injury Prevention: Youth
Knowledge: Infant Care			
DEFINITION: Extent of understanding conveyed about caring for a baby from birth to first birthday	Teaching: Infant Nutrition Teaching: Infant Safety Parent Education: Infant	Anticipatory Guidance Infant Care Newborn Care Teaching: Infant Stimulation	Childbirth Preparation Circumcision Care Lactation Counseling

Outcome	Major Interventions	Suggested Interventions	Optional Interventions
Knowledge: Parenting			
DEFINITION: Extent of understanding conveyed about provision of a nurturing and constructive environment for a child from 1 year through 17 years of age	Parent Education: Adolescent Parent Education: Childrearing Family Parent Education: Infant	Lactation Counseling Teaching: Infant Nutrition Teaching: Infant Safety Teaching: Infant Stimulation Teaching: Toddler Nutrition Teaching: Toddler Safety Teaching: Toilet Training	Bowel Incontinence Care: Encopresis Parenting Promotion Resiliency Promotion Urinary Incontinence Care: Enuresis
Parenting Performance			
DEFINITION: Parental actions to provide a child a nurturing and constructive physical, emotional, and social environment	Developmental Enhancement: Adolescent Developmental Enhancement: Child Parenting Promotion	Attachment Promotion Infant Care Resiliency Promotion Role Enhancement	Environmental Management: Safety Family Integrity Promotion: Childbearing Family
Parenting: Psychosocial Safety			
DEFINITION: Parental actions to protect a child from social contacts that might cause harm or injury	Developmental Enhancement: Adolescent Developmental Enhancement: Child Parent Education: Adolescent Parent Education: Childrearing Family	Environmental Management: Safety Parenting Promotion Role Enhancement	Abuse Protection Support: Child Risk Identification: Childbearing Family

NURSING DIAGNOSIS: Personal Identity, Disturbed

DEFINITION: Inability to distinguish between self and nonself.

Outcome	Major Interventions	Suggested Interventions	Optional Interventions
Distorted Thought Self-Control			
DEFINITION: Self-restraint of disruptions in perception, thought processes, and thought content	Delusion Management Hallucination Management	Anxiety Reduction Cognitive Restructuring Delirium Management Dementia Management Medication Management Reality Orientation	Active Listening Art Therapy Body Image Enhancement Environmental Management
Identity			
DEFINITION: Distinguishes between self and nonself and characterizes one's essence	Self-Awareness Enhancement Self-Esteem Enhancement	Anticipatory Guidance Body Image Enhancement Counseling Developmental Enhancement: Adolescent Developmental Enhancement: Child Medication Management Mutual Goal Setting Reality Orientation Sexual Counseling Socialization Enhancement Substance Use Prevention	Assertiveness Training Cognitive Restructuring Complex Relationship Building Delirium Management Delusion Management Dementia Management Eating Disorders Management Hallucination Management Hypnosis Substance Use Treatment Therapy Group Values Clarification

Outcome	Major Interventions	Suggested Interventions	Optional Interventions
Self-Mutilation Restraint			
DEFINITION: Personal actions to refrain from intentional self-inflicted injury (nonlethal)	Behavior Management: Self-Harm Environmental Management: Violence Prevention	Anger Control Assistance Anxiety Reduction Behavior Management Behavior Modification Cognitive Restructuring Coping Enhancement Counseling Emotional Support Environmental Management: Safety Impulse Control Training Limit Setting Mood Management Mutual Goal Setting Patient Contracting Physical Restraint Seclusion Security Enhancement Self-Responsibility Facilitation Suicide Prevention Surveillance: Safety	Active Listening Calming Technique Delusion Management Hallucination Management Substance Use Treatment

NURSING DIAGNOSIS: Post-Trauma Syndrome

DEFINITION: Maladaptive response to a traumatic, overwhelming event.

Outcome	Major Interventions	Suggested Interventions	Optional Interventions
Abuse Recovery: Emotional			
DEFINITION: Extent of healing of psychological injuries due to abuse	Counseling Support System Enhancement	Anger Control Assistance Anxiety Reduction Coping Enhancement Emotional Support Forgiveness Facilitation Mood Management Self-Esteem Enhancement Socialization Enhancement Suicide Prevention Support Group	Assertiveness Training Behavior Management: Self-Harm Family Support Security Enhancement Simple Relaxation Therapy Spiritual Support Therapy Group Trauma Therapy: Child
Abuse Recovery: Financial			
DEFINITION: Extent of control of monetary and legal matters following financial exploitation	Coping Enhancement Counseling Financial Resource Assistance	Assertiveness Training Decision-Making Support Patient Rights Protection Security Enhancement Support System Enhancement	Self-Esteem Enhancement Support Group

Outcome	Major Interventions	Suggested Interventions	Optional Interventions
Abuse Recovery: Sexual			
DEFINITION: Extent of healing of physical and psychological injuries due to sexual abuse or exploitation	Counseling Rape-Trauma Treatment Support System Enhancement	Active Listening Anger Control Assistance Anxiety Reduction Coping Enhancement Emotional Support Forgiveness Facilitation Guilt Work Facilitation Self-Esteem Enhancement Sexual Counseling Simple Relaxation Therapy Substance Use Prevention Trauma Therapy: Child	Assertiveness Training Behavior Management: Self-Harm Behavior Management: Sexual Grief Work Facilitation Hope Instillation Mood Management Presence Self-Awareness Enhancement Socialization Enhancement Spiritual Support Support Group Suicide Prevention
Anxiety Level			
DEFINITION: Severity of manifested apprehension, tension, or uneasiness arising from an unidentifiable source	Anxiety Reduction	Abuse Protection Support Coping Enhancement Environmental Management Security Enhancement Simple Relaxation Therapy	Animal-Assisted Therapy Exercise Promotion Music Therapy Progressive Muscle Relaxation

Continued

Outcome	Major Interventions	Suggested Interventions	Optional Interventions
Coping			
DEFINITION: Personal actions to manage stressors that tax an individual's resources	Coping Enhancement Counseling	Anxiety Reduction Emotional Support Grief Work Facilitation Hope Instillation Progressive Muscle Relaxation Simple Relaxation Therapy Spiritual Support Support Group Support System Enhancement	Behavior Management: Self-Harm Mood Management Reminiscence Therapy Sibling Support Socialization Enhancement Trauma Therapy: Child
Depression Level			
DEFINITION: Severity of melancholic mood and loss of interest in life events	Mood Management Suicide Prevention	Counseling Forgiveness Facilitation Grief Work Facilitation Guilt Work Facilitation Medication Administration Milieu Therapy Self-Esteem Enhancement	Animal-Assisted Therapy Anxiety Reduction Patient Contracting Socialization Enhancement Substance Use Prevention
Fear Level			
DEFINITION: Severity of manifested apprehension, tension, or uneasiness arising from an identifiable source	Coping Enhancement Security Enhancement	Calming Technique Crisis Intervention Emotional Support Environmental Management: Safety Rape-Trauma Treatment Simple Relaxation Therapy	Family Presence Facilitation Truth Telling

Outcome	Major Interventions	Suggested Interventions	Optional Interventions
Fear Level: Child			
DEFINITION: Severity of manifested apprehension, tension, or uneasiness arising from an identifiable source in a child from 1 year through 17 years of age	Trauma Therapy: Child	Abuse Protection Support: Child Calming Technique Coping Enhancement Emotional Support Environmental Management: Safety Security Enhancement	Animal-Assisted Therapy Distraction Family Presence Facilitation Truth Telling Visitation Facilitation
Impulse Self-Control			
DEFINITION: Self-restraint of compulsive or impulsive behaviors	Impulse Control Training	Anger Control Assistance Anxiety Reduction Behavior Management: Self-Harm Environmental Management: Safety Mutual Goal Setting Patient Contracting	Coping Enhancement Emotional Support Mood Management Security Enhancement Substance Use Prevention Suicide Prevention Support Group Support System Enhancement

Continued

Outcome	Major Interventions	Suggested Interventions	Optional Interventions
Self-Mutilation Restraint			
DEFINITION: Personal actions to refrain from intentional self-inflicted injury (nonlethal)	Behavior Management: Self-Harm Counseling	Anger Control Assistance Anxiety Reduction Behavior Management Behavior Modification Cognitive Restructuring Coping Enhancement Environmental Management: Safety Impulse Control Training Limit Setting Mood Management Mutual Goal Setting Patient Contracting Security Enhancement Suicide Prevention Surveillance: Safety	Area Restriction Emotional Support Environmental Management Milieu Therapy Reality Orientation

NURSING DIAGNOSIS: Powerlessness

DEFINITION: Perception that one's own actions will not significantly affect an outcome; a perceived lack of control over a current situation or immediate happening.

Outcome	Major Interventions	Suggested Interventions	Optional Interventions
Depression Self-Control			
DEFINITION: Personal actions to minimize melancholy and maintain interest in life events	Cognitive Restructuring Mood Management Self-Esteem Enhancement	Activity Therapy Animal-Assisted Therapy Art Therapy Complex Relationship Building Emotional Support Hope Instillation Presence Self-Awareness Enhancement Support Group	Coping Enhancement Crisis Intervention Grief Work Facilitation Guilt Work Facilitation Humor Meditation Facilitation Reminiscence Therapy Therapy Group
Family Participation in Professional Care			
DEFINITION: Family involvement in decision-making, delivery, and evaluation of care provided by health care personnel	Decision-Making Support Family Involvement Promotion	Family Planning: Unplanned Pregnancy Family Presence Facilitation Family Support Health Care Information Exchange Health System Guidance	Anticipatory Guidance Culture Brokerage Health Education Insurance Authorization Normalization Promotion Patient Rights Protection Risk Identification

Continued

Outcome	Major Interventions	Suggested Interventions	Optional Interventions
Health Beliefs			
DEFINITION: Personal convictions that influence health behaviors	Health Education Values Clarification	Cognitive Restructuring Hope Instillation Risk Identification Self-Awareness Enhancement Self-Esteem Enhancement Self-Modification Assistance	Culture Brokerage Health System Guidance Learning Facilitation Mutual Goal Setting Patient Contracting Spiritual Support Teaching: Individual
Health Beliefs: Perceived Ability to Perform			
DEFINITION: Personal conviction that one can carry out a given health behavior	Mutual Goal Setting Self-Esteem Enhancement	Health System Guidance Patient Contracting Risk Identification Self-Awareness Enhancement Self-Modification Assistance Teaching: Individual Values Clarification	Culture Brokerage Coping Enhancement Learning Facilitation Self-Care Assistance Support System Enhancement
Health Beliefs: Perceived Control			
DEFINITION: Personal conviction that one can influence a health outcome	Decision-Making Support Self-Responsibility Facilitation	Emotional Support Health System Guidance Patient Rights Protection Self-Esteem Enhancement Self-Modification Assistance Support System Enhancement Teaching: Individual Values Clarification	Assertiveness Training Counseling Culture Brokerage Hope Instillation

Outcome	Major Interventions	Suggested Interventions	Optional Interventions
Health Beliefs: Perceived Resources			
DEFINITION: Personal conviction that one has adequate means to carry out a health behavior	Financial Resource Assistance Health System Guidance	Culture Brokerage Health Care Information Exchange Insurance Authorization Patient Rights Protection Referral Support System Enhancement Sustenance Support	Environmental Management Teaching: Individual
Hope			
DEFINITION: Optimism that is personally satisfying and life-supporting	Emotional Support Hope Instillation	Coping Enhancement Decision-Making Support Grief Work Facilitation Grief Work Facilitation: Perinatal Death Presence Security Enhancement Self-Esteem Enhancement Spiritual Support	Crisis Intervention Health System Guidance Reminiscence Therapy Self-Responsibility Facilitation Support System Enhancement

Continued

Outcome	Major Interventions	Suggested Interventions	Optional Interventions
Participation in Health Care Decisions			
DEFINITION: Personal involvement in selecting and evaluating health care options to achieve desired outcome	Decision-Making Support Health System Guidance Self-Responsibility Facilitation	Active Listening Admission Care Assertiveness Training Complex Relationship Building Culture Brokerage Discharge Planning Patient Rights Protection Values Clarification	Anticipatory Guidance Anxiety Reduction Coping Enhancement Family Involvement Promotion Health Care Information Exchange Patient Rights Protection Referral
Personal Autonomy			
DEFINITION: Personal actions of a competent individual to exercise governance in life decisions	Decision-Making Support Patient Rights Protection Self-Responsibility Facilitation	Anticipatory Guidance Assertiveness Training Health System Guidance Mutual Goal Setting Self-Esteem Enhancement	Culture Brokerage Health Care Information Exchange Relocation Stress Reduction

NURSING DIAGNOSIS: Protection, Ineffective

DEFINITION: Decrease in the ability to guard the self from internal or external threats such as illness or injury.

Outcome	Major Interventions	Suggested Interventions	Optional Interventions
Abuse Protection			
DEFINITION: Protection of self or dependent others from abuse	Abuse Protection Support Abuse Protection Support: Child Abuse Protection Support: Domestic Partner Abuse Protection Support: Elder	Environmental Management: Safety Environmental Management: Violence Prevention Risk Identification Security Enhancement Self-Awareness Enhancement Surveillance: Safety	Caregiver Support Coping Enhancement Decision-Making Support Emotional Support Self-Responsibility Facilitation
Blood Coagulation			
DEFINITION: Extent to which blood clots within normal period of time	Bleeding Precautions	Bleeding Reduction Blood Products Administration Emergency Care Hemorrhage Control	Autotransfusion Surgical Precautions
Community Violence Level			
DEFINITION: Incidence of violent acts compared with local, state, or national values	Environmental Management: Community	Community Health Development Environmental Risk Protection Surveillance: Community	Bioterrorism Preparedness Program Development

Continued

Outcome	Major Interventions	Suggested Interventions	Optional Interventions
Fetal Status: Antepartum			
DEFINITION: Extent to which fetal signs are within normal limits from conception to the onset of labor	Electronic Fetal Monitoring: Antepartum Ultrasonography: Limited Obstetric	High-Risk Pregnancy Care Surveillance: Late Pregnancy	Labor Suppression Prenatal Care Resuscitation: Fetus
Fetal Status: Intrapartum			
DEFINITION: Extent to which fetal signs are within normal limits from onset of labor to delivery	Electronic Fetal Monitoring: Intrapartum	Amnioinfusion Intrapartal Care: High-Risk Delivery	Intrapartal Care Labor Induction
Health Promoting Behavior			
DEFINITION: Personal actions to sustain or increase wellness	Health Education Self-Modification Assistance	Coping Enhancement Exercise Promotion Health Screening Nutrition Management Oral Health Promotion Risk Identification Self-Responsibility Facilitation Weight Management	Energy Management Nutrition Therapy Pressure Ulcer Prevention Sleep Enhancement Smoking Cessation Assistance Substance Use Prevention Teaching: Foot Care Teaching: Safe Sex

Outcome	Major Interventions	Suggested Interventions	Optional Interventions
Immune Hypersensitivity Response			
DEFINITION: Severity of inappropriate immune responses	Infection Protection Risk Identification	Allergy Management Asthma Management Infection Control Pruritus Management Respiratory Monitoring Skin Care: Topical Treatments Skin Surveillance Teaching: Disease Process Teaching: Individual Teaching: Prescribed Medication	Coping Enhancement Health Education Self-Modification Assistance Self-Responsibility Facilitation Temperature Regulation
Immune Status			
DEFINITION: Natural and acquired appropriately targeted resistance to internal and external antigens	Allergy Management Infection Protection	Health Education Infection Control Latex Precautions Medication Administration Risk Identification Surveillance Teaching: Individual Teaching: Prescribed Medication	Chemotherapy Management Pruritus Management Radiation Therapy Management

Continued

Outcome	Major Interventions	Suggested Interventions	Optional Interventions
Immunization Behavior			
DEFINITION: Personal actions to obtain immunization to prevent a communicable disease	Immunization/ Vaccination Management Risk Identification	Anticipatory Guidance Decision-Making Support Health Education Health System Guidance Infection Protection	Parent Education: Infant
Nutritional Status			
DEFINITION: Extent to which nutrients are available to meet metabolic needs	Nutrition Therapy Nutritional Counseling	Fluid/Electrolyte Management Nutrition Management Nutritional Monitoring Self-Care Assistance: Feeding Teaching: Prescribed Diet Weight Management	Diet Staging Eating Disorders Management Enteral Tube Feeding Gastrointestinal Intubation Prenatal Care Total Parenteral Nutrition (TPN) Administration

NURSING DIAGNOSIS: Rape-Trauma Syndrome

DEFINITION: Sustained maladaptive response to a forced, violent sexual penetration against the victim's will and consent.

Outcome	Major Interventions	Suggested Interventions	Optional Interventions
Abuse Protection			
DEFINITION: Protection of self or dependent others from abuse	Abuse Protection Support Abuse Protection Support: Child Abuse Protection Support: Domestic Partner Abuse Protection Support: Elder	Counseling Environmental Management: Safety Environmental Management: Violence Prevention Risk Identification Security Enhancement Surveillance: Safety	Anticipatory Guidance Caregiver Support Decision-Making Support Documentation Emotional Support Self-Awareness Enhancement
Abuse Recovery: Emotional			
DEFINITION: Extent of healing of psychological injuries due to abuse	Counseling Rape-Trauma Treatment Trauma Therapy: Child	Coping Enhancement Crisis Intervention Emotional Support Mood Management Self-Esteem Enhancement Support Group Therapy Group	Abuse Protection Support Anger Control Assistance Anxiety Reduction Family Support Security Enhancement Self-Awareness Enhancement Spiritual Support Support System Enhancement

Continued

Outcome	Major Interventions	Suggested Interventions	Optional Interventions
Abuse Recovery: Sexual			
DEFINITION: Extent of healing of physical and psychological injuries due to sexual abuse or exploitation	Counseling Rape-Trauma Treatment Trauma Therapy: Child	Anger Control Assistance Anxiety Reduction Calming Technique Crisis Intervention Decision-Making Support Emotional Support Hope Instillation Presence Referral Self-Esteem Enhancement Sexual Counseling Specimen Management Support Group Support System Enhancement Therapeutic Play Therapy Group	Abuse Protection Support Anticipatory Guidance Art Therapy Behavior Management: Self-Harm Behavior Management: Sexual Coping Enhancement Family Therapy Grief Work Facilitation Guilt Work Facilitation Health System Guidance Pain Management Role Enhancement Security Enhancement Sleep Enhancement Spiritual Support Substance Use Prevention

Outcome	Major Interventions	Suggested Interventions	Optional Interventions
Coping			
DEFINITION: Personal actions to manage stressors that tax an individual's resources	Coping Enhancement Crisis Intervention Rape-Trauma Treatment	Anxiety Reduction Behavior Management: Self-Harm Calming Technique Counseling Emotional Support Family Support Grief Work Facilitation Guilt Work Facilitation Hope Instillation Presence Simple Relaxation Therapy Spiritual Support Support Group	Art Therapy Cognitive Restructuring Decision-Making Support Family Therapy Support System Enhancement Therapeutic Play Therapy Group
Sexual Functioning			
DEFINITION: Integration of physical, socioemotional, and intellectual aspects of sexual expression and performance	Behavior Management: Sexual Sexual Counseling	Anxiety Reduction Grief Work Facilitation Guilt Work Facilitation Self-Awareness Enhancement Self-Esteem Enhancement Self-Modification Assistance	Forgiveness Facilitation Impulse Control Training Self-Responsibility Facilitation Substance Use Prevention

NURSING DIAGNOSIS: Rape-Trauma Syndrome: Compound Reaction

DEFINITION: Forced violent sexual penetration against the victim's will and consent. The trauma syndrome that develops from this attack or attempted attack includes an acute phase of disorganization of the victim's lifestyle and a long-term process or reorganization of lifestyle.

Outcome	Major Interventions	Suggested Interventions	Optional Interventions
Abuse Protection			
DEFINITION: Protection of self or dependent others from abuse	Abuse Protection Support	Assertiveness Training	Anticipatory Guidance
	Abuse Protection Support: Child	Counseling	Caregiver Support
	Abuse Protection Support: Domestic Partner	Environmental Management: Safety	Decision-Making Support
	Abuse Protection Support: Elder	Environmental Management: Violence Prevention	Documentation
		Risk Identification	Emotional Support
		Security Enhancement	Self-Awareness Enhancement
		Self-Esteem Enhancement	Self-Responsibility Facilitation
		Surveillance: Safety	Values Clarification

Outcome	Major Interventions	Suggested Interventions	Optional Interventions
Abuse Recovery: Emotional			
DEFINITION: Extent of healing of psychological injuries due to abuse	Coping Enhancement Counseling Rape-Trauma Treatment	Assertiveness Training Crisis Intervention Emotional Support Mood Management Self-Esteem Enhancement Socialization Enhancement Suicide Prevention Support Group Therapy Group Trauma Therapy: Child	Abuse Protection Support Anger Control Assistance Anxiety Reduction Behavior Management: Self-Harm Behavior Modification: Social Skills Complex Relationship Building Family Support Forgiveness Facilitation Hope Instillation Role Enhancement Security Enhancement Self-Awareness Enhancement Spiritual Support Support System Enhancement
Abuse Recovery: Physical			
DEFINITION: Extent of healing of physical injuries due to abuse	Abuse Protection Support Rape-Trauma Treatment	Bowel Incontinence Care Environmental Management: Comfort Environmental Management: Safety Health Screening Health System Guidance Heat/Cold Application Infection Protection Pain Management Skin Surveillance	Coping Enhancement Counseling Crisis Intervention Grief Work Facilitation Medication Administration Security Enhancement

Continued

Outcome	Major Interventions	Suggested Interventions	Optional Interventions
Abuse Recovery: Sexual			
DEFINITION: Extent of healing of physical and psychological injuries due to sexual abuse or exploitation	Crisis Intervention Rape-Trauma Treatment	Anger Control Assistance Anticipatory Guidance Anxiety Reduction Calming Technique Coping Enhancement Counseling Emotional Support Grief Work Facilitation Guilt Work Facilitation Hope Instillation Mood Management Presence Referral Self-Esteem Enhancement Sexual Counseling Substance Use Prevention Support Group Support System Enhancement Therapy Group Trauma Therapy: Child	Abuse Protection Support Activity Therapy Animal-Assisted Therapy Art Therapy Assertiveness Training Behavior Management: Self-Harm Behavior Management: Sexual Body Image Enhancement Complex Relationship Building Decision-Making Support Eating Disorders Management Family Therapy Forgiveness Facilitation Forgiveness Facilitation Health System Guidance Hypnosis Music Therapy Simple Relaxation Therapy Socialization Enhancement Spiritual Support Suicide Prevention Therapeutic Play

Outcome	Major Interventions	Suggested Interventions	Optional Interventions
Coping			
DEFINITION: Personal actions to manage stressors that tax an individual's resources	Coping Enhancement Crisis Intervention Rape-Trauma Treatment	Anxiety Reduction Calming Technique Counseling Decision-Making Support Emotional Support Family Support Grief Work Facilitation Guilt Work Facilitation Hope Instillation Pain Management Presence Simple Relaxation Therapy Spiritual Support Support Group	Animal-Assisted Therapy Art Therapy Behavior Management: Self-Harm Bibliotherapy Body Image Enhancement Cognitive Restructuring Family Therapy Hypnosis Mood Management Music Therapy Recreation Therapy Sibling Support Support System Enhancement Therapeutic Play Therapy Group
Personal Autonomy			
DEFINITION: Personal actions of a competent individual to exercise governance in life decisions	Decision-Making Support Rape-Trauma Treatment	Anger Control Assistance Assertiveness Training Behavior Modification Cognitive Restructuring Hope Instillation Self-Responsibility Facilitation	Anxiety Reduction Coping Enhancement Forgiveness Facilitation Grief Work Facilitation Guilt Work Facilitation Mood Management

Continued

Outcome	Major Interventions	Suggested Interventions	Optional Interventions
Self-Esteem			
DEFINITION: Personal judgment of self-worth	Rape-Trauma Treatment Self-Esteem Enhancement	Body Image Enhancement Cognitive Restructuring Counseling Guilt Work Facilitation Self-Awareness Enhancement Support Group	Assertiveness Training Behavior Modification Complex Relationship Building Self-Modification Assistance
Sexual Functioning			
DEFINITION: Integration of physical, socioemotional, and intellectual aspects of sexual expression and performance	Rape-Trauma Treatment Sexual Counseling	Anger Control Assistance Anxiety Reduction Coping Enhancement Self-Awareness Enhancement Self-Modification Assistance Support Group	Grief Work Facilitation Guilt Work Facilitation Referral Therapy Group

NURSING DIAGNOSIS: Rape-Trauma Syndrome: Silent Reaction

DEFINITION: Forced violent sexual penetration against the victim's will and consent. The trauma syndrome that develops from this attack or attempted attack includes an acute phase of disorganization of the victim's lifestyle and a long-term process of reorganization of lifestyle.

Outcome	Major Interventions	Suggested Interventions	Optional Interventions
Abuse Protection			
DEFINITION: Protection of self or dependent others from abuse	Abuse Protection Support Abuse Protection Support: Child Abuse Protection Support: Domestic Partner Abuse Protection Support: Elder	Assertiveness Training Counseling Environmental Management: Safety Environmental Management: Violence Prevention Risk Identification Security Enhancement Surveillance: Safety	Anticipatory Guidance Caregiver Support Decision-Making Support Documentation Emotional Support Self-Awareness Enhancement Self-Responsibility Facilitation Values Clarification
Abuse Recovery: Emotional			
DEFINITION: Extent of healing of psychological injuries due to abuse	Abuse Protection Support Coping Enhancement Counseling Rape-Trauma Treatment	Assertiveness Training Crisis Intervention Emotional Support Mood Management Self-Esteem Enhancement Socialization Enhancement Support Group Therapy Group	Anger Control Assistance Anxiety Reduction Behavior Management: Self-Harm Behavior Modification: Social Skills Complex Relationship Building Family Support Role Enhancement Security Enhancement Self-Awareness Enhancement Spiritual Support Support System Enhancement

Continued

Outcome	Major Interventions	Suggested Interventions	Optional Interventions
Abuse Recovery: Sexual			
DEFINITION: Extent of healing of physical and psychological injuries due to sexual abuse or exploitation	Behavior Management: Sexual Rape-Trauma Treatment Sexual Counseling	Anger Control Assistance Anticipatory Guidance Anxiety Reduction Art Therapy Calming Technique Coping Enhancement Counseling Crisis Intervention Decision-Making Support Emotional Support Hope Instillation Presence Referral Security Enhancement Support Group Support System Enhancement Therapy Group Trauma Therapy: Child	Abuse Protection Support Animal-Assisted Therapy Body Image Enhancement Complex Relationship Building Family Therapy Grief Work Facilitation Guilt Work Facilitation Health System Guidance Self-Esteem Enhancement Simple Relaxation Therapy Socialization Enhancement Spiritual Support Substance Use Prevention Therapeutic Play
Anxiety Level			
DEFINITION: Severity of manifested apprehension, tension, or uneasiness arising from an unidentifiable source	Anxiety Reduction Rape-Trauma Treatment	Active Listening Calming Technique Crisis Intervention Security Enhancement Simple Relaxation Therapy	Abuse Protection Support Coping Enhancement Emotional Support

Outcome	Major Interventions	Suggested Interventions	Optional Interventions
Anxiety Self-Control			
DEFINITION: Personal actions to eliminate or reduce feelings of apprehension, tension, or uneasiness from an unidentifiable source	Anxiety Reduction	Coping Enhancement Counseling Grief Work Facilitation Guilt Work Facilitation Progressive Muscle Relaxation Simple Relaxation Therapy Spiritual Support Support System Enhancement	Animal-Assisted Therapy Biofeedback Exercise Promotion Medication Administration Medication Prescribing Music Therapy Support Group
Sexual Functioning			
DEFINITION: Integration of physical, socioemotional, and intellectual aspects of sexual expression and performance	Sexual Counseling	Anger Control Assistance Behavior Management: Sexual Complex Relationship Building Decision-Making Support Emotional Support Self-Modification Assistance Self-Responsibility Facilitation Substance Use Prevention	Anxiety Reduction Assertiveness Training Grief Work Facilitation Guilt Work Facilitation Impulse Control Training

NURSING DIAGNOSIS: Religiosity, Impaired

DEFINITION: Impaired ability to exercise reliance on beliefs and/or participate in rituals of a particular faith tradition.

Outcome	Major Interventions	Suggested Interventions	Optional Interventions
Spiritual Health DEFINITION: Connectedness with self, others, higher power, all life, nature, and the universe that transcends and empowers the self	Spiritual Growth Facilitation Spiritual Support Values Clarification	Active Listening Coping Enhancement Emotional Support Forgiveness Facilitation Grief Work Facilitation Guilt Work Facilitation Hope Instillation Meditation Facilitation Religious Addiction Prevention Religious Ritual Enhancement	Anxiety Reduction Bibliotherapy Counseling Culture Brokerage Decision-Making Support Dying Care Family Support Family Therapy Security Enhancement Support System Enhancement

NURSING DIAGNOSIS: Religiosity, Readiness for Enhanced

DEFINITION: Ability to increase reliance on religious beliefs and/or participate in rituals of a particular faith tradition.

Outcome	Major Interventions	Suggested Interventions	Optional Interventions
Personal Well-Being			
DEFINITION: Extent of positive perception of one's health status and life circumstances	Spiritual Growth Facilitation Spiritual Support	Decision-Making Support Emotional Support Forgiveness Facilitation Self-Awareness Enhancement Values Clarification	Counseling Self-Esteem Enhancement Self-Modification Assistance Self-Responsibility Facilitation
Spiritual Health			
DEFINITION: Connectedness with self, others, higher power, all life, nature, and the universe that transcends and empowers the self	Religious Ritual Enhancement Spiritual Growth Facilitation	Emotional Support Forgiveness Facilitation Guilt Work Facilitation Meditation Facilitation Self-Awareness Enhancement Spiritual Support Values Clarification	Abuse Protection Support: Religious Presence Religious Addiction Prevention Reminiscence Therapy Resiliency Promotion

NURSING DIAGNOSIS: Relocation Stress Syndrome

DEFINITION: Physiological and/or psychosocial disturbances following transfer from one environment to another.

Outcome	Major Interventions	Suggested Interventions	Optional Interventions
Anxiety Level DEFINITION: Severity of manifested apprehension, tension, or uneasiness arising from an unidentifiable source	Anxiety Reduction Relocation Stress Reduction	Active Listening Animal-Assisted Therapy Anticipatory Guidance Calming Technique Coping Enhancement Presence Security Enhancement Simple Massage Simple Relaxation Therapy Spiritual Support Support System Enhancement Touch	Decision-Making Support Environmental Management Family Mobilization Grief Work Facilitation Progressive Muscle Relaxation Simple Guided Imagery Sleep Enhancement Support Group Truth Telling Visitation Facilitation

Outcome	Major Interventions	Suggested Interventions	Optional Interventions
Child Adaptation to Hospitalization			
DEFINITION: Adaptive response of a child from 3 years through 17 years of age to hospitalization	Coping Enhancement Security Enhancement Trauma Therapy: Child	Active Listening Admission Care Culture Brokerage Emotional Support Environmental Management Family Integrity Promotion Family Involvement Promotion Family Mobilization Family Process Maintenance Family Support Patient Rights Protection Self-Care Assistance Sibling Support Sleep Enhancement Support System Enhancement Therapeutic Play Touch Truth Telling Visitation Facilitation	Animal-Assisted Therapy Anticipatory Guidance Anxiety Reduction Art Therapy Calming Technique Developmental Enhancement: Child Family Presence Facilitation Humor Limit Setting Music Therapy Preparatory Sensory Information Presence Spiritual Support Support Group Teaching: Individual Teaching: Procedure/ Treatment

Continued

Outcome	Major Interventions	Suggested Interventions	Optional Interventions
Coping			
DEFINITION: Personal actions to manage stressors that tax an individual's resources	Coping Enhancement Relocation Stress Reduction	Active Listening Anticipatory Guidance Anxiety Reduction Calming Technique Caregiver Support Counseling Emotional Support Family Support Family Mobilization Hope Instillation Humor Presence Recreation Therapy Resiliency Promotion Self-Responsibility Facilitation Spiritual Support Support Group Touch	Animal-Assisted Therapy Art Therapy Family Support Mood Management Music Therapy Reminiscence Therapy Sibling Support Simple Guided Imagery Simple Massage Simple Relaxation Therapy Support System Enhancement Therapeutic Play Therapy Group Visitation Facilitation
Depression Level			
DEFINITION: Severity of melancholic mood and loss of interest in life events	Hope Instillation Mood Management	Counseling Emotional Support Exercise Promotion Medication Management Nutritional Monitoring Self-Modification Assistance Sleep Enhancement	Activity Therapy Anger Control Assistance Animal-Assisted Therapy Nutrition Management Recreation Therapy Spiritual Support Support System Enhancement

Outcome	Major Interventions	Suggested Interventions	Optional Interventions
Discharge Readiness: Independent Living DEFINITION: Readiness of a patient to relocate from a health care institution to living independently	Discharge Planning Health System Guidance Relocation Stress Reduction	Anticipatory Guidance Decision-Making Support Mutual Goal Setting Self-Responsibility Facilitation Teaching: Disease Process Teaching: Prescribed Activity/Exercise Teaching: Prescribed Diet Teaching: Prescribed Medication Teaching: Procedure/Treatment	Cardiac Care: Rehabilitative Chemotherapy Management Coping Enhancement Exercise Promotion Family Involvement Promotion Health Education Self-Care Assistance: IADL Self-Modification Assistance
Loneliness Severity DEFINITION: Severity of emotional, social, or existential isolation response	Family Involvement Promotion Socialization Enhancement Spiritual Support	Active Listening Activity Therapy Animal-Assisted Therapy Emotional Support Environmental Management Presence Recreation Therapy Support System Enhancement Therapeutic Play Touch Visitation Facilitation	Art Therapy Bibliotherapy Music Therapy Patient Rights Protection Risk Identification

Continued

Outcome	Major Interventions	Suggested Interventions	Optional Interventions
Psychosocial Adjustment: Life Change			
DEFINITION: Adaptive psychosocial response of an individual to a significant life change	Coping Enhancement Relocation Stress Reduction	Active Listening Anger Control Assistance Anticipatory Guidance Counseling Discharge Planning Emotional Support Family Involvement Promotion Health Education Resiliency Promotion Role Enhancement	Decision-Making Support Dementia Management Family Integrity Promotion Family Mobilization Family Process Maintenance Humor Spiritual Support
Quality of Life			
DEFINITION: Extent of positive perception of current life circumstances	Relocation Stress Reduction Values Clarification	Active Listening Coping Enhancement Decision-Making Support Emotional Support Family Integrity Promotion Family Involvement Promotion Family Support Hope Instillation Humor Role Enhancement Security Enhancement Socialization Enhancement Spiritual Support Support System Enhancement	Culture Brokerage Mood Management Patient Rights Protection Reminiscence Therapy Support Group Truth Telling

Outcome	Major Interventions	Suggested Interventions	Optional Interventions
Stress Level DEFINITION: Severity of manifested physical or mental tension resulting from factors that alter an existing equilibrium	Coping Enhancement Relocation Stress Reduction	Anger Control Assistance Anxiety Reduction Emotional Support Family Involvement Promotion Nutritional Monitoring Presence Security Enhancement Sleep Enhancement Spiritual Support Support System Enhancement	Active Listening Animal-Assisted Therapy Decision-Making Support Music Therapy Socialization Enhancement

R

NURSING DIAGNOSIS: Role Performance, Ineffective

DEFINITION: Patterns of behavior and self-expression do not match the environmental context, norms, and expectations.

Outcome	Major Interventions	Suggested Interventions	Optional Interventions
Caregiver Lifestyle Disruption DEFINITION: Severity of disturbances in the lifestyle of a family member due to caregiving	Coping Enhancement Role Enhancement	Anticipatory Guidance Caregiver Support Decision-Making Support Emotional Support Family Support Health System Guidance Mutual Goal Setting Support Group Support System Enhancement	Family Involvement Promotion Insurance Authorization
Coping DEFINITION: Personal actions to manage stressors that tax an individual's resources	Anticipatory Guidance Coping Enhancement	Caregiver Support Counseling Decision-Making Support Emotional Support Family Support Role Enhancement Spiritual Support Support Group Teaching: Individual Values Clarification	Body Image Enhancement Cognitive Restructuring Family Therapy Mood Management Normalization Promotion Socialization Enhancement Spiritual Support Substance Use Prevention Support Group Support System Enhancement

Outcome	Major Interventions	Suggested Interventions	Optional Interventions
Depression Level			
DEFINITION: Severity of melancholic mood and loss of interest in life events	Hope Instillation Mood Management	Activity Therapy Cognitive Restructuring Counseling Emotional Support Exercise Promotion Medication Management Patient Contracting Self-Awareness Enhancement Self-Esteem Enhancement Self-Modification Assistance Sleep Enhancement Support Group Therapy Group	Mutual Goal Setting Spiritual Support Support System Enhancement
Parenting Performance			
DEFINITION: Parental actions to provide a child a nurturing and constructive physical, emotional, and social environment	Parenting Promotion Role Enhancement	Anticipatory Guidance Attachment Promotion Childbirth Preparation Coping Enhancement Parent Education: Adolescent Parent Education: Childrearing Family Parent Education: Infant Support System Enhancement	Environmental Management: Attachment Process Family Planning: Contraception Teaching: Infant Nutrition Teaching: Infant Safety Teaching: Infant Stimulation Teaching: Toddler Nutrition Teaching: Toddler Safety Teaching: Toilet Training

Continued

Outcome	Major Interventions	Suggested Interventions	Optional Interventions
Psychosocial Adjustment: Life Change			
DEFINITION: Adaptive psychosocial response of an individual to a significant life change	Anticipatory Guidance Coping Enhancement	Counseling Emotional Support Parent Education: Adolescent Parent Education: Childrearing Family Parent Education: Infant Role Enhancement	Decision-Making Support Family Mobilization Family Process Maintenance Family Therapy Humor Spiritual Support
Role Performance			
DEFINITION: Congruence of an individual's role behavior with role expectations	Role Enhancement	Anticipatory Guidance Caregiver Support Cognitive Restructuring Complex Relationship Building Emotional Support Self-Awareness Enhancement Self-Esteem Enhancement Values Clarification	Active Listening Attachment Promotion Body Image Enhancement Counseling Decision-Making Support Family Therapy Normalization Promotion Support Group Support System Enhancement Teaching: Sexuality

NURSING DIAGNOSIS: Self-Care Deficit: Bathing/Hygiene

DEFINITION: Impaired ability to perform or complete bathing/hygiene activities for oneself.

Outcome	Major Interventions	Suggested Interventions	Optional Interventions
Ostomy Self-Care			
DEFINITION: Personal actions to maintain ostomy for elimination	Ostomy Care Self-Care Assistance: Bathing/Hygiene	Bowel Management Flatulence Reduction Skin Surveillance	Bowel Irrigation Incision Site Care
Self-Care: Activities of Daily Living (ADL)			
DEFINITION: Ability to perform the most basic physical tasks and personal care activities independently with or without assistive device	Self-Care Assistance: Bathing/Hygiene	Energy Management Self-Care Assistance Self-Responsibility Facilitation Teaching: Individual	Behavior Modification Exercise Promotion Exercise Promotion: Stretching Exercise Therapy: Ambulation Exercise Therapy: Balance Exercise Therapy: Joint Mobility Exercise Therapy: Muscle Control Fall Prevention
Self-Care: Bathing			
DEFINITION: Ability to cleanse own body independently with or without assistive device	Self-Care Assistance: Bathing/Hygiene	Bathing Ear Care Foot Care Hair Care Nail Care Perineal Care Teaching: Individual	Energy Management Environmental Management: Comfort Environmental Management: Safety Exercise Promotion Fall Prevention

Continued

Outcome	Major Interventions	Suggested Interventions	Optional Interventions
Self-Care: Hygiene			
DEFINITION: Ability to maintain own personal cleanliness and kempt appearance independently with or without assistive device	Self-Care Assistance: Bathing/Hygiene	Bathing Ear Care Oral Health Maintenance Perineal Care Teaching: Individual	Contact Lens Care Energy Management Foot Care Hair Care Nail Care Oral Health Promotion Oral Health Restoration
Self-Care: Oral Hygiene			
DEFINITION: Ability to care for own mouth and teeth independently with or without assistive device	Oral Health Maintenance	Oral Health Promotion Oral Health Restoration Self-Care Assistance: Bathing/Hygiene Teaching: Individual	Nutrition Management Nutritional Monitoring

NURSING DIAGNOSIS: Self-Care Deficit: Dressing/Grooming

DEFINITION: An impaired ability to perform or complete dressing and grooming activities for oneself.

Outcome	Major Interventions	Suggested Interventions	Optional Interventions
Self-Care: Activities of Daily Living (ADL)			
DEFINITION: Ability to perform the most basic physical tasks and personal care activities independently with or without assistive device	Self-Care Assistance: Dressing/ Grooming	Energy Management Environmental Management Self-Care Assistance Teaching: Individual	Exercise Promotion Exercise Promotion: Stretching Exercise Therapy: Ambulation Exercise Therapy: Balance Exercise Therapy: Joint Mobility Exercise Therapy: Muscle Control Fall Prevention Pain Management
Self-Care: Dressing			
DEFINITION: Ability to dress self independently with or without assistive device	Dressing Self-Care Assistance: Dressing/ Grooming	Environmental Management Self-Care Assistance Teaching: Individual	Communication Enhancement: Visual Deficit Energy Management Environmental Management: Comfort Environmental Management: Safety Exercise Promotion Fall Prevention
Self-Care: Hygiene			
DEFINITION: Ability to maintain own personal cleanliness and kempt appearance independently with or without assistive device	Hair Care Self-Care Assistance: Dressing/ Grooming	Bathing Dressing Nail Care Self-Care Assistance: Bathing/Hygiene Teaching: Individual	Contact Lens Care Energy Management Oral Health Maintenance Oral Health Promotion

NURSING DIAGNOSIS: Self-Care Deficit: Feeding

DEFINITION: Impaired ability to perform or complete feeding activities.

Outcome	Major Interventions	Suggested Interventions	Optional Interventions
Nutritional Status			
DEFINITION: Extent to which nutrients are available to meet metabolic needs	Nutrition Management Nutritional Counseling Nutritional Monitoring	Feeding Nutrition Therapy Self-Care Assistance: Feeding Teaching: Individual	Enteral Tube Feeding Gastrointestinal Intubation Sustenance Support Total Parenteral Nutrition (TPN) Administration Weight Management
Nutritional Status: Food & Fluid Intake			
DEFINITION: Amount of food and fluid taken into the body over a 24-hour period	Feeding Nutritional Monitoring	Fluid Management Fluid Monitoring Nutrition Management Self-Care Assistance: Feeding Teaching: Individual Teaching: Prescribed Diet	Enteral Tube Feeding Intravenous (IV) Therapy Oral Health Maintenance Swallowing Therapy Total Parenteral Nutrition (TPN) Administration Weight Management
Self-Care: Activities of Daily Living (ADL)			
DEFINITION: Ability to perform the most basic physical tasks and personal care activities independently with or without assistive device	Self-Care Assistance: Feeding	Feeding Self-Care Assistance Teaching: Individual	Energy Management Environmental Management Exercise Promotion Exercise Therapy: Joint Mobility Exercise Therapy: Muscle Control Family Involvement Promotion

Outcome	Major Interventions	Suggested Interventions	Optional Interventions
Self-Care: Eating			
DEFINITION: Ability to prepare and ingest food and fluid independently with or without assistive device	Self-Care Assistance: Feeding	Environmental Management Feeding Nutrition Management Nutritional Monitoring Positioning	Aspiration Precautions Family Involvement Promotion Oral Health Maintenance Pain Management Swallowing Therapy
Swallowing Status			
DEFINITION: Safe passage of fluids and/or solids from the mouth to the stomach	Referral Swallowing Therapy	Aspiration Precautions Feeding Nutritional Monitoring Positioning Self-Care Assistance: Feeding Teaching: Individual	Anxiety Reduction Enteral Tube Feeding Family Involvement Promotion Nutrition Management Oral Health Maintenance Total Parenteral Nutrition (TPN) Administration

NURSING DIAGNOSIS: Self-Care Deficit: Toileting

DEFINITION: An impaired ability to perform or complete own toileting activities.

Outcome	Major Interventions	Suggested Interventions	Optional Interventions
Knowledge: Ostomy Care DEFINITION: Extent of understanding conveyed about maintenance of an ostomy for elimination	Ostomy Care Teaching: Individual	Teaching: Prescribed Activity/Exercise Teaching: Prescribed Diet Teaching: Procedure/Treatment Teaching: Psychomotor Skill	Learning Facilitation Teaching: Disease Process Teaching: Prescribed Medication
Ostomy Self-Care DEFINITION: Personal actions to maintain ostomy for elimination	Bowel Management Ostomy Care	Flatulence Reduction Nutritional Counseling Self-Care Assistance: Bathing/Hygiene Skin Care: Topical Treatments Teaching: Prescribed Diet	Bowel Irrigation Diarrhea Management Incision Site Care Weight Management Wound Care

Outcome	Major Interventions	Suggested Interventions	Optional Interventions
Self-Care: Activities of Daily Living (ADL)			
DEFINITION: Ability to perform the most basic physical tasks and personal care activities independently with or without assistive device	Self-Care Assistance: Toileting	Energy Management Environmental Management Self-Care Assistance	Exercise Promotion Exercise Promotion: Stretching Exercise Therapy: Ambulation Exercise Therapy: Balance Exercise Therapy: Joint Mobility Exercise Therapy: Muscle Control Fall Prevention
Self-Care: Hygiene			
DEFINITION: Ability to maintain own personal cleanliness and kempt appearance independently with or without assistive device	Self-Care Assistance: Bathing/Hygiene	Bathing Patient Contracting Perineal Care Self-Care Assistance: Toileting Teaching: Individual	Bowel Irrigation Ostomy Care Skin Surveillance
Self-Care: Toileting			
DEFINITION: Ability to toilet self independently with or without assistive device	Bowel Management Self-Care Assistance: Toileting	Bowel Incontinence Care: Encopresis Bowel Training Exercise Promotion Medication Management Urinary Elimination Management	Constipation/Impaction Management Perineal Care Promoted Voiding Skin Surveillance Urinary Incontinence Care

NURSING DIAGNOSIS: Self-Concept, Readiness for Enhanced

DEFINITION: A pattern of perceptions or ideas about the self that is sufficient for well-being and can be strengthened.

Outcome	Major Interventions	Suggested Interventions	Optional Interventions
Body Image			
DEFINITION: Perception of own appearance and body functions	Body Image Enhancement	Anticipatory Guidance Developmental Enhancement: Adolescent Developmental Enhancement: Child Self-Awareness Enhancement Self-Esteem Enhancement	Amputation Care Role Enhancement Self-Modification Assistance Weight Management
Personal Autonomy			
DEFINITION: Personal actions of a competent individual to exercise governance in life decisions	Self-Awareness Enhancement	Assertiveness Training Role Enhancement Self-Esteem Enhancement Self-Responsibility Facilitation	Coping Enhancement Decision-Making Support Developmental Enhancement: Adolescent
Self-Esteem			
DEFINITION: Personal judgment of self-worth	Self-Esteem Enhancement	Body Image Enhancement Emotional Support Self-Awareness Enhancement Socialization Enhancement	Assertiveness Training Developmental Enhancement: Adolescent Developmental Enhancement: Child Self-Modification Assistance Weight Management

NURSING DIAGNOSIS: Self-Esteem: Chronic Low

DEFINITION: Long standing negative self-evaluation/feelings about self or self-capabilities.

Outcome	Major Interventions	Suggested Interventions	Optional Interventions
Depression Level DEFINITION: Severity of melancholic mood and loss of interest in life events	Hope Instillation Mood Management	Behavior Management: Self-Harm Counseling Emotional Support Grief Work Facilitation Guilt Work Facilitation Milieu Therapy Self-Awareness Enhancement Self-Esteem Enhancement Self-Modification Assistance Support Group Therapy Group	Crisis Intervention Spiritual Support Substance Use Prevention Suicide Prevention Support System Enhancement Therapeutic Play
Quality of Life DEFINITION: Extent of positive perception of current life circumstances	Self-Esteem Enhancement Values Clarification	Active Listening Body Image Enhancement Coping Enhancement Counseling Decision-Making Support Emotional Support Role Enhancement Self-Awareness Enhancement Socialization Enhancement Spiritual Support Support System Enhancement	Anxiety Reduction Culture Brokerage Genetic Counseling Grief Work Facilitation Guilt Work Facilitation Hope Instillation Mood Management Security Enhancement Support Group

Continued

Outcome	Major Interventions	Suggested Interventions	Optional Interventions
Self-Esteem			
DEFINITION: Personal judgment of self-worth	Self-Esteem Enhancement	Body Image Enhancement Cognitive Restructuring Counseling Developmental Enhancement: Adolescent Developmental Enhancement: Child Emotional Support Resiliency Promotion Self-Awareness Enhancement Socialization Enhancement Support System Enhancement	Active Listening Assertiveness Training Complex Relationship Building Coping Enhancement Eating Disorders Management Family Mobilization Role Enhancement Security Enhancement Self-Modification Assistance Spiritual Support Substance Use Prevention Suicide Prevention Support Group Weight Management

NURSING DIAGNOSIS: Self-Esteem: Situational Low

DEFINITION: Development of a negative perception of self worth in response to a current situation (specify).

Outcome	Major Interventions	Suggested Interventions	Optional Interventions
Adaptation to Physical Disability			
DEFINITION: Adaptive response to a significant functional challenge due to a physical disability	Body Image Enhancement Self-Esteem Enhancement	Amputation Care Coping Enhancement Counseling Grief Work Facilitation Mood Management Substance Use Prevention	Animal-Assisted Therapy Emotional Support Role Enhancement Support System Enhancement
Grief Resolution			
DEFINITION: Adjustment to actual or impending loss	Grief Work Facilitation Grief Work Facilitation: Perinatal Death	Active Listening Coping Enhancement Counseling Emotional Support Hope Installation Substance Use Prevention Support Group	Animal-Assisted Therapy Bibliotherapy Decision-Making Support Guilt Work Facilitation Sibling Support Spiritual Support

Continued

Outcome	Major Interventions	Suggested Interventions	Optional Interventions
Psychosocial Adjustment: Life Change			
DEFINITION: Adaptive psychosocial response of an individual to a significant life change	Anticipatory Guidance Coping Enhancement	Body Image Enhancement Cognitive Restructuring Counseling Decision-Making Support Emotional Support Resiliency Promotion Role Enhancement Self-Esteem Enhancement	Childbirth Preparation Complex Relationship Building Decision-Making Support Family Planning: Unplanned Pregnancy Hormone Replacement Therapy Reproductive Technology Management Therapy Group
Self-Esteem			
DEFINITION: Personal judgment of self-worth	Self-Esteem Enhancement	Active Listening Body Image Enhancement Cognitive Restructuring Coping Enhancement Counseling Developmental Enhancement: Adolescent Developmental Enhancement: Child Emotional Support Mood Management Self-Awareness Enhancement Socialization Enhancement Support Group	Assertiveness Training Complex Relationship Building Grief Work Facilitation Guilt Work Facilitation Role Enhancement Security Enhancement Self-Care Assistance Self-Modification Assistance Spiritual Support Urinary Incontinence Care: Enuresis Weight Management

NURSING DIAGNOSIS: Self-Mutilation

DEFINITION: Deliberate self-injurious behavior causing tissue damage with the intent of causing nonfatal injury to attain relief of tension.

Outcome	Major Interventions	Suggested Interventions	Optional Interventions
Identity			
DEFINITION: Distinguishes between self and non-self and characterizes one's essence	Cognitive Restructuring Self-Awareness Enhancement	Body Image Enhancement Counseling Mood Management Self-Esteem Enhancement Socialization Enhancement	Developmental Enhancement: Adolescent Developmental Enhancement: Child Eating Disorders Management Hallucination Management
Impulse Self-Control			
DEFINITION: Self-restraint of compulsive or impulsive behaviors	Impulse Control Training	Anger Control Assistance Anxiety Reduction Area Restriction Behavior Management: Self-Harm Behavior Modification Limit Setting Self-Modification Assistance Self-Responsibility Facilitation	Behavior Management Environmental Management: Safety Environmental Management: Violence Prevention Milieu Therapy Patient Contracting Seclusion

Continued

Outcome	Major Interventions	Suggested Interventions	Optional Interventions
Self-Mutilation Restraint			
DEFINITION: Personal actions to refrain from intentional self-inflicted injury (non-lethal)	Behavior Management: Self-Harm Impulse Control Training Wound Care	Activity Therapy Anger Control Assistance Area Restriction Behavior Modification Calming Technique Chemical Restraint Counseling Environmental Management: Safety Limit Setting Mutual Goal Setting Physical Restraint Risk Identification Self-Responsibility Facilitation Surveillance: Safety	Animal-Assisted Therapy Anxiety Reduction Behavior Management Family Therapy Medication Administration Patient Contracting Suicide Prevention Therapy Group

NURSING DIAGNOSIS: Sensory Perception: Auditory, Disturbed

DEFINITION: Change in the amount or patterning of incoming stimuli accompanied by a diminished, exaggerated, distorted, or impaired response to such stimuli.

Outcome	Major Interventions	Suggested Interventions	Optional Interventions
Cognitive Orientation DEFINITION: Ability to identify person, place, and time accurately	Cognitive Stimulation Reality Orientation	Cerebral Perfusion Promotion Cognitive Restructuring Communication Enhancement: Hearing Deficit Communication Enhancement: Speech Deficit Delirium Management Delusion Management Dementia Management Hallucination Management Medication Management	Activity Therapy Environmental Management Neurologic Monitoring Sleep Enhancement Surveillance: Safety
Communication: Receptive DEFINITION: Reception and interpretation of verbal and/or non-verbal messages	Communication Enhancement: Hearing Deficit	Active Listening Communication Enhancement: Speech Deficit Learning Readiness Enhancement	Cognitive Stimulation Delusion Management Dementia Management Ear Care Environmental Management Reality Orientation

Continued

Outcome	Major Interventions	Suggested Interventions	Optional Interventions
Distorted Thought Self-Control			
DEFINITION: Self-restraint of disruptions in perception, thought processes, and thought content	Delusion Management Hallucination Management	Anxiety Reduction Cognitive Restructuring Delirium Management Dementia Management Medication Management Milieu Therapy Reality Orientation Therapy Group	Active Listening Activity Therapy Animal-Assisted Therapy Cognitive Stimulation Communication Enhancement: Hearing Deficit Communication Enhancement: Speech Deficit Environmental Management
Hearing Compensation Behavior			
DEFINITION: Personal actions to identify, monitor, and compensate for hearing loss	Communication Enhancement: Hearing Deficit	Cognitive Stimulation Communication Enhancement: Speech Deficit Ear Care Emotional Support Environmental Management Exercise Therapy: Balance Medication Administration: Ear Positioning	Activity Therapy Fall Prevention Fluid Management Self-Esteem Enhancement Sleep Enhancement

Outcome	Major Interventions	Suggested Interventions	Optional Interventions
Neurological Status: Cranial/ Sensory Motor Function			
DEFINITION: Ability of the cranial nerves to convey sensory and motor impulses	Communication Enhancement: Hearing Deficit Neurologic Monitoring	Cerebral Edema Management Cerebral Perfusion Promotion Environmental Management: Safety Risk Identification Surveillance: Safety	Ear Care Medication Administration Medication Management Surveillance
Sensory Function: Hearing			
DEFINITION: Extent to which sounds are correctly sensed	Communication Enhancement: Hearing Deficit	Ear Care Environmental Management Medication Administration: Ear	Cerebral Perfusion Promotion Environmental Management: Safety Risk Identification

NURSING DIAGNOSIS: Sensory Perception: Gustatory, Disturbed

DEFINITION: Change in the amount or patterning of incoming stimuli accompanied by a diminished, exaggerated, distorted, or impaired response to such stimuli.

Outcome	Major Interventions	Suggested Interventions	Optional Interventions
Appetite			
DEFINITION: Desire to eat when ill or receiving treatment	Nausea Management Nutrition Management	Environmental Management Feeding Fluid Management Oral Health Maintenance Oral Health Promotion Self-Care Assistance: Feeding Vomiting Management	Delusion Management Dementia Management Medication Management Oral Health Restoration Pain Management
Nutritional Status: Food & Fluid Intake			
DEFINITION: Amount of food and fluid taken into the body over a 24-hour period	Fluid Monitoring Nausea Management Nutritional Monitoring	Feeding Fluid Management Nutrition Management Self-Care Assistance: Feeding Vomiting Management	Bottle Feeding Medication Management Oral Health Restoration Swallowing Therapy Weight Gain Assistance Weight Management

Outcome	Major Interventions	Suggested Interventions	Optional Interventions
Sensory Function: Taste & Smell			
DEFINITION: Extent to which chemicals inhaled or dissolved in saliva are correctly sensed	Nausea Management Nutrition Management	Cerebral Perfusion Promotion Cognitive Stimulation Electrolyte Monitoring Environmental Management Feeding Fluid Management Fluid Monitoring Nutrition Management Vomiting Management Weight Management	Medication Management Neurologic Monitoring Nutritional Monitoring Swallowing Therapy

S

NURSING DIAGNOSIS: Sensory Perception: Kinesthetic, Disturbed

DEFINITION: Change in the amount or patterning of incoming stimuli accompanied by a diminished, exaggerated, distorted, or impaired response to such stimuli.

Outcome	Major Interventions	Suggested Interventions	Optional Interventions
Balance			
DEFINITION: Ability to maintain body equilibrium	Exercise Therapy: Balance Exercise Therapy: Muscle Control	Body Mechanics Promotion Energy Management Exercise Therapy: Ambulation Exercise Therapy: Joint Mobility Fall Prevention Surveillance: Safety	Environmental Management: Safety Exercise Promotion Positioning Teaching: Prescribed Activity/Exercise
Body Positioning: Self-Initiated			
DEFINITION: Ability to change own body position independently with or without assistive device	Body Mechanics Promotion Exercise Promotion: Strength Training	Exercise Promotion Exercise Promotion: Stretching Exercise Therapy: Balance Exercise Therapy: Joint Mobility Exercise Therapy: Muscle Control Self-Care Assistance	Energy Management Fall Prevention Pain Management Peripheral Sensation Management Positioning Self-Modification Assistance Unilateral Neglect Management

Outcome	Major Interventions	Suggested Interventions	Optional Interventions
Coordinated Movement DEFINITION: Ability of muscles to work together voluntarily for purposeful movement	Body Mechanics Promotion Exercise Therapy: Muscle Control	Activity Therapy Exercise Promotion Exercise Promotion: Strength Training Exercise Promotion: Stretching Exercise Therapy: Ambulation Exercise Therapy: Balance Exercise Therapy: Joint Mobility	Sleep Enhancement Medication Management Nutrition Management
Neurological Status: Central Motor Control DEFINITION: Ability of the central nervous system to coordinate skeletal muscle activity for body movement	Neurologic Monitoring	Cerebral Perfusion Promotion Electrolyte Management Electrolyte Monitoring Energy Management Environmental Management Exercise Promotion: Stretching Exercise Promotion: Strength Training Exercise Therapy: Balance Exercise Therapy: Muscle Control Medication Administration Medication Management Surveillance	Dysreflexia Management Exercise Therapy: Joint Mobility Surveillance: Safety

Continued

Outcome	Major Interventions	Suggested Interventions	Optional Interventions
Sensory Function: Proprioception			
DEFINITION: Extent to which the position and movement of the head and body are correctly sensed	Body Mechanics Promotion Exercise Therapy: Balance	Activity Therapy Exercise Promotion Exercise Promotion: Strength Training Exercise Therapy: Ambulation Exercise Therapy: Muscle Control Positioning Neurologic Monitoring	Cerebral Perfusion Promotion Developmental Enhancement: Child Exercise Promotion: Stretching Fluid Management Fluid Monitoring

NURSING DIAGNOSIS: Sensory Perception: Olfactory, Disturbed

DEFINITION: Change in the amount or patterning of incoming stimuli accompanied by a diminished, exaggerated, distorted, or impaired response to such stimuli.

Outcome	Major Interventions	Suggested Interventions	Optional Interventions
Appetite			
DEFINITION: Desire to eat when ill or receiving treatment	Environmental Management	Fluid Management Fluid Monitoring Medication Management Nausea Management Nutrition Management Vomiting Management	Dementia Management Weight Management
Neurological Status: Cranial/ Sensory Motor Function			
DEFINITION: Ability of the cranial nerves to convey sensory and motor impulses	Environmental Management Neurologic Monitoring	Aromatherapy Cerebral Edema Management Cerebral Perfusion Promotion	Delusion Management Medication Management Nausea Management Surveillance
Nutritional Status: Food & Fluid Intake			
DEFINITION: Amount of food and fluid taken into the body over a 24-hour period	Nutrition Management	Environmental Management Feeding Fluid Management Fluid Monitoring Nausea Management Nutritional Monitoring Vomiting Management	Bottle Feeding Medication Management Oral Health Restoration Weight Management

Continued

Outcome	Major Interventions	Suggested Interventions	Optional Interventions
Sensory Function: Taste & Smell			
DEFINITION: Extent to which chemicals inhaled or dissolved in saliva are correctly sensed	Nutrition Management	Aromatherapy Cerebral Perfusion Promotion Environmental Management Feeding Nausea Management Nutritional Monitoring Weight Management	Delusion Management Dementia Management Fluid Management Fluid Monitoring Medication Management Neurologic Monitoring

NURSING DIAGNOSIS: Sensory Perception: Tactile, Disturbed

DEFINITION: Change in the amount or patterning of incoming stimuli accompanied by a diminished, exaggerated, distorted, or impaired response to such stimuli.

Outcome	Major Interventions	Suggested Interventions	Optional Interventions
Distorted Thought Self-Control			
DEFINITION: Self-restraint of disruptions in perception, thought processes, and thought content	Delusion Management Hallucination Management	Anxiety Reduction Dementia Management Medication Management Reality Orientation Sleep Enhancement Therapy Group	Active Listening Activity Therapy Body Image Enhancement Cognitive Stimulation Environmental Management
Neurological Status: Spinal Sensory/Motor Function			
DEFINITION: Ability of the spinal nerves to convey sensory and motor impulses	Environmental Management: Safety Peripheral Sensation Management	Cerebral Perfusion Promotion Dysreflexia Management Electrolyte Monitoring Laboratory Data Interpretation Medication Administration Medication Management Neurologic Monitoring Pressure Ulcer Prevention Skin Surveillance Surveillance Traction/ Immobilization Care	Exercise Promotion: Stretching Exercise Therapy: Ambulation Exercise Therapy: Balance Risk Identification Skin Care: Topical Treatments Splinting

Continued

Outcome	Major Interventions	Suggested Interventions	Optional Interventions
Sensory Function: Cutaneous			
DEFINITION: Extent to which stimulation of the skin is correctly sensed	Lower Extremity Monitoring	Amputation Care	Emotional Support
	Peripheral Sensation Management	Cutaneous Stimulation	Exercise Therapy: Ambulation
		Electrolyte Management	Exercise Therapy: Balance
		Environmental Management	Medication Management
		Neurologic Monitoring	Prosthesis Care
		Pain Management	Transcutaneous Electrical Nerve Stimulation (TENS)
		Positioning	
		Pressure Management	
		Skin Surveillance	
		Surveillance: Safety	
		Teaching: Foot Care	
		Touch	

NURSING DIAGNOSIS: Sensory Perception: Visual, Disturbed

DEFINITION: Change in the amount or patterning of incoming stimuli accompanied by a diminished, exaggerated, distorted, or impaired response to such stimuli.

Outcome	Major Interventions	Suggested Interventions	Optional Interventions
Distorted Thought Self-Control			
DEFINITION: Self-restraint of disruptions in perception, thought processes, and thought content	Delusion Management Hallucination Management	Anxiety Reduction Cognitive Restructuring Delirium Management Dementia Management Medication Management Reality Orientation	Activity Therapy Body Image Enhancement Cognitive Stimulation Communication Enhancement: Visual Deficit Environmental Management Music Therapy Recreation Therapy
Neurological Status: Cranial/ Sensory Motor Function			
DEFINITION: Ability of the cranial nerves to convey sensory and motor impulses	Communication Enhancement: Visual Deficit Neurologic Monitoring	Cerebral Edema Management Cerebral Perfusion Promotion Environmental Management Environmental Management: Safety Hallucination Management Risk Identification Surveillance: Safety	Eye Care Medication Management Surveillance

Continued

Outcome	Major Interventions	Suggested Interventions	Optional Interventions
Sensory Function: Vision			
DEFINITION: Extent to which visual images are correctly sensed	Communication Enhancement: Visual Deficit	Cerebral Perfusion Promotion Cognitive Stimulation Environmental Management Eye Care Medication Administration: Eye Surveillance: Safety	Cerebral Edema Management Developmental Enhancement: Child Emotional Support Hallucination Management Medication Management Neurologic Monitoring Self-Esteem Enhancement
Vision Compensation Behavior			
DEFINITION: Personal actions to compensate for visual impairment	Communication Enhancement: Visual Deficit Environmental Management	Cognitive Restructuring Cognitive Stimulation Emotional Support Exercise Therapy: Balance Fall Prevention Feeding Medication Administration: Eye Positioning Surveillance: Safety	Activity Therapy Contact Lens Care Exercise Therapy: Ambulation Medication Management

NURSING DIAGNOSIS: Sexual Dysfunction			
DEFINITION: Change in sexual function that is viewed as unsatisfying, unrewarding, or inadequate.			

Outcome	Major Interventions	Suggested Interventions	Optional Interventions
Abuse Recovery: Sexual DEFINITION: Extent of healing of physical and psychological injuries due to sexual abuse or exploitation	Abuse Protection Support Coping Enhancement Counseling Sexual Counseling	Abuse Protection Support: Child Abuse Protection Support: Domestic Partner Abuse Protection Support: Elder Active Listening Emotional Support Health System Guidance Self-Awareness Enhancement Self-Esteem Enhancement Teaching: Sexuality	Anxiety Reduction Behavior Management: Sexual Body Image Enhancement Decision-Making Support Family Therapy Guilt Work Facilitation Resiliency Promotion Role Enhancement Simple Relaxation Therapy Spiritual Support Substance Use Prevention Support Group Support System Enhancement Therapy Group

Continued

Outcome	Major Interventions	Suggested Interventions	Optional Interventions
Physical Aging DEFINITION: Normal physical changes that occur with the natural aging process	Sexual Counseling	Anxiety Reduction Circulatory Care: Arterial Insufficiency Emotional Support Exercise Promotion Hormone Replacement Therapy Medication Management Self-Esteem Enhancement Self-Modification Assistance Substance Use Prevention Teaching: Sexuality	Body Image Enhancement Complex Relationship Building Energy Management Substance Use Treatment
Risk Control: Sexually Transmitted Diseases (STD) DEFINITION: Personal actions to prevent, eliminate, or reduce behaviors associated with sexually transmitted diseases	Behavior Modification Infection Protection Risk Identification Teaching: Safe Sex	Active Listening Anticipatory Guidance Behavior Management: Sexual Health Screening Health System Guidance Patient Contracting Self-Awareness Enhancement Self-Modification Assistance Self-Responsibility Facilitation Sexual Counseling Teaching: Sexuality Values Clarification	Assertiveness Training Emotional Support Family Involvement Promotion Fertility Preservation Impulse Control Training Self-Esteem Enhancement Substance Use Prevention Substance Use Treatment Support Group Support System Enhancement

Outcome	Major Interventions	Suggested Interventions	Optional Interventions
Sexual Functioning			
DEFINITION: Integration of physical, socioemotional, and intellectual aspects of sexual expression and performance	Sexual Counseling	Behavior Management: Sexual Childbirth Preparation Self-Awareness Enhancement Self-Esteem Enhancement Self-Responsibility Facilitation Teaching: Safe Sex Teaching: Sexuality Values Clarification	Circulatory Care: Arterial Insufficiency Energy Management Family Planning: Contraception Family Planning: Infertility Medication Management Premenstrual Syndrome (PMS) Management Prenatal Care Reproductive Technology Management Substance Use Treatment
Sexual Identity			
DEFINITION: Acknowledgment and acceptance of own sexual identity	Self-Awareness Enhancement Sexual Counseling	Counseling Emotional Support Role Enhancement Self-Esteem Enhancement Teaching: Sexuality Values Clarification	Anxiety Reduction Decision-Making Support Family Process Maintenance

NURSING DIAGNOSIS: Sexuality Patterns, Ineffective

DEFINITION: Expressions of concern regarding own sexuality.

Outcome	Major Interventions	Suggested Interventions	Optional Interventions
Abuse Recovery: Sexual DEFINITION: Extent of healing of physical and psychological injuries due to sexual abuse or exploitation	Coping Enhancement Self-Esteem Enhancement Sexual Counseling	Abuse Protection Support Active Listening Anger Control Assistance Anxiety Reduction Counseling Teaching: Sexuality Therapy Group	Behavior Management: Sexual Body Image Enhancement Complex Relationship Building Decision-Making Support Guilt Work Facilitation Self-Awareness Enhancement Spiritual Support Support Group Support System Enhancement
Body Image DEFINITION: Perception of own appearance and body functions	Body Image Enhancement	Active Listening Anticipatory Guidance Emotional Support Self-Awareness Enhancement Self-Esteem Enhancement Values Clarification	Cognitive Restructuring Coping Enhancement Counseling Postpartal Care Prenatal Care

Outcome	Major Interventions	Suggested Interventions	Optional Interventions
Physical Maturation: Female			
DEFINITION: Normal physical changes in the female that occur with the transition from childhood to adulthood	Teaching: Safe Sex Teaching: Sexuality	Anticipatory Guidance Anxiety Reduction Body Image Enhancement Self-Awareness Enhancement Self-Esteem Enhancement	Behavior Management: Sexual Parent Education: Adolescent Premenstrual Syndrome (PMS) Management
Physical Maturation: Male			
DEFINITION: Normal physical changes in the male that occur with the transition from childhood to adulthood	Teaching: Safe Sex Teaching: Sexuality	Anticipatory Guidance Anxiety Reduction Body Image Enhancement Self-Awareness Enhancement Self-Esteem Enhancement	Behavior Management: Sexual Parent Education: Adolescent
Role Performance			
DEFINITION: Congruence of an individual's role behavior with role expectations	Role Enhancement Teaching: Safe Sex	Anticipatory Guidance Behavior Modification Childbirth Preparation Counseling Family Planning: Contraception Self-Awareness Enhancement Sexual Counseling Values Clarification	Active Listening Fertility Preservation Reproductive Technology Management Self-Esteem Enhancement Support Group Support System Enhancement Teaching: Sexuality

Continued

Outcome	Major Interventions	Suggested Interventions	Optional Interventions
Self-Esteem			
DEFINITION: Personal judgment of self-worth	Self-Esteem Enhancement	Active Listening Body Image Enhancement Counseling Developmental Enhancement: Adolescent Developmental Enhancement: Child Self-Awareness Enhancement Support Group	Assertiveness Training Complex Relationship Building Coping Enhancement Fertility Preservation
Sexual Identity			
DEFINITION: Acknowledgment and acceptance of own sexual identity	Sexual Counseling	Anxiety Reduction Body Image Enhancement Developmental Enhancement: Adolescent Hormone Replacement Therapy Role Enhancement Self-Awareness Enhancement Self-Esteem Enhancement Values Clarification	Anticipatory Guidance Behavior Management: Sexual Coping Enhancement Counseling Premenstrual Syndrome (PMS) Management Support System Enhancement Teaching: Sexuality

NURSING DIAGNOSIS: Skin Integrity, Impaired

DEFINITION: Altered epidermis and/or dermis.

Outcome	Major Interventions	Suggested Interventions	Optional Interventions
Allergic Response: Localized DEFINITION: Severity of localized hypersensitive immune response to a specific environmental (exogenous) antigen	Latex Precautions Medication Administration Pruritus Management	Medication Administration: Eye Medication Administration: Intravenous (IV) Medication Administration: Nasal Medication Administration: Skin Skin Care: Topical Treatments Skin Surveillance	Infection Protection Vital Signs Monitoring Wound Care
Hemodialysis Access DEFINITION: Functionality of a dialysis access site	Dialysis Access Maintenance	Bleeding Reduction Circulatory Precautions Incision Site Care Infection Protection Skin Surveillance Splinting	Fluid Management Teaching: Procedure/ Treatment

Continued

Outcome	Major Interventions	Suggested Interventions	Optional Interventions
Tissue Integrity: Skin & Mucous Membranes			
DEFINITION: Structural intactness and normal physiological function of skin and mucous membranes	Pressure Management Pressure Ulcer Care Skin Surveillance	Bathing Bed Rest Care Circulatory Care: Arterial Insufficiency Circulatory Precautions Cutaneous Stimulation Fluid Management Foot Care Infection Protection Medication Administration: Skin Medication Management Nutrition Management Positioning Pressure Ulcer Prevention Radiation Therapy Management Skin Care: Topical Treatments Urinary Incontinence Care	Amputation Care Cast Care: Maintenance Diarrhea Management Exercise Promotion Fluid/Electrolyte Management Ostomy Care Perineal Care Positioning: Wheelchair Self-Care Assistance: Bathing/Hygiene Self-Care Assistance: Toileting Simple Massage Traction/Immobilization Care

Outcome	Major Interventions	Suggested Interventions	Optional Interventions
Wound Healing: Primary Intention			
DEFINITION: Extent of regeneration of cells and tissue following intentional closure	Incision Site Care Wound Care	Bleeding Reduction: Wound Circulatory Precautions Fluid/Electrolyte Management Infection Control: Intraoperative Infection Protection Lower Extremity Monitoring Medication Administration Medication Administration: Skin Nutrition Management Nutrition Therapy Skin Care: Donor Site Skin Care: Graft Site Skin Care: Topical Treatments Skin Surveillance Splinting Suturing Teaching: Procedure/Treatment Wound Care: Closed Drainage	Amputation Care Bathing Bed Rest Care Cesarean Section Care Infection Control Perineal Care Teaching: Psychomotor Skill

Continued

Outcome	Major Interventions	Suggested Interventions	Optional Interventions
Wound Healing: Secondary Intention			
DEFINITION: Extent of regeneration of cells and tissue in an open wound	Pressure Ulcer Care Wound Care	Circulatory Care: Arterial Insufficiency Circulatory Care: Venous Insufficiency Circulatory Precautions Fluid Management Infection Control Infection Protection Medication Administration Medication Administration: Skin Nutrition Therapy Skin Care: Topical Treatments Skin Surveillance Splinting Transcutaneous Electrical Nerve Stimulation (TENS) Wound Irrigation	Bathing Cutaneous Stimulation Hyperglycemia Management Leech Therapy Lower Extremity Monitoring Nutrition Management Positioning Teaching: Procedure/ Treatment Teaching: Psychomotor Skill Total Parenteral Nutrition (TPN) Administration

NURSING DIAGNOSIS: Sleep Deprivation

DEFINITION: Prolonged periods of time without sleep (sustained natural, periodic suspension of relative consciousness).

Outcome	Major Interventions	Suggested Interventions	Optional Interventions
Mood Equilibrium			
DEFINITION: Appropriate adjustment of prevailing emotional tone in response to circumstances	Medication Management Mood Management Sleep Enhancement	Anxiety Reduction Coping Enhancement Energy Management Environmental Management: Comfort Meditation Facilitation Phototherapy: Mood/Sleep Regulation Simple Relaxation Therapy Surveillance: Safety	Animal-Assisted Therapy Music Therapy Progressive Muscle Relaxation Reminiscence Therapy Simple Guided Imagery
Rest			
DEFINITION: Quantity and pattern of diminished activity for mental and physical rejuvenation	Energy Management Sleep Enhancement	Autogenic Training Biofeedback Exercise Promotion Meditation Facilitation Pain Management Simple Guided Imagery Simple Relaxation Therapy	Environmental Management: Comfort Music Therapy Progressive Muscle Relaxation Surveillance: Safety

Continued

Outcome	Major Interventions	Suggested Interventions	Optional Interventions
Sleep DEFINITION: Natural periodic suspension of consciousness during which the body is restored	Sleep Enhancement	Anxiety Reduction Environmental Management Environmental Management: Comfort Medication Management Meditation Facilitation Pain Management Progressive Muscle Relaxation Simple Guided Imagery Simple Massage	Dementia Management Exercise Promotion Music Therapy Nausea Management Phototherapy: Mood/Sleep Regulation Simple Relaxation Therapy Urinary Incontinence Care: Enuresis Vomiting Management
Symptom Severity DEFINITION: Severity of perceived adverse changes in physical, emotional, and social functioning	Sleep Enhancement	Anxiety Reduction Coping Enhancement Energy Management Medication Administration Medication Management Pain Management Positioning	Progressive Muscle Relaxation Simple Guided Imagery Simple Massage Simple Relaxation Therapy

NURSING DIAGNOSIS: Sleep Pattern, Disturbed

DEFINITION: Time-limited disruption of sleep (natural, periodic suspension of consciousness) amount and quality.

Outcome	Major Interventions	Suggested Interventions	Optional Interventions
Personal Well-Being			
DEFINITION: Extent of positive perception of one's health status and life circumstances	Coping Enhancement Sleep Enhancement	Autogenic Training Emotional Support Environmental Management Meditation Facilitation Pain Management Security Enhancement Simple Guided Imagery Simple Relaxation Therapy	Abuse Protection Support Dying Care Energy Management Exercise Promotion Hormone Replacement Therapy Phototherapy: Mood/Sleep Regulation Substance Use Prevention
Sleep			
DEFINITION: Natural periodic suspension of consciousness during which the body is restored	Environmental Management: Comfort Sleep Enhancement	Calming Technique Environmental Management Exercise Promotion Medication Administration Medication Management Medication Prescribing Music Therapy Pain Management Phototherapy: Mood/Sleep Regulation Security Enhancement Simple Massage Simple Relaxation Therapy	Anxiety Reduction Autogenic Training Bathing Dementia Management Energy Management Hormone Replacement Therapy Kangaroo Care Meditation Facilitation Positioning Progressive Muscle Relaxation Touch Urinary Incontinence Care: Enuresis

NURSING DIAGNOSIS: Sleep, Readiness for Enhanced

DEFINITION: A pattern of natural, periodic suspension of consciousness that provides adequate rest, sustains a desired lifestyle, and can be strengthened.

Outcome	Major Interventions	Suggested Interventions	Optional Interventions
Comfort Level DEFINITION: Extent of positive perception of physical and psychological ease	Environmental Management: Comfort Sleep Enhancement	Anxiety Reduction Medication Management Nausea Management Pain Management Progressive Muscle Relaxation Simple Massage Simple Relaxation Therapy	Energy Management Exercise Promotion Hormone Replacement Therapy Premenstrual Syndrome (PMS) Management Security Enhancement
Rest DEFINITION: Quantity and pattern of diminished activity for mental and physical rejuvenation	Energy Management Sleep Enhancement	Autogenic Training Biofeedback Environmental Management: Comfort Exercise Promotion Simple Guided Imagery Simple Relaxation Therapy	Anxiety Reduction Coping Enhancement Meditation Facilitation Music Therapy Pain Management Progressive Muscle Relaxation Self-Care Assistance

Outcome	Major Interventions	Suggested Interventions	Optional Interventions
Sleep			
DEFINITION: Natural periodic suspension of consciousness during which the body is restored	Sleep Enhancement	Anxiety Reduction Autogenic Training Environmental Management: Comfort Phototherapy: Mood/Sleep Regulation Progressive Muscle Relaxation Security Enhancement Simple Massage Simple Relaxation Therapy	Calming Technique Hormone Replacement Therapy Medication Management Music Therapy Nausea Management Pain Management Premenstrual Syndrome (PMS) Management

NURSING DIAGNOSIS: Social Interaction, Impaired

DEFINITION: Insufficient or excessive quantity or ineffective quality of social exchange.

Outcome	Major Interventions	Suggested Interventions	Optional Interventions
Child Development: Middle Childhood DEFINITION: Milestones of physical, cognitive, and psychosocial progression from 6 years through 11 years of age	Developmental Enhancement: Child	Anticipatory Guidance Behavior Management: Overactivity/ Inattention Behavior Modification: Social Skills Family Integrity Promotion Family Involvement Promotion Learning Facilitation Mutual Goal Setting Self-Awareness Enhancement Self-Esteem Enhancement Socialization Enhancement Substance Use Prevention	Abuse Protection Support: Child Behavior Management Behavior Modification Counseling Family Process Maintenance Family Support Family Therapy Therapeutic Play

Outcome	Major Interventions	Suggested Interventions	Optional Interventions
Child Development: Adolescence			
DEFINITION: Milestones of physical, cognitive, and psychosocial progression from 12 years through 17 years of age	Developmental Enhancement: Adolescent Self-Esteem Enhancement Socialization Enhancement	Anticipatory Guidance Behavior Management: Sexual Behavior Modification: Social Skills Family Integrity Promotion Family Involvement Promotion Mutual Goal Setting Role Enhancement Self-Awareness Enhancement Self-Responsibility Facilitation Spiritual Support Substance Use Prevention Values Clarification	Abuse Protection Support Behavior Management Behavior Modification Counseling Eating Disorders Management Family Process Maintenance Family Support Family Therapy Sexual Counseling Support Group Support System Enhancement
Family Social Climate			
DEFINITION: Supportive milieu as characterized by family member relationships and goals	Family Integrity Promotion Family Process Maintenance	Abuse Protection Support: Child Abuse Protection Support: Domestic Partner Abuse Protection Support: Elder Counseling Family Support Normalization Promotion Resiliency Promotion	Attachment Promotion Behavior Management: Overactivity/Inattention Caregiver Support Family Therapy Support System Enhancement

Continued

Outcome	Major Interventions	Suggested Interventions	Optional Interventions
Leisure Participation			
DEFINITION: Use of relaxing, interesting, and enjoyable activities to promote well-being	Recreation Therapy Socialization Enhancement	Anxiety Reduction Behavior Modification: Social Skills Self-Esteem Enhancement	Activity Therapy Animal-Assisted Therapy Exercise Promotion
Play Participation			
DEFINITION: Use of activities by a child from 1 year through 11 years of age to promote enjoyment, entertainment, and development	Socialization Enhancement Therapeutic Play	Behavior Modification: Social Skills Normalization Promotion Recreation Therapy	Activity Therapy Anger Control Assistance Animal-Assisted Therapy Family Support Family Therapy

Outcome	Major Interventions	Suggested Interventions	Optional Interventions
Social Interaction Skills			
DEFINITION: Personal behaviors that promote effective relationships	Behavior Modification: Social Skills Complex Relationship Building	Assertiveness Training Behavior Management: Sexual Counseling Dementia Management Developmental Enhancement: Adolescent Developmental Enhancement: Child Recreation Therapy Resiliency Promotion Self-Awareness Enhancement Self-Esteem Enhancement Support Group Support System Enhancement Therapy Group	Active Listening Anger Control Assistance Anxiety Reduction Communication Enhancement: Hearing Deficit Communication Enhancement: Speech Deficit Coping Enhancement Family Therapy Humor Impulse Control Training Pass Facilitation Reminiscence Therapy Visitation Facilitation

Continued

Outcome	Major Interventions	Suggested Interventions	Optional Interventions
Social Involvement			
DEFINITION: Social interactions with persons, groups, or organizations	Socialization Enhancement	Animal-Assisted Therapy Developmental Enhancement: Adolescent Developmental Enhancement: Child Recreation Therapy Relocation Stress Reduction Reminiscence Therapy Self-Awareness Enhancement Self-Esteem Enhancement Substance Use Treatment Therapeutic Play Values Clarification Visitation Facilitation	Active Listening Assertiveness Training Behavior Management Communication Enhancement: Hearing Deficit Communication Enhancement: Speech Deficit Complex Relationship Building Family Therapy Milieu Therapy Mutual Goal Setting Normalization Promotion Pass Facilitation Substance Use Treatment: Alcohol Withdrawal Substance Use Treatment: Drug Withdrawal Support Group Support System Enhancement

NURSING DIAGNOSIS: Social Isolation

DEFINITION: Aloneness experienced by the individual and perceived as imposed by others and as a negative or threatening state.

Outcome	Major Interventions	Suggested Interventions	Optional Interventions
Family Social Climate			
DEFINITION: Supportive milieu as characterized by family member relationships and goals	Family Integrity Promotion	Abuse Protection Support: Child Abuse Protection Support: Domestic Partner Abuse Protection Support: Elder Behavior Modification: Social Skills Caregiver Support Counseling Family Process Maintenance Family Therapy Normalization Promotion Resiliency Promotion	Attachment Promotion Family Support Grief Work Facilitation: Perinatal Death Support System Enhancement
Leisure Participation			
DEFINITION: Use of relaxing, interesting, and enjoyable activities to promote well-being	Recreation Therapy	Activity Therapy Animal-Assisted Therapy Exercise Promotion Socialization Enhancement Therapeutic Play	Art Therapy Music Therapy Reminiscence Therapy

Continued

Outcome	Major Interventions	Suggested Interventions	Optional Interventions
Loneliness Severity			
DEFINITION: Severity of emotional, social, or existential isolation response	Socialization Enhancement Support System Enhancement	Active Listening Activity Therapy Animal-Assisted Therapy Complex Relationship Building Counseling Developmental Enhancement: Adolescent Developmental Enhancement: Child Emotional Support Hope Instillation Milieu Therapy Presence Relocation Stress Reduction Self-Esteem Enhancement Spiritual Growth Facilitation Therapy Group Touch Visitation Facilitation	Abuse Protection Support: Child Abuse Protection Support: Domestic Partner Abuse Protection Support: Elder Communication Enhancement: Hearing Deficit Communication Enhancement: Speech Deficit Environmental Management Family Therapy Grief Work Facilitation Self-Awareness Enhancement Support Group

Outcome	Major Interventions	Suggested Interventions	Optional Interventions
Mood Equilibrium			
DEFINITION: Appropriate adjustment of prevailing emotional tone in response to circumstances	Mood Management	Active Listening Coping Enhancement Counseling Emotional Support Grief Work Facilitation Guilt Work Facilitation Hope Instillation Medication Management Presence Self-Esteem Enhancement Spiritual Support Support System Enhancement Touch	Animal-Assisted Therapy Anxiety Reduction Art Therapy Bibliotherapy Environmental Management Exercise Promotion Family Support Humor Music Therapy Socialization Enhancement Support Group Therapeutic Play Therapy Group Visitation Facilitation
Personal Well-Being			
DEFINITION: Extent of positive perception of one's health status and life circumstances	Coping Enhancement Self-Awareness Enhancement	Counseling Emotional Support Family Support Hope Instillation Humor Self-Esteem Enhancement Socialization Enhancement Spiritual Support Support System Enhancement Visitation Facilitation	Abuse Protection Support Communication Enhancement: Hearing Deficit Communication Enhancement: Speech Deficit Communication Enhancement: Visual Deficit Dying Care Exercise Promotion Normalization Promotion Pain Management Substance Use Prevention Weight Management

Continued

Outcome	Major Interventions	Suggested Interventions	Optional Interventions
Play Participation			
DEFINITION: Use of activities by a child from 1 year through 11 years of age to promote enjoyment, entertainment, and development	Socialization Enhancement Therapeutic Play	Exercise Promotion Recreation Therapy	Activity Therapy Animal-Assisted Therapy Art Therapy Environmental Management Music Therapy
Social Interaction Skills			
DEFINITION: Personal behaviors that promote effective relationships	Behavior Modification: Social Skills Complex Relationship Building	Counseling Developmental Enhancement: Adolescent Developmental Enhancement: Child Family Integrity Promotion Normalization Promotion Recreation Therapy Self-Awareness Enhancement Self-Esteem Enhancement Touch	Anger Control Assistance Anxiety Reduction Communication Enhancement: Hearing Deficit Communication Enhancement: Speech Deficit Family Therapy Humor Therapy Group

Outcome	Major Interventions	Suggested Interventions	Optional Interventions
Social Involvement			
DEFINITION: Social interactions with persons, groups, or organizations	Socialization Enhancement	Activity Therapy Animal-Assisted Therapy Complex Relationship Building Forgiveness Facilitation Pass Facilitation Recreation Therapy Self-Awareness Enhancement Self-Esteem Enhancement Therapeutic Play Visitation Facilitation	Active Listening Art Therapy Communication Enhancement: Hearing Deficit Communication Enhancement: Speech Deficit Counseling Culture Brokerage Developmental Enhancement: Adolescent Developmental Enhancement: Child Emotional Support Family Therapy Milieu Therapy Mood Management Normalization Promotion Presence Support Group Support System Enhancement Urinary Elimination Management
Social Support			
DEFINITION: Perceived availability and actual provision of reliable assistance from others	Family Involvement Promotion Support System Enhancement	Caregiver Support Family Support Referral Socialization Enhancement Support Group	Coping Enhancement Emotional Support Spiritual Support Therapy Group

NURSING DIAGNOSIS: Sorrow: Chronic

DEFINITION: Cyclical, recurring, and potentially progressive pattern of pervasive sadness experienced (by a parent, caregiver, or individual with chronic illness or disability) in response to continual loss, throughout the trajectory of an illness or disability.

Outcome	Major Interventions	Suggested Interventions	Optional Interventions
Acceptance: Health Status			
DEFINITION: Reconciliation to significant change in health circumstances	Coping Enhancement Hope Instillation	Counseling Decision-Making Support Emotional Support Grief Work Facilitation Presence Resiliency Promotion Spiritual Support Support Group Values Clarification	Active Listening Genetic Counseling Normalization Promotion Risk Identification: Genetic Truth Telling
Depression Level			
DEFINITION: Severity of melancholic mood and loss of interest in life events	Hope Instillation Mood Management	Bibliotherapy Cognitive Restructuring Counseling Emotional Support Exercise Promotion Forgiveness Facilitation Grief Work Facilitation Guilt Work Facilitation Resiliency Promotion Self-Modification Assistance Sleep Enhancement Support Group	Activity Therapy Animal-Assisted Therapy Spiritual Support Substance Use Prevention Support System Enhancement

Outcome	Major Interventions	Suggested Interventions	Optional Interventions
Depression Self-Control			
DEFINITION: Personal actions to minimize melancholy and maintain interest in life events	Mood Management	Activity Therapy Behavior Management Energy Management Exercise Promotion Medication Management Resiliency Promotion Self-Modification Assistance Sleep Enhancement	Grief Work Facilitation Guilt Work Facilitation Substance Use Prevention
Grief Resolution			
DEFINITION: Adjustment to actual or impending loss	Grief Work Facilitation Grief Work Facilitation: Perinatal Death	Active Listening Coping Enhancement Dying Care Emotional Support Hope Instillation Reminiscence Therapy Spiritual Support Support Group	Animal-Assisted Therapy Bibliotherapy Decision-Making Support Forgiveness Facilitation Guilt Work Facilitation Music Therapy Presence Visitation Facilitation
Hope			
DEFINITION: Optimism that is personally satisfying and life-supporting	Hope Instillation Spiritual Support	Coping Enhancement Emotional Support Resiliency Promotion Self-Awareness Enhancement Support Group Support System Enhancement	Counseling Family Mobilization Forgiveness Facilitation Milieu Therapy Presence Touch

Continued

Outcome	Major Interventions	Suggested Interventions	Optional Interventions
Mood Equilibrium			
DEFINITION: Appropriate adjustment of prevailing emotional tone in response to circumstances	Mood Management	Active Listening Coping Enhancement Counseling Emotional Support Grief Work Facilitation Hope Instillation Medication Management Presence Resiliency Promotion Socialization Enhancement Spiritual Support Support Group	Activity Therapy Anger Control Assistance Animal-Assisted Therapy Bibliotherapy Exercise Promotion Family Support Forgiveness Facilitation Humor Meditation Facilitation Music Therapy Sleep Enhancement Support System Enhancement
Psychosocial Adjustment: Life Change			
DEFINITION: Adaptive psychosocial response of an individual to a significant life change	Coping Enhancement Grief Work Facilitation	Counseling Decision-Making Support Emotional Support Hope Instillation Mood Management Socialization Enhancement Spiritual Support Support Group	Anger Control Assistance Dying Care Family Mobilization Truth Telling

NURSING DIAGNOSIS: Spiritual Distress

DEFINITION: Impaired ability to experience and integrate meaning and purpose in life through a person's connectedness with self, others, art, music, literature, nature, or a power greater than oneself.

Outcome	Major Interventions	Suggested Interventions	Optional Interventions
Dignified Life Closure DEFINITION: Personal actions to maintain control during approaching end of life	Dying Care Emotional Support Spiritual Support	Active Listening Anticipatory Guidance Anxiety Reduction Bibliotherapy Coping Enhancement Decision-Making Support Family Involvement Promotion Forgiveness Facilitation Grief Work Facilitation Guilt Work Facilitation Hope Instillation Presence Reminiscence Therapy Security Enhancement Spiritual Growth Facilitation Support System Enhancement Touch Truth Telling Values Clarification	Anger Control Assistance Animal-Assisted Therapy Caregiver Support Culture Brokerage Health System Guidance Meditation Facilitation Music Therapy Referral Resiliency Promotion Self-Awareness Enhancement

Continued

Outcome	Major Interventions	Suggested Interventions	Optional Interventions
Hope DEFINITION: Optimism that is personally satisfying and life-supporting	Hope Instillation Spiritual Growth Facilitation Spiritual Support	Coping Enhancement Emotional Support Self-Awareness Enhancement Support Group Support System Enhancement Values Clarification	Counseling Family Support Presence Touch
Spiritual Health DEFINITION: Connectedness with self, others, higher power, all life, nature, and the universe that transcends and empowers the self	Spiritual Growth Facilitation Spiritual Support	Active Listening Coping Enhancement Emotional Support Forgiveness Facilitation Grief Work Facilitation Guilt Work Facilitation Hope Instillation Meditation Facilitation Resiliency Promotion Self-Awareness Enhancement Support Group Values Clarification	Abuse Protection Support: Religious Art Therapy Bibliotherapy Counseling Dying Care Family Support Music Therapy Referral Religious Addiction Prevention Reminiscence Therapy Self-Esteem Enhancement Socialization Enhancement Touch

NURSING DIAGNOSIS: Spiritual Well-Being, Readiness for Enhanced

DEFINITION: Ability to experience and integrate meaning and purpose in life through connectedness with self, others, art, music, literature, nature, or a power greater than oneself.

Outcome	Major Interventions	Suggested Interventions	Optional Interventions
Hope DEFINITION: Optimism that is personally satisfying and life-supporting	Hope Instillation Spiritual Growth Facilitation Spiritual Support	Coping Enhancement Emotional Support Self-Awareness Enhancement Self-Esteem Enhancement Support Group Values Clarification	Art Therapy Bibliotherapy Counseling Family Support Music Therapy Presence Touch
Personal Well-Being DEFINITION: Extent of positive perception of one's health status and life circumstances	Self-Awareness Enhancement Self-Esteem Enhancement Spiritual Growth Facilitation	Active Listening Coping Enhancement Counseling Hope Instillation Meditation Facilitation Religious Ritual Enhancement Resiliency Promotion Role Enhancement Self-Modification Assistance Self-Responsibility Facilitation Spiritual Support Values Clarification	Autogenic Training Bibliotherapy Family Support Simple Guided Imagery

Continued

Outcome	Major Interventions	Suggested Interventions	Optional Interventions
Quality of Life			
DEFINITION: Extent of positive perception of current life circumstances	Values Clarification	Coping Enhancement Emotional Support Hope Instillation Humor Self-Awareness Enhancement Self-Esteem Enhancement Self-Responsibility Facilitation Spiritual Support	Active Listening Culture Brokerage Decision-Making Support Family Support Resiliency Promotion Reminiscence Therapy Support Group
Spiritual Health			
DEFINITION: Connectedness with self, others, higher power, all life, nature, and the universe that transcends and empowers the self	Spiritual Growth Facilitation Spiritual Support	Bibliotherapy Meditation Facilitation Religious Ritual Enhancement Resiliency Promotion Role Enhancement Self-Awareness Enhancement Self-Esteem Enhancement Self-Modification Assistance Values Clarification	Counseling Family Support Music Therapy Religious Addiction Prevention Simple Guided Imagery Touch

NURSING DIAGNOSIS: Surgical Recovery, Delayed

DEFINITION: Extension of the number of postoperative days required to initiate and perform activities that maintain life, health, and well-being.

Outcome	Major Interventions	Suggested Interventions	Optional Interventions
Ambulation			
DEFINITION: Ability to walk from place to place independently with or without assistive device	Exercise Therapy: Ambulation	Energy Management Exercise Promotion: Stretching Exercise Therapy Joint Mobility Teaching: Prescribed Activity/Exercise	Fluid Management Nutrition Management Nutrition Therapy
Blood Loss Severity			
DEFINITION: Severity of internal or external bleeding/ hemorrhage	Bleeding Reduction Fluid Management Hypovolemia Management	Bleeding Precautions Blood Products Administration Electrolyte Management Fluid/Electrolyte Management Fluid Monitoring Intravenous (IV) Insertion Intravenous (IV) Therapy Shock Prevention Vital Signs Monitoring	Capillary Blood Sample Hemodynamic Regulation Phlebotomy: Arterial Blood Sample Phlebotomy: Venous Blood Sample Shock Management: Volume

Continued

Outcome	Major Interventions	Suggested Interventions	Optional Interventions

Endurance
 	
DEFINITION:
  Capacity to
  sustain activity
	Energy
	  Management
		Exercise Promotion
		Exercise Promotion:
		  Strength Training
		Nutrition
		  Management
		Sleep Enhancement
			Environmental
			  Management
			Environmental
			  Management:
			  Comfort
			Exercise Therapy:
			  Ambulation
			Exercise Therapy:
			  Muscle Control
			Self-Care Assistance

Fluid Overload Severity
 	
DEFINITION:
  Severity of excess
  fluids in the
  intracellular and
  extracellular
  compartments of
  the body
	Fluid Management
	Hypervolemia
	  Management
		Electrolyte
		  Monitoring
		Fluid/Electrolyte
		  Management
		Fluid Monitoring
		Hemodynamic
		  Regulation
		Medication
		  Administration
		Medication
		  Management
		Vital Signs Monitoring
			Hemodialysis Therapy
			Neurologic Monitoring
			Skin Surveillance

Outcome	Major Interventions	Suggested Interventions	Optional Interventions
Immobility Consequences: Physiological DEFINITION: Severity of compromise in physiological functioning due to impaired physical mobility	Bed Rest Care Embolus Precautions Exercise Therapy: Joint Mobility	Bowel Management Case Management Circulatory Precautions Constipation/ Impaction Management Cough Enhancement Exercise Promotion: Stretching Flatulence Reduction Lower Extremity Monitoring Positioning Simple Massage Skin Surveillance Teaching: Prescribed Activity/Exercise Urinary Elimination Management Urinary Retention Care	Airway Management Aspiration Precautions Discharge Planning Environmental Management: Home Preparation Feeding Fever Treatment Insurance Authorization Multidisciplinary Care Conference Oral Health Maintenance Respiratory Monitoring Vital Signs Monitoring
Infection Severity DEFINITION: Severity of infection and associated symptoms	Incision Site Care Infection Control	Fluid Management Infection Protection Nutrition Therapy Temperature Regulation Vital Signs Monitoring Wound Care Wound Care: Closed Drainage Wound Irrigation	Amputation Care Discharge Planning Fever Treatment Skin Care: Donor Site Skin Care: Graft Site Skin Surveillance

Continued

Outcome	Major Interventions	Suggested Interventions	Optional Interventions
Nausea & Vomiting Severity			
DEFINITION: Severity of nausea, retching, and vomiting symptoms	Nausea Management Vomiting Management	Diet Staging Fluid/Electrolyte Management Fluid Management Fluid Monitoring Medication Administration Nutrition Management	Enteral Tube Feeding Total Parenteral Nutrition (TPN) Administration
Pain Level			
DEFINITION: Severity of observed or reported pain	Pain Management	Analgesic Administration Analgesic Administration: Intraspinal Environmental Management: Comfort Medication Administration Medication Management Positioning Sleep Enhancement Splinting Surveillance Transcutaneous Electrical Nerve Stimulation (TENS) Vital Signs Monitoring	Energy Management Music Therapy Simple Massage

Outcome	Major Interventions	Suggested Interventions	Optional Interventions
Post Procedure Recovery Status			
DEFINITION: Extent to which an individual returns to baseline function following a procedure(s) requiring anesthesia or sedation	Incision Site Care Pain Management Vital Signs Monitoring	Airway Management Analgesic Administration Fluid Management Infection Protection Nausea Management Respiratory Monitoring Temperature Regulation Urinary Elimination Management Wound Care: Closed Drainage	Bed Rest Care Cough Enhancement Oral Health Maintenance Positioning Sleep Enhancement
Self-Care: Activities of Daily Living (ADL)			
DEFINITION: Ability to perform the most basic physical tasks and personal care activities independently with or without assistive device	Self-Care Assistance	Energy Management Exercise Therapy: Ambulation Self-Care Assistance: Bathing/Hygiene Self-Care Assistance: Dressing/Grooming Self-Care Assistance: Feeding Self-Care Assistance: Toileting	Caregiver Support Discharge Planning Environmental Management: Home Preparation Environmental Management: Safety Exercise Promotion Exercise Therapy: Joint Mobility Fall Prevention Health Care Information Exchange Health System Guidance Home Maintenance Assistance Multidisciplinary Care Conference Telephone Consultation

Continued

Outcome	Major Interventions	Suggested Interventions	Optional Interventions
Wound Healing: Primary Intention			
DEFINITION: Extent of regeneration of cells and tissue following intentional closure	Incision Site Care Nutrition Management Wound Care	Circulatory Precautions Fever Treatment Fluid Management Infection Control Infection Control: Intraoperative Infection Protection Medication Administration Nutrition Therapy Skin Surveillance Splinting Temperature Regulation Wound Care: Closed Drainage	Bathing Cesarean Section Care Hyperglycemia Management Perineal Care Wound Irrigation

NURSING DIAGNOSIS: Swallowing, Impaired

DEFINITION: Abnormal functioning of the swallowing mechanism associated with deficits in oral, pharyngeal, or esophageal structure or function.

Outcome	Major Interventions	Suggested Interventions	Optional Interventions
Aspiration Prevention			
DEFINITION: Personal actions to prevent the passage of fluid and solid particles into the lung	Aspiration Precautions	Airway Management Airway Suctioning Positioning Risk Identification Surveillance Swallowing Therapy	Anxiety Reduction Cough Enhancement Enteral Tube Feeding
Swallowing Status			
DEFINITION: Safe passage of fluids and/or solids from the mouth to the stomach	Aspiration Precautions Swallowing Therapy	Airway Suctioning Progressive Muscle Relaxation Surveillance	Anxiety Reduction Emotional Support Enteral Tube Feeding Feeding Medication Management Nutrition Management Positioning Referral
Swallowing Status: Esophageal Phase			
DEFINITION: Safe passage of fluids and/or solids from the pharynx to the stomach	Positioning	Anxiety Reduction Aspiration Precautions Progressive Muscle Relaxation Surveillance Swallowing Therapy	Airway Suctioning Enteral Tube Feeding

Continued

Outcome	Major Interventions	Suggested Interventions	Optional Interventions
Swallowing Status: Oral Phase			
DEFINITION: Preparation, containment, and posterior movement of fluids and/or solids in the mouth	Swallowing Therapy	Aspiration Precautions Feeding Positioning Self-Care Assistance: Feeding Surveillance	Nutrition Management Nutrition Therapy Oral Health Maintenance Oral Health Restoration
Swallowing Status: Pharyngeal Phase			
DEFINITION: Safe passage of fluids and/or solids from the mouth to the esophagus	Aspiration Precautions Swallowing Therapy	Airway Suctioning Positioning Progressive Muscle Relaxation Surveillance	Anxiety Reduction Emotional Support Referral

NURSING DIAGNOSIS: Therapeutic Regimen Management, Effective

DEFINITION: Pattern of regulating and integrating into daily living a program for treatment of illness and its sequelae that are satisfactory for meeting specific health goals.

Outcome	Major Interventions	Suggested Interventions	Optional Interventions
Adherence Behavior			
DEFINITION: Self-initiated actions to promote wellness, recovery, and rehabilitation	Anticipatory Guidance Health Education Health System Guidance	Decision-Making Support Health Screening Learning Facilitation Learning Readiness Enhancement Risk Identification Self-Modification Assistance	Culture Brokerage Referral Teaching: Individual Telephone Consultation Telephone Follow-up

Continued

Outcome	Major Interventions	Suggested Interventions	Optional Interventions
Compliance Behavior			
DEFINITION: Personal actions to promote wellness, recovery, and rehabilitation based on professional advice	Mutual Goal Setting Patient Contracting	Health System Guidance Learning Facilitation Learning Readiness Enhancement Self-Modification Assistance Support System Enhancement Surveillance Teaching: Individual Teaching: Prescribed Activity/Exercise Teaching: Prescribed Diet Teaching: Prescribed Medication Teaching: Procedure/ Treatment Teaching: Psychomotor Skill Teaching: Safe Sex Telephone Consultation Telephone Follow-up Values Clarification	Culture Brokerage Patient Rights Protection Smoking Cessation Assistance Substance Use Prevention
Family Participation in Professional Care			
DEFINITION: Family involvement in decision-making, delivery, and evaluation of care provided by health care personnel	Family Involvement Promotion	Family Mobilization Health Education Health System Guidance Mutual Goal Setting	Caregiver Support Culture Brokerage Family Process Maintenance Family Support Fiscal Resource Management

Outcome	Major Interventions	Suggested Interventions	Optional Interventions
Knowledge: Treatment Regimen			
DEFINITION: Extent of understanding conveyed about a specific treatment regimen	Teaching: Procedure/ Treatment	Allergy Management Anticipatory Guidance Asthma Management Chemotherapy Management Learning Facilitation Learning Readiness Enhancement Medication Management Nutritional Counseling Radiation Therapy Management Teaching: Group Teaching: Individual Teaching: Prescribed Activity/Exercise Teaching: Prescribed Diet Teaching: Prescribed Medication Teaching: Psychomotor Skill	Health System Guidance Nausea Management Teaching: Disease Process Vomiting Management Weight Gain Assistance Weight Management Weight Reduction Assistance

Continued

Outcome	Major Interventions	Suggested Interventions	Optional Interventions
Participation in Health Care Decisions			
DEFINITION: Personal involvement in selecting and evaluating health care options to achieve desired outcome	Decision-Making Support Health System Guidance	Anticipatory Guidance Assertiveness Training Culture Brokerage Discharge Planning Mutual Goal Setting Patient Rights Protection Self-Responsibility Facilitation Telephone Consultation Values Clarification	Caregiver Support Family Involvement Promotion Health Care Information Exchange Referral
Risk Control			
DEFINITION: Personal actions to prevent, eliminate, or reduce modifiable health threats	Health Education Risk Identification Self-Modification Assistance	Health Screening Health System Guidance Learning Facilitation Learning Readiness Enhancement Surveillance Surveillance: Late Pregnancy Surveillance: Remote Electronic Surveillance: Safety	Environmental Management: Safety Environmental Management: Worker Safety Immunization/ Vaccination Management Infection Protection Laser Precautions Latex Precautions Vehicle Safety Promotion

Outcome	Major Interventions	Suggested Interventions	Optional Interventions
Symptom Control			
DEFINITION: Personal actions to minimize perceived adverse changes in physical and emotional functioning	Anticipatory Guidance Self-Modification Assistance	Anxiety Reduction Health Education Health Screening Health System Guidance Learning Facilitation Learning Readiness Enhancement Teaching: Disease Process Teaching: Individual	Allergy Management Asthma Management Coping Enhancement Emotional Support Family Involvement Promotion Nausea Management Pain Management Vomiting Management
Treatment Behavior: Illness or Injury			
DEFINITION: Personal actions to palliate or eliminate pathology	Anticipatory Guidance Decision-Making Support	Asthma Management Cardiac Care: Rehabilitative Chemotherapy Management Medication Management Self-Modification Assistance Self-Responsibility Facilitation Teaching: Disease Process Teaching: Prescribed Activity/Exercise Teaching: Prescribed Diet Teaching: Prescribed Medication Teaching: Procedure/ Treatment Teaching: Psychomotor Skill	Health Screening Weight Gain Assistance Weight Reduction Assistance

NURSING DIAGNOSIS: Therapeutic Regimen Management, Ineffective

DEFINITION: Pattern of regulating and integrating into daily living a program for treatment of illness and the sequelae of illness that is unsatisfactory for meeting specific health goals.

Outcome	Major Interventions	Suggested Interventions	Optional Interventions
Blood Glucose Level DEFINITION: Extent to which glucose levels in plasma and urine are maintained in normal range	Hyperglycemia Management Hypoglycemia Management	Bedside Laboratory Testing Capillary Blood Sample Medication Administration: Intradermal Medication Administration: Oral Medication Management Nutritional Counseling Teaching: Disease Process Teaching: Prescribed Diet Teaching: Prescribed Medication Teaching: Procedure/ Treatment Teaching: Psychomotor Skill	Acid-Base Management: Metabolic Acidosis Acid-Base Monitoring Intravenous (IV) Insertion Intravenous (IV) Therapy Learning Facilitation Learning Readiness Enhancement Self-Responsibility Facilitation

Outcome	Major Interventions	Suggested Interventions	Optional Interventions
Cardiac Disease Self-Management			
DEFINITION: Personal actions to manage heart disease and prevent disease progression	Cardiac Precautions Teaching: Disease Process Teaching: Prescribed Activity/Exercise Teaching: Prescribed Diet Teaching: Prescribed Medication	Cardiac Care: Rehabilitative Counseling Embolus Precautions Health Education Medication Management Nutrition Management Nutritional Counseling	Anger Control Assistance Coping Enhancement Mutual Goal Setting Peripheral Sensation Management Self-Modification Assistance Self-Responsibility Facilitation

Continued

Outcome	Major Interventions	Suggested Interventions	Optional Interventions
Compliance Behavior			
DEFINITION: Personal actions to promote wellness, recovery, and rehabilitation based on professional advice	Behavior Modification	Case Management	Bibliotherapy
	Mutual Goal Setting	Cognitive Restructuring	Consultation
	Patient Contracting	Coping Enhancement	Exercise Promotion
	Self-Modification Assistance	Counseling	Family Involvement Promotion
		Culture Brokerage	Family Mobilization
		Emotional Support	Financial Resource Assistance
		Family Support	Patient Rights Protection
		Health System Guidance	Self-Awareness Enhancement
		Learning Facilitation	Self-Esteem Enhancement
		Learning Readiness Enhancement	Smoking Cessation Assistance
		Nutritional Counseling	Support Group
		Risk Identification	Surveillance
		Self-Responsibility Facilitation	Teaching: Prescribed Activity/Exercise
		Support System Enhancement	Teaching: Prescribed Diet
		Teaching: Disease Process	Teaching: Prescribed Medication
		Teaching: Procedure/Treatment	Teaching: Safe Sex
		Teaching: Psychomotor Skill	
		Telephone Consultation	
		Telephone Follow-up	
		Values Clarification	

Outcome	Major Interventions	Suggested Interventions	Optional Interventions
Diabetes Self-Management			
DEFINITION: Personal actions to manage diabetes mellitus and prevent disease progression	Teaching: Disease Process Teaching: Prescribed Diet Teaching: Prescribed Medication	Anticipatory Guidance Capillary Blood Sample Coping Enhancement Hyperglycemia Management Hypoglycemia Management Medication Administration: Intradermal Medication Administration: Oral Medication Management Nutritional Counseling Teaching: Foot Care Teaching: Group Teaching: Individual Teaching: Psychomotor Skill	Anxiety Reduction Emotional Support Health Education Lower Extremity Monitoring Self-Modification Assistance Self-Responsibility Facilitation Skin Surveillance
Knowledge: Diet			
DEFINITION: Extent of understanding conveyed about recommended diet	Teaching: Prescribed Diet	Health System Guidance Learning Facilitation Nutritional Counseling Self-Responsibility Facilitation	Culture Brokerage Fluid Management Weight Gain Assistance Weight Management Weight Reduction Assistance

Continued

Outcome	Major Interventions	Suggested Interventions	Optional Interventions
Knowledge: Treatment Regimen DEFINITION: Extent of understanding conveyed about a specific treatment regimen	Teaching: Procedure/ Treatment	Active Listening Chemotherapy Management Learning Facilitation Learning Readiness Enhancement Medication Management Nutrition Management Radiation Therapy Management Teaching: Disease Process Teaching: Group Teaching: Individual Teaching: Prescribed Activity/Exercise Teaching: Prescribed Diet Teaching: Prescribed Medication Teaching: Psychomotor Skill	Family Involvement Promotion Health System Guidance High-Risk Pregnancy Care Prenatal Care Weight Gain Assistance Weight Management Weight Reduction Assistance

Outcome	Major Interventions	Suggested Interventions	Optional Interventions
Medication Response			
DEFINITION: Therapeutic and adverse effects of prescribed medication	Teaching: Individual Teaching: Prescribed Medication	Hormone Replacement Therapy Learning Readiness Facilitation Medication Administration Medication Management Teaching: Disease Process	Allergy Management Asthma Management Chemotherapy Management Health Education
Participation in Health Care Decisions			
DEFINITION: Personal involvement in selecting and evaluating health care options to achieve desired outcome	Decision-Making Support Health System Guidance	Active Listening Assertiveness Training Counseling Culture Brokerage Discharge Planning Patient Rights Protection Self-Responsibility Facilitation Telephone Consultation Values Clarification	Behavior Modification Bibliotherapy Coping Enhancement Family Involvement Promotion Health Care Information Exchange Referral

Continued

Outcome	Major Interventions	Suggested Interventions	Optional Interventions
Self-Care: Non-Parenteral Medication			
DEFINITION: Ability to administer oral and topical medications to meet therapeutic goals independently with or without assistive device	Self-Care Assistance Teaching: Prescribed Medication	Learning Facilitation Medication Administration: Ear Medication Administration: Enteral Medication Administration: Eye Medication Administration: Inhalation Medication Administration: Nasal Medication Administration: Oral Medication Administration: Rectal Medication Administration: Skin Medication Administration: Vaginal Medication Management Teaching: Disease Process	Asthma Management Chemotherapy Management Self-Modification Assistance Self-Responsibility Facilitation Skin Care: Topical Treatments

Outcome	Major Interventions	Suggested Interventions	Optional Interventions
Self-Care: Parenteral Medication			
DEFINITION: Ability to administer parenteral medications to meet therapeutic goals independently with or without assistive device	Teaching: Prescribed Medication Teaching: Psychomotor Skill	Learning Facilitation Medication Administration: Intradermal Medication Administration: Intramuscular (IM) Medication Administration: Intravenous (IV) Medication Administration: Subcutaneous Patient-Controlled Analgesia (PCA) Assistance Teaching: Disease Process	Anticipatory Guidance Anxiety Reduction Emotional Support Intravenous (IV) Therapy Self-Responsibility Facilitation
Symptom Control			
DEFINITION: Personal actions to minimize perceived adverse changes in physical and emotional functioning	Self-Modification Assistance Teaching: Disease Process	Active Listening Behavior Modification Crisis Intervention Nutritional Counseling Teaching: Prescribed Activity/Exercise Teaching: Prescribed Medication Self-Responsibility Facilitation	Coping Enhancement Exercise Promotion Financial Resource Assistance

Continued

Outcome	Major Interventions	Suggested Interventions	Optional Interventions
Systemic Toxin Clearance: Dialysis			
DEFINITION: Clearance of toxins from the body with peritoneal or hemodialysis	Hemodialysis Therapy Hemofiltration Therapy Peritoneal Dialysis Therapy	Acid-Base Management Acid-Base Monitoring Electrolyte Management Electrolyte Management: Hypercalcemia Electrolyte Management: Hyperkalemia Electrolyte Management: Hypermagnesemia Electrolyte Management: Hypernatremia Electrolyte Management: Hyperphosphatemia Electrolyte Monitoring Fluid/Electrolyte Management Vital Signs Monitoring	Bedside Laboratory Testing Laboratory Data Interpretation Medication Management Teaching: Procedure/ Treatment Teaching: Psychomotor Skill

Outcome	Major Interventions	Suggested Interventions	Optional Interventions
Treatment Behavior: Illness or Injury DEFINITION: Personal actions to palliate or eliminate pathology	Behavior Modification Self-Responsibility Facilitation Teaching: Disease Process	Cognitive Restructuring Coping Enhancement Counseling Emotional Support Learning Facilitation Mutual Goal Setting Patient Contracting Self-Modification Assistance Support Group Support System Enhancement Teaching: Individual Teaching: Prescribed Activity/Exercise Teaching: Prescribed Diet Teaching: Prescribed Medication Teaching: Procedure/ Treatment Teaching: Psychomotor Skill Telephone Consultation Telephone Follow-up Values Clarification	Active Listening Crisis Intervention Family Involvement Promotion Family Mobilization Self-Awareness Enhancement Self-Care Assistance Smoking Cessation Assistance Substance Use Treatment Surveillance Weight Gain Assistance Weight Reduction Assistance

NURSING DIAGNOSIS: Therapeutic Regimen Management, Readiness for Enhanced

DEFINITION: A pattern of regulating and integrating into daily living a program(s) for treatment of illness and its sequelae that is sufficient for meeting health-related goals and can be strengthened.

Outcome	Major Interventions	Suggested Interventions	Optional Interventions
Adherence Behavior			
DEFINITION: Self-initiated actions to promote wellness, recovery, and rehabilitation	Anticipatory Guidance Health Education	Decision-Making Support Learning Facilitation Learning Readiness Enhancement Self-Modification Assistance	Culture Brokerage Health System Guidance Smoking Cessation Assistance
Compliance Behavior			
DEFINITION: Personal actions to promote wellness, recovery, and rehabilitation based on professional advice	Mutual Goal Setting Self-Modification Assistance	Health System Guidance Learning Facilitation Learning Readiness Enhancement Nutritional Counseling Patient Contracting Teaching: Individual Teaching: Prescribed Activity/Exercise Teaching: Prescribed Diet Teaching: Prescribed Medication	Culture Brokerage Patient Rights Protection Telephone Consultation

Outcome	Major Interventions	Suggested Interventions	Optional Interventions
Knowledge: Treatment Regimen			
DEFINITION: Extent of understanding conveyed about a specific treatment regimen	Teaching: Individual	Learning Facilitation Learning Readiness Enhancement Nutritional Counseling Teaching: Prescribed Activity/Exercise Teaching: Prescribed Diet Teaching: Prescribed Medication Teaching: Procedure/ Treatment	Teaching: Disease Process Teaching: Group Teaching: Psychomotor Skill
Participation in Health Care Decisions			
DEFINITION: Personal involvement in selecting and evaluating health care options to achieve desired outcome	Decision-Making Support Health System Guidance	Anticipatory Guidance Assertiveness Training Culture Brokerage Mutual Goal Setting Self-Responsibility Facilitation	Family Involvement Promotion Organ Procurement

Continued

Outcome	Major Interventions	Suggested Interventions	Optional Interventions
Risk Control			
DEFINITION: Personal actions to prevent, eliminate, or reduce modifiable health threats	Health Education Risk Identification	Health Screening Surveillance Surveillance: Late Pregnancy Surveillance: Safety	Immunization/ Vaccination Management Infection Control
Treatment Behavior: Illness or Injury			
DEFINITION: Personal actions to palliate or eliminate pathology	Anticipatory Guidance Self-Modification Assistance	Decision-Making Support Learning Readiness Enhancement Teaching: Disease Process Teaching: Prescribed Activity/Exercise Teaching: Prescribed Diet Teaching: Prescribed Medication Teaching: Procedure/ Treatment	Infection Protection Nutritional Counseling Teaching: Psychomotor Skill

NURSING DIAGNOSIS: Thermoregulation, Ineffective

DEFINITION: Temperature fluctuation between hypothermia and hyperthermia.

Outcome	Major Interventions	Suggested Interventions	Optional Interventions
Thermoregulation			
DEFINITION: Balance among heat production, heat gain, and heat loss	Temperature Regulation Temperature Regulation: Intraoperative	Environmental Management Fever Treatment Fluid Management Fluid Monitoring Heat Exposure Treatment Hypothermia Treatment Malignant Hyperthermia Precautions Medication Administration Vital Signs Monitoring	Bathing Emergency Care Hemodynamic Regulation Shock Management
Thermoregulation: Newborn			
DEFINITION: Balance among heat production, heat gain, and heat loss during the first 28 days of life	Newborn Care Temperature Regulation	Environmental Management Fluid Management Fluid Monitoring Medication Administration Newborn Monitoring Vital Signs Monitoring	Acid-Base Management Bathing Dressing Fever Treatment Heat Exposure Treatment Hypoglycemia Management Hypothermia Treatment Phototherapy: Neonate

NURSING DIAGNOSIS: Thought Processes, Disturbed

DEFINITION: Disruption in cognitive operations and activities.

Outcome	Major Interventions	Suggested Interventions	Optional Interventions
Cognition DEFINITION: Ability to execute complex mental processes	Dementia Management Environmental Management: Safety	Cognitive Restructuring Elopement Precautions Environmental Management Medication Management Memory Training Milieu Therapy Reminiscence Therapy	Area Restriction Cognitive Stimulation Mood Management Patient Rights Protection Reality Orientation
Cognitive Orientation DEFINITION: Ability to identify person, place, and time accurately	Reality Orientation	Cognitive Stimulation Delirium Management Delusion Management Dementia Management Elopement Precautions Hallucination Management Medication Management Surveillance	Animal-Assisted Therapy Area Restriction Calming Technique Environmental Management Milieu Therapy Neurologic Monitoring Reminiscence Therapy Substance Use Treatment

Outcome	Major Interventions	Suggested Interventions	Optional Interventions
Concentration			
DEFINITION: Ability to focus on a specific stimulus	Anxiety Reduction Behavior Management: Overactivity/ Inattention	Analgesic Administration Cerebral Perfusion Promotion Delirium Management Hallucination Management Hypoglycemia Management Medication Management Milieu Therapy Substance Use Treatment Touch	Active Listening Calming Technique Cognitive Restructuring Cognitive Stimulation Delusion Management Dementia Management Environmental Management Reality Orientation
Decision-Making			
DEFINITION: Ability to make judgments and choose between two or more alternatives	Decision-Making Support	Counseling Emotional Support Patient Rights Protection Support System Enhancement	Family Support Security Enhancement Self-Esteem Enhancement

Continued

Outcome	Major Interventions	Suggested Interventions	Optional Interventions
Distorted Thought Self-Control			
DEFINITION: Self-restraint of disruptions in perception, thought processes, and thought content	Delusion Management Hallucination Management	Anxiety Reduction Behavior Management Behavior Modification Cognitive Restructuring Delirium Management Dementia Management Environmental Management: Safety Medication Management Milieu Therapy Reality Orientation Surveillance: Safety Therapy Group	Animal-Assisted Therapy Cognitive Stimulation Environmental Management Memory Training Music Therapy Recreation Therapy Sleep Enhancement
Identity			
DEFINITION: Distinguishes between self and non-self and characterizes one's essence	Cognitive Restructuring Self-Awareness Enhancement Self-Esteem Enhancement	Counseling Developmental Enhancement: Adolescent Developmental Enhancement: Child Medication Management	Bibliotherapy Delirium Management Delusion Management Dementia Management Family Therapy Hallucination Management Milieu Therapy Reminiscence Therapy Therapy Group

Outcome	Major Interventions	Suggested Interventions	Optional Interventions
Information Processing			
DEFINITION: Ability to acquire, organize, and use information	Cognitive Stimulation	Anxiety Reduction Calming Technique Energy Management Learning Facilitation Learning Readiness Enhancement Medication Management Memory Training Pain Management Sleep Enhancement	Cerebral Edema Management Cerebral Perfusion Promotion Cognitive Restructuring Delirium Management Delusion Management Dementia Management Environmental Management Hallucination Management Milieu Therapy Music Therapy Oxygen Therapy Reminiscence Therapy
Memory			
DEFINITION: Ability to cognitively retrieve and report previously stored information	Dementia Management Memory Training	Active Listening Cognitive Restructuring Cognitive Stimulation Elopement Precautions Environmental Management: Safety Learning Facilitation Milieu Therapy Reminiscence Therapy	Bibliotherapy Coping Enhancement Medication Management Patient Rights Protection Reality Orientation

Continued

Outcome	Major Interventions	Suggested Interventions	Optional Interventions
Neurological Status: Consciousness			
DEFINITION: Arousal, orientation, and attention to the environment	Cerebral Perfusion Promotion Environmental Management: Safety Neurologic Monitoring	Cerebral Edema Management Cognitive Stimulation Delirium Management Dementia Management Environmental Management Fluid Resuscitation Intracranial Pressure (ICP) Monitoring Medication Administration Medication Management Surveillance Vital Signs Monitoring	Family Support Patient Rights Protection Physical Restraint Substance Use Treatment Substance Use Treatment: Alcohol Withdrawal Substance Use Treatment: Drug Withdrawal Substance Use Treatment: Overdose Temperature Regulation Touch

NURSING DIAGNOSIS: Tissue Integrity, Impaired

DEFINITION: Damage to mucous membrane, corneal, integumentary, or subcutaneous tissues.

Outcome	Major Interventions	Suggested Interventions	Optional Interventions
Allergic Response: Localized DEFINITION: Severity of localized hypersensitive immune response to a specific environmental (exogenous) antigen	Skin Care: Topical Treatments Skin Surveillance	Allergy Management Infection Protection Latex Precautions Medication Administration Medication Administration: Eye Medication Administration: Skin Wound Care	Infection Control Medication Management
Ostomy Self-Care DEFINITION: Personal actions to maintain ostomy for elimination	Ostomy Care Skin Surveillance	Fluid Management Nutrition Management Skin Care: Topical Treatments Teaching: Individual Teaching: Procedure/ Treatment Teaching: Psychomotor Skill	Bathing Flatulence Reduction Infection Control Infection Protection Latex Precautions Pressure Management

Continued

Outcome	Major Interventions	Suggested Interventions	Optional Interventions
Tissue Integrity: Skin & Mucous Membranes			
DEFINITION: Structural intactness and normal physiological function of skin and mucous membranes	Oral Health Maintenance Pressure Ulcer Prevention Wound Care	Bleeding Reduction: Gastrointestinal Bleeding Reduction: Nasal Bleeding Reduction: Postpartum Uterus Circulatory Precautions Eye Care Infection Protection Lower Extremity Monitoring Medication Administration: Ear Medication Administration: Eye Medication Administration: Rectal Medication Administration: Vaginal Nutrition Management Oral Health Restoration Pressure Management Radiation Therapy Management Rectal Prolapse Management Simple Massage Skin Surveillance	Amputation Care Bathing Bed Rest Care Blood Products Administration Cast Care: Maintenance Diarrhea Management Fluid Management Fluid Monitoring Medication Management Perineal Care Positioning Pressure Ulcer Care Teaching: Foot Care Traction/Immobilization Care Urinary Incontinence Care Urinary Incontinence Care: Enuresis Vital Signs Monitoring

Outcome	Major Interventions	Suggested Interventions	Optional Interventions
Wound Healing: Primary Intention			
DEFINITION: Extent of regeneration of cells and tissue following intentional closure	Incision Site Care Infection Protection Wound Care	Amputation Care Circulatory Precautions Fluid Management Infection Control: Intraoperative Medication Administration Nutrition Management Skin Care: Graft Site Splinting Suturing Wound Care: Closed Drainage	Cesarean Section Care Infection Control Perineal Care
Wound Healing: Secondary Intention			
DEFINITION: Extent of regeneration of cells and tissue in an open wound	Wound Care	Circulatory Care: Arterial Insufficiency Circulatory Precautions Fluid Management Infection Control Infection Protection Medication Administration Nutrition Management Skin Care: Donor Site Splinting Transcutaneous Electrical Nerve Stimulation (TENS) Wound Irrigation	Bathing Cutaneous Stimulation Leech Therapy Lower Extremity Monitoring Pressure Ulcer Care Total Parenteral Nutrition (TPN) Administration

NURSING DIAGNOSIS: Tissue Perfusion: Cardiopulmonary, Ineffective

DEFINITION: Decrease in oxygen resulting in the failure to nourish the tissues at the capillary level.

Outcome	Major Interventions	Suggested Interventions	Optional Interventions
Cardiac Pump Effectiveness DEFINITION: Adequacy of blood volume ejected from the left ventricle to support systemic perfusion pressure	Cardiac Care: Acute Dysrhythmia Management Hemodynamic Regulation Shock Management: Cardiac	Cardiac Care Cardiac Care: Rehabilitative Cardiac Precautions Circulatory Precautions Emergency Care Fluid/Electrolyte Management Fluid Management Hypovolemia Management Invasive Hemodynamic Monitoring Laboratory Data Interpretation Vital Signs Monitoring	Blood Products Administration Embolus Precautions Fluid Monitoring Intravenous (IV) Insertion Intravenous (IV) Therapy Lower Extremity Monitoring Medication Administration: Intravenous (IV) Resuscitation: Neonate Shock Management Shock Prevention Temperature Regulation Temporary Pacemaker Management

Outcome	Major Interventions	Suggested Interventions	Optional Interventions
Circulation Status			
DEFINITION: Unobstructed, unidirectional blood flow at an appropriate pressure through large vessels of the systemic and pulmonary circuits	Cardiac Care: Acute Hemodynamic Regulation	Circulatory Care: Mechanical Assist Device Embolus Care: Peripheral Embolus Care: Pulmonary Embolus Precautions Fluid Management Fluid Monitoring Hemorrhage Control Hypovolemia Management Medication Administration Shock Prevention	Bleeding Reduction Blood Products Administration Fluid Resuscitation Invasive Hemodynamic Monitoring Laboratory Data Interpretation Resuscitation Resuscitation: Neonate Shock Management: Cardiac Shock Management: Vasogenic
Respiratory Status: Gas Exchange			
DEFINITION: Alveolar exchange of carbon dioxide and oxygen to maintain arterial blood gas concentrations	Acid-Base Monitoring Oxygen Therapy Respiratory Monitoring	Acid-Base Management: Respiratory Acidosis Acid-Base Management: Respiratory Alkalosis Bedside Laboratory Testing Embolus Care: Pulmonary Fluid/Electrolyte Management Neurologic Monitoring Phlebotomy: Arterial Blood Sample	Circulatory Care: Arterial Insufficiency Circulatory Care: Venous Insufficiency Intravenous (IV) Insertion Intravenous (IV) Therapy Medication Administration Resuscitation

Continued

T

Outcome	Major Interventions	Suggested Interventions	Optional Interventions
Tissue Perfusion: Cardiac			
DEFINITION: Adequacy of blood flow through the coronary vasculature to maintain heart function	Cardiac Care: Acute Hemodynamic Regulation Shock Management: Cardiac	Acid-Base Management Acid-Base Monitoring Cardiac Care Cardiac Precautions Circulatory Precautions Dysrhythmia Management Emergency Care Fluid/Electrolyte Management Fluid Management Fluid Monitoring Fluid Resuscitation Hypovolemia Management Invasive Hemodynamic Monitoring Medication Administration Oxygen Therapy Pain Management Respiratory Monitoring Shock Management Technology Management Vital Signs Monitoring	Acid-Base Management: Metabolic Acidosis Acid-Base Management: Metabolic Alkalosis Bedside Laboratory Testing Bleeding Reduction Blood Products Administration Code Management Electronic Fetal Monitoring: Intrapartum Embolus Precautions Hemorrhage Control Laboratory Data Interpretation Medication Management Phlebotomy: Arterial Blood Sample Phlebotomy: Venous Blood Sample Resuscitation Resuscitation: Neonate Shock Management: Vasogenic Smoking Cessation Assistance Substance Use Treatment

Outcome	Major Interventions	Suggested Interventions	Optional Interventions
Tissue Perfusion: Pulmonary			
DEFINITION: Adequacy of blood flow through pulmonary vasculature to perfuse alveoli/ capillary unit	Acid-Base Management: Respiratory Acidosis Acid-Base Management: Respiratory Alkalosis Embolus Care: Pulmonary	Acid-Base Monitoring Cardiac Care: Acute Fluid Management Hemodynamic Regulation Intravenous (IV) Insertion Intravenous (IV) Therapy Invasive Hemodynamic Monitoring Medication Administration Medication Management Oxygen Therapy Respiratory Monitoring Vital Signs Monitoring	Electrolyte Management Emergency Care Hemorrhage Control Mechanical Ventilation Resuscitation Resuscitation: Neonate Shock Management Shock Prevention

Continued

Outcome	Major Interventions	Suggested Interventions	Optional Interventions
Vital Signs			
DEFINITION: Extent to which temperature, pulse, respiration, and blood pressure are within normal range	Hemodynamic Regulation	Acid-Base Management	Blood Products Administration
	Vital Signs Monitoring	Cardiac Care	Emergency Care
		Dysrhythmia Management	Hemorrhage Control
		Electrolyte Management	Oxygen Therapy
		Fluid Management	Pain Management
		Hypovolemia Management	Resuscitation
		Intravenous (IV) Therapy	
		Medication Administration	
		Medication Management	
		Respiratory Monitoring	
		Shock Management	
		Shock Prevention	
		Surveillance	
		Temperature Regulation	

NURSING DIAGNOSIS: Tissue Perfusion: Cerebral, Ineffective

DEFINITION: Decrease in oxygen resulting in the failure to nourish the tissues at the capillary level.

Outcome	Major Interventions	Suggested Interventions	Optional Interventions
Circulation Status			
DEFINITION: Unobstructed, unidirectional blood flow at an appropriate pressure through large vessels of the systemic and pulmonary circuits	Cerebral Perfusion Promotion	Bleeding Precautions Bleeding Reduction Embolus Care: Peripheral Embolus Precautions Fluid Monitoring Hemodynamic Regulation Hypovolemia Management Laboratory Data Interpretation Shock Management Shock Prevention	Bedside Laboratory Testing Blood Products Administration Fluid Resuscitation Intravenous (IV) Insertion Intravenous (IV) Therapy Invasive Hemodynamic Monitoring Phlebotomy: Arterial Blood Sample Phlebotomy: Venous Blood Sample Shock Management: Vasogenic Shock Management: Volume Subarachnoid Hemorrhage Precautions
Cognition			
DEFINITION: Ability to execute complex mental processes	Cerebral Perfusion Promotion Neurologic Monitoring	Acid-Base Management Fluid/Electrolyte Management Fluid Management Hypovolemia Management Intracranial Pressure (ICP) Monitoring Oxygen Therapy	Nutrition Management Seizure Precautions Shock Management Medication Management

Continued

Outcome	Major Interventions	Suggested Interventions	Optional Interventions
Neurological Status			
DEFINITION: Ability of the peripheral and central nervous system to receive, process, and respond to internal and external stimuli	Cerebral Perfusion Promotion Intracranial Pressure (ICP) Monitoring Neurologic Monitoring	Acid-Base Management Acid-Base Monitoring Bedside Laboratory Testing Cerebral Edema Management Code Management Electrolyte Management Electrolyte Monitoring Fluid Management Invasive Hemodynamic Monitoring Laboratory Data Interpretation Medication Administration Medication Management Oxygen Therapy Peripheral Sensation Management Positioning: Neurologic Respiratory Monitoring Resuscitation Seizure Management Seizure Precautions Subarachnoid Hemorrhage Precautions Surveillance Vital Signs Monitoring	Acid-Base Management: Metabolic Acidosis Acid-Base Management: Metabolic Alkalosis Acid-Base Management: Respiratory Acidosis Acid-Base Management: Respiratory Alkalosis Electronic Fetal Monitoring: Intrapartum Emergency Care Pain Management Peripherally Inserted Central (PIC) Catheter Care Resuscitation: Fetus Resuscitation: Neonate

Outcome	Major Interventions	Suggested Interventions	Optional Interventions
Neurological Status: Consciousness			
DEFINITION: Arousal, orientation, and attention to the environment	Cerebral Perfusion Promotion Neurologic Monitoring	Cerebral Edema Management Fluid/Electrolyte Management Fluid Management Hypovolemia Management Intracranial Pressure (ICP) Monitoring Oxygen Therapy Positioning: Neurologic	Resuscitation Seizure Management Seizure Precautions Subarachnoid Hemorrhage Precautions

Continued

Outcome	Major Interventions	Suggested Interventions	Optional Interventions
Tissue Perfusion: Cerebral			
DEFINITION: Adequacy of blood flow through the cerebral vasculature to maintain brain function	Cerebral Perfusion Promotion Intracranial Pressure (ICP) Monitoring Neurologic Monitoring	Acid-Base Management Acid-Base Monitoring Bedside Laboratory Testing Bleeding Reduction Cerebral Edema Management Fluid Management Fluid Monitoring Fluid Resuscitation Hemorrhage Control Hypovolemia Management Laboratory Data Interpretation Medication Administration Medication Administration: Intravenous (IV) Medication Administration: Ventricular Reservoir Medication Management Oxygen Therapy Positioning Seizure Management Seizure Precautions Shock Management Subarachnoid Hemorrhage Precautions Surveillance Vital Signs Monitoring	Blood Products Administration Code Management Electrolyte Management Electrolyte Monitoring Electronic Fetal Monitoring: Intrapartum Embolus Precautions Intravenous (IV) Insertion Intravenous (IV) Therapy Phlebotomy: Arterial Blood Sample Phlebotomy: Cannulated Vessel Phlebotomy: Venous Blood Sample Resuscitation Resuscitation: Neonate Shock Management: Vasogenic Shock Management: Volume Technology Management

NURSING DIAGNOSIS: Tissue Perfusion: Gastrointestinal, Ineffective

DEFINITION: Decrease in oxygen resulting in the failure to nourish the tissues at the capillary level.

Outcome	Major Interventions	Suggested Interventions	Optional Interventions
Circulation Status			
DEFINITION: Unobstructed, unidirectional blood flow at an appropriate pressure through large vessels of the systemic and pulmonary circuits	Hemodynamic Regulation Hypovolemia Management	Bleeding Precautions Bleeding Reduction: Gastrointestinal Fluid Monitoring Fluid Resuscitation Hemorrhage Control Intravenous (IV) Insertion Intravenous (IV) Therapy Shock Management Vital Signs Monitoring	Bedside Laboratory Testing Blood Products Administration Invasive Hemodynamic Monitoring Laboratory Data Interpretation Peripherally Inserted Central (PIC) Catheter Care Phlebotomy: Arterial Blood Sample Phlebotomy: Venous Blood Sample
Electrolyte & Acid/Base Balance			
DEFINITION: Balance of the electrolytes and non-electrolytes in the intracellular and extracellular compartments of the body	Electrolyte Management Fluid/Electrolyte Management	Acid-Base Management Acid-Base Monitoring Electrolyte Monitoring Fluid Management Fluid Monitoring Intravenous (IV) Insertion Intravenous (IV) Therapy Laboratory Data Interpretation Vital Signs Monitoring	Phlebotomy: Arterial Blood Sample Total Parenteral Nutrition (TPN) Administration

Continued

Outcome	Major Interventions	Suggested Interventions	Optional Interventions
Fluid Balance DEFINITION: Water balance in the intracellular and extracellular compartments of the body	Fluid/Electrolyte Management Fluid Management	Bedside Laboratory Testing Diarrhea Management Electrolyte Management Electrolyte Monitoring Fluid Monitoring Fluid Resuscitation Hypovolemia Management Intravenous (IV) Insertion Intravenous (IV) Therapy Laboratory Data Interpretation Medication Administration Medication Management Nutrition Management Nutritional Monitoring Total Parenteral Nutrition (TPN) Administration Vital Signs Monitoring	Enteral Tube Feeding Hemodynamic Regulation Invasive Hemodynamic Monitoring Shock Management Venous Access Device (VAD) Maintenance

Outcome	Major Interventions	Suggested Interventions	Optional Interventions
Hydration DEFINITION: Adequate water in the intracellular and extracellular compartments of the body	Fluid/Electrolyte Management Hypovolemia Management	Diarrhea Management Electrolyte Management Electrolyte Monitoring Fluid Management Fluid Monitoring Fluid Resuscitation Intravenous (IV) Insertion Intravenous (IV) Therapy Nutrition Management Nutritional Monitoring Vital Signs Monitoring	Peripherally Inserted Central (PIC) Catheter Care Shock Management Temperature Regulation Total Parenteral Nutrition (TPN) Administration

Continued

Outcome	Major Interventions	Suggested Interventions	Optional Interventions
Tissue Perfusion: Abdominal Organs			
DEFINITION: Adequacy of blood flow through the small vessels of the abdominal viscera to maintain organ function	Hypovolemia Management Intravenous (IV) Therapy	Acid-Base Management Acid-Base Monitoring Bedside Laboratory Testing Electrolyte Management Electrolyte Monitoring Flatulence Reduction Fluid/Electrolyte Management Fluid Management Fluid Monitoring Gastrointestinal Intubation Laboratory Data Interpretation Medication Administration: Enteral Medication Management Nausea Management Nutrition Management Oxygen Therapy Pain Management Shock Management Tube Care: Gastrointestinal Vital Signs Monitoring	Bleeding Reduction: Gastrointestinal Bowel Management Enteral Tube Feeding Medication Administration: Intravenous (IV) Resuscitation

NURSING DIAGNOSIS: Tissue Perfusion: Peripheral, Ineffective

DEFINITION: Decrease in oxygen resulting in the failure to nourish the tissues at the capillary level.

Outcome	Major Interventions	Suggested Interventions	Optional Interventions
Circulation Status DEFINITION: Unobstructed, unidirectional blood flow at an appropriate pressure through large vessels of the systemic and pulmonary circuits	Circulatory Care: Arterial Insufficiency Circulatory Care: Venous Insufficiency	Acid-Base Management Acid-Base Monitoring Circulatory Care: Mechanical Assist Device Circulatory Precautions Fluid/Electrolyte Management Fluid Management Fluid Monitoring Hemodynamic Regulation Hypovolemia Management Peripheral Sensation Management Vital Signs Monitoring	Emergency Care Fluid Resuscitation Invasive Hemodynamic Monitoring Laboratory Data Interpretation Lower Extremity Monitoring Neurologic Monitoring Oxygen Therapy Peripherally Inserted Central (PIC) Catheter Care Resuscitation Resuscitation: Neonate Shock Management

Continued

Outcome	Major Interventions	Suggested Interventions	Optional Interventions
Fluid Overload Severity			
DEFINITION: Severity of excess fluids in the intracellular and extracellular compartments of the body	Fluid/Electrolyte Management Fluid Management Hypervolemia Management	Acid-Base Management Acid-Base Monitoring Circulatory Care: Venous Insufficiency Fluid Monitoring Lower Extremity Monitoring Medication Administration Medication Management Positioning Pressure Management Skin Surveillance	Cardiac Care Hemodialysis Therapy Leech Therapy Oxygen Therapy Peritoneal Dialysis Therapy Pressure Ulcer Prevention
Sensory Function: Cutaneous			
DEFINITION: Extent to which stimulation of the skin is correctly sensed	Neurologic Monitoring Peripheral Sensation Management	Circulatory Care: Arterial Insufficiency Circulatory Care: Venous Insufficiency Cutaneous Stimulation Positioning Pressure Ulcer Prevention Skin Surveillance	Foot Care Pain Management Temperature Regulation

Outcome	Major Interventions	Suggested Interventions	Optional Interventions
Tissue Integrity: Skin & Mucous Membranes			
DEFINITION: Structural intactness and normal physiological function of skin and mucous membranes	Circulatory Care: Arterial Insufficiency Circulatory Care: Venous Insufficiency Skin Surveillance	Bed Rest Care Circulatory Precautions Foot Care Medication Administration: Skin Nutrition Management Positioning Pressure Management Pressure Ulcer Prevention	Amputation Care Cast Care: Maintenance Cutaneous Stimulation Fluid Management Fluid Monitoring Medication Management Total Parenteral Nutrition (TPN) Administration

Continued

Outcome	Major Interventions	Suggested Interventions	Optional Interventions
Tissue Perfusion: Peripheral			
DEFINITION: Adequacy of blood flow through the small vessels of the extremities to maintain tissue function	Circulatory Care: Arterial Insufficiency Circulatory Care: Venous Insufficiency Embolus Care: Peripheral	Bedside Laboratory Testing Circulatory Care: Mechanical Assist Device Circulatory Precautions Embolus Precautions Fluid/Electrolyte Management Fluid Management Hypovolemia Management Lower Extremity Monitoring Medication Administration Medication Management Pneumatic Tourniquet Precautions Positioning Pressure Ulcer Prevention Shock Management Shock Management: Cardiac Shock Management: Vasogenic Shock Management: Volume Skin Surveillance	Emergency Care Exercise Promotion Intravenous (IV) Insertion Intravenous (IV) Therapy Laboratory Data Interpretation Phlebotomy: Arterial Blood Sample Phlebotomy: Venous Blood Sample Positioning: Wheelchair Resuscitation Resuscitation: Neonate

NURSING DIAGNOSIS: Tissue Perfusion: Renal, Ineffective

DEFINITION: Decrease in oxygen resulting in the failure to nourish the tissues at the capillary level.

Outcome	Major Interventions	Suggested Interventions	Optional Interventions
Circulation Status			
DEFINITION: Unobstructed, unidirectional blood flow at an appropriate pressure through large vessels of the systemic and pulmonary circuits	Hypovolemia Management	Bleeding Precautions Bleeding Reduction Fluid Monitoring Hemorrhage Control Laboratory Data Interpretation Shock Management Shock Management: Vasogenic Shock Management: Volume Shock Prevention	Bedside Laboratory Testing Blood Products Administration Fluid Resuscitation Hemodynamic Regulation Intravenous (IV) Insertion Intravenous (IV) Therapy Invasive Hemodynamic Monitoring Oxygen Therapy Resuscitation

Continued

Outcome	Major Interventions	Suggested Interventions	Optional Interventions
Electrolyte & Acid/Base Balance			
DEFINITION: Balance of the electrolytes and non-electrolytes in the intracellular and extracellular compartments of the body	Electrolyte Management Fluid/Electrolyte Management	Acid-Base Management Acid-Base Management: Metabolic Acidosis Acid-Base Management: Metabolic Alkalosis Acid-Base Monitoring Electrolyte Monitoring Emergency Care Fluid Management Fluid Monitoring Hemodialysis Therapy Hemodynamic Regulation Hemofiltration Therapy Hypovolemia Management Laboratory Data Interpretation Peritoneal Dialysis Therapy Vital Signs Monitoring	Electrolyte Management: Hypercalcemia Electrolyte Management: Hyperkalemia Electrolyte Management: Hypermagnesemia Electrolyte Management: Hypernatremia Intravenous (IV) Insertion Intravenous (IV) Therapy Medication Administration Medication Management Phlebotomy: Arterial Blood Sample Phlebotomy: Venous Blood Sample Specimen Management Total Parenteral Nutrition (TPN) Administration

Outcome	Major Interventions	Suggested Interventions	Optional Interventions
Fluid Balance			
DEFINITION: Water balance in the intracellular and extracellular compartments of the body	Fluid/Electrolyte Management Fluid Management Hemodialysis Therapy Peritoneal Dialysis Therapy	Bedside Laboratory Testing Electrolyte Management Electrolyte Monitoring Fluid Monitoring Fluid Resuscitation Hemofiltration Therapy Hypervolemia Management Hypovolemia Management Intravenous (IV) Insertion Intravenous (IV) Therapy Laboratory Data Interpretation Medication Administration Medication Management Urinary Elimination Management Vital Signs Monitoring	Hemodynamic Regulation Invasive Hemodynamic Monitoring Peripherally Inserted Central (PIC) Catheter Care Shock Management Shock Management: Volume Shock Prevention Surveillance Total Parenteral Nutrition (TPN) Administration Venous Access Device (VAD) Maintenance

Continued

Outcome	Major Interventions	Suggested Interventions	Optional Interventions
Fluid Overload Severity			
DEFINITION: Severity of excess fluids in the intracellular and extracellular compartments of the body	Fluid/Electrolyte Management Hemodialysis Therapy Hemofiltration Therapy Peritoneal Dialysis Therapy	Acid-Base Management Acid-Base Monitoring Dialysis Access Maintenance Emergency Care Fluid Management Fluid Monitoring Hypervolemia Management Vital Signs Monitoring	Hemodynamic Regulation Invasive Hemodynamic Monitoring Laboratory Data Interpretation Medication Administration Nutrition Management
Kidney Function			
DEFINITION: Filtration of blood and elimination of metabolic waste products through the formation of urine	Acid-Base Monitoring Electrolyte Management Fluid/Electrolyte Management	Acid-Base Management Bedside Laboratory Testing Electrolyte Management: Hypercalcemia Electrolyte Management: Hyperkalemia Electrolyte Management: Hypermagnesemia Electrolyte Management: Hypernatremia Electrolyte Management: Hyperphosphatemia Fluid Management Fluid Monitoring Laboratory Data Interpretation	Dialysis Access Maintenance Hemodialysis Therapy Nutrition Management Medication Management Peritoneal Dialysis Therapy Teaching: Disease Process Teaching: Prescribed Diet Teaching: Prescribed Medication Teaching: Procedure/ Treatment Urinary Catheterization

Outcome	Major Interventions	Suggested Interventions	Optional Interventions
Tissue Perfusion: Abdominal Organs			
DEFINITION: Adequacy of blood flow through the small vessels of the abdominal viscera to maintain organ function	Fluid/Electrolyte Management Hypovolemia Management	Acid-Base Management Acid-Base Monitoring Electrolyte Management Electrolyte Monitoring Fluid Resuscitation Intravenous (IV) Insertion Intravenous (IV) Therapy Laboratory Data Interpretation Medication Management Shock Management Shock Management: Volume Shock Prevention Vital Signs Monitoring	Bleeding Reduction: Gastrointestinal Emergency Care Hemorrhage Control Oxygen Therapy Specimen Management

NURSING DIAGNOSIS: Transfer Ability, Impaired

DEFINITION: Limitation of independent movement between two nearby surfaces.

Outcome	Major Interventions	Suggested Interventions	Optional Interventions
Balance			
DEFINITION: Ability to maintain body equilibrium	Exercise Therapy: Balance Fall Prevention	Body Mechanics Promotion Energy Management Exercise Therapy: Joint Mobility Exercise Therapy: Muscle Control	Environmental Management: Safety Exercise Promotion Positioning Teaching: Prescribed Activity/Exercise Weight Management
Body Positioning: Self-Initiated			
DEFINITION: Ability to change own body position independently with or without assistive device	Exercise Promotion: Strength Training Exercise Therapy: Muscle Control	Body Mechanics Promotion Exercise Promotion Exercise Promotion: Stretching Exercise Therapy: Ambulation Exercise Therapy: Balance Exercise Therapy: Joint Mobility Self-Care Assistance: Transfer Teaching: Prescribed Activity/Exercise	Energy Management Fall Prevention Pain Management Positioning Self-Care Assistance: Toileting Unilateral Neglect Management

Outcome	Major Interventions	Suggested Interventions	Optional Interventions
Coordinated Movement DEFINITION: Ability of muscles to work together voluntarily for purposeful movement	Exercise Promotion: Strength Training Exercise Therapy: Balance Exercise Therapy: Muscle Control	Body Mechanics Promotion Energy Management Exercise Promotion Exercise Promotion: Stretching Self-Care Assistance: Transfer	Medication Management Nutrition Management Pain Management Sleep Enhancement Weight Management
Mobility DEFINITION: Ability to move purposefully in own environment independently with or without assistive device	Exercise Therapy: Ambulation Exercise Therapy: Balance Exercise Therapy: Joint Mobility Exercise Therapy: Muscle Control	Body Mechanics Promotion Energy Management Exercise Promotion: Strength Training Exercise Promotion: Stretching Fall Prevention Positioning: Wheelchair	Analgesic Administration Environmental Management: Safety Exercise Promotion Medication Management Mutual Goal Setting Nutrition Management Pain Management Simple Relaxation Therapy Sleep Enhancement Teaching: Prescribed Activity/Exercise

Continued

Outcome	Major Interventions	Suggested Interventions	Optional Interventions
Transfer Performance			
DEFINITION: Ability to change body location independently with or without assistive device	Exercise Promotion: Strength Training Self-Care Assistance: Transfer	Body Mechanics Promotion Energy Management Exercise Promotion Exercise Promotion: Stretching Exercise Therapy: Balance Exercise Therapy: Joint Mobility Exercise Therapy: Muscle Control Fall Prevention Positioning Positioning: Wheelchair Teaching: Prescribed Activity/Exercise Teaching: Psychomotor Skill	Environmental Management: Safety Pain Management Self-Care Assistance Self-Care Assistance: Toileting Surveillance: Safety Weight Management

NURSING DIAGNOSIS: Unilateral Neglect

DEFINITION: Lack of awareness and attention to one side of the body.

Outcome	Major Interventions	Suggested Interventions	Optional Interventions
Adaptation to Physical Disability DEFINITION: Adaptive response to a significant functional challenge due to a physical disability	Anticipatory Guidance Coping Enhancement Unilateral Neglect Management	Amputation Care Body Image Enhancement Emotional Support Environmental Management: Safety Self-Care Assistance Touch	Caregiver Support Mutual Goal Setting Support System Enhancement Teaching: Disease Process Teaching: Individual
Body Positioning: Self-Initiated DEFINITION: Ability to change own body position independently with or without assistive device	Self-Care Assistance Unilateral Neglect Management	Body Mechanics Promotion Exercise Promotion Exercise Promotion: Stretching Exercise Therapy: Ambulation Exercise Therapy: Balance Exercise Therapy: Joint Mobility Exercise Therapy: Muscle Control Teaching: Individual	Fall Prevention Lower Extremity Monitoring Pain Management Peripheral Sensation Management Positioning

Continued

Outcome	Major Interventions	Suggested Interventions	Optional Interventions
Coordinated Movement DEFINITION: Ability of muscles to work together voluntarily for purposeful movement	Exercise Therapy: Muscle Control Unilateral Neglect Management	Environmental Management: Safety Exercise Promotion: Stretching Exercise Therapy: Balance Exercise Therapy: Muscle Control Self-Care Assistance	Cerebral Perfusion Promotion Communication Enhancement: Visual Deficit Fall Prevention
Self-Care: Activities of Daily Living (ADL) DEFINITION: Ability to perform the most basic physical tasks and personal care activities independently with or without assistive device	Self-Care Assistance	Self-Care Assistance: Bathing/Hygiene Self-Care Assistance: Dressing/Grooming Self-Care Assistance: Feeding Self-Care Assistance: Toileting	Environmental Management: Safety Exercise Promotion Exercise Promotion: Stretching Exercise Therapy: Ambulation Exercise Therapy: Balance Exercise Therapy: Joint Mobility Exercise Therapy: Muscle Control Fall Prevention Home Maintenance Assistance

NURSING DIAGNOSIS: Urinary Elimination, Impaired

DEFINITION: Disturbance in urine elimination.

Outcome	Major Interventions	Suggested Interventions	Optional Interventions
Urinary Continence DEFINITION: Control of elimination of urine from the bladder	Urinary Bladder Training Urinary Elimination Management	Fluid Management Fluid Monitoring Medication Administration Medication Management Medication Prescribing Pelvic Muscle Exercise Pessary Management Prompted Voiding Self-Care Assistance: Toileting Teaching: Prescribed Medication Teaching: Procedure/ Treatment Urinary Catheterization Urinary Catheterization: Intermittent Urinary Habit Training Urinary Incontinence Care Urinary Incontinence Care: Enuresis	Anxiety Reduction Biofeedback Bladder Irrigation Environmental Management Infection Control Infection Protection Perineal Care Postpartal Care Skin Surveillance Tube Care: Urinary Urinary Retention Care

Continued

Outcome	Major Interventions	Suggested Interventions	Optional Interventions
Urinary Elimination			
DEFINITION: Collection and discharge of urine	Urinary Elimination Management	Fluid Management Fluid Monitoring Medication Administration Medication Management Medication Prescribing Specimen Management Teaching: Prescribed Medication Urinary Catheterization Urinary Catheterization: Intermittent Urinary Incontinence Care Urinary Incontinence Care: Enuresis	Hemodialysis Therapy Pain Management Pelvic Muscle Exercise Prompted Voiding Tube Care: Urinary Urinary Retention Care Weight Management

NURSING DIAGNOSIS: Urinary Elimination, Readiness for Enhanced

DEFINITION: A pattern of urinary functions that is sufficient for meeting eliminatory needs and can be strengthened.

Outcome	Major Interventions	Suggested Interventions	Optional Interventions
Urinary Elimination			
DEFINITION: Collection and discharge of urine	Urinary Elimination Management	Environmental Management	Pain Management
		Fluid Management	Postpartal Care
		Infection Protection	
		Medication Management	
		Pelvic Muscle Exercise	
		Self-Care Assistance: Toileting	
		Weight Management	

NURSING DIAGNOSIS: Urinary Incontinence: Functional

DEFINITION: Inability of usually continent person to reach toilet in time to avoid unintentional loss of urine.

Outcome	Major Interventions	Suggested Interventions	Optional Interventions
Self-Care: Toileting			
DEFINITION: Ability to toilet self independently with or without assistive device	Self-Care Assistance: Toileting	Environmental Management Prompted Voiding Urinary Habit Training	Perineal Care Urinary Incontinence Care
Urinary Continence			
DEFINITION: Control of elimination of urine from the bladder	Prompted Voiding Urinary Habit Training	Environmental Management Fluid Management Pelvic Muscle Exercise Self-Care Assistance: Toileting Urinary Elimination Management Urinary Incontinence Care	Bathing Communication Enhancement: Visual Deficit Dressing Exercise Promotion Exercise Therapy: Ambulation Perineal Care Self-Awareness Enhancement Surveillance: Safety
Urinary Elimination			
DEFINITION: Collection and discharge of urine	Urinary Elimination Management	Prompted Voiding Self-Care Assistance: Toileting Urinary Habit Training	Fluid Management Perineal Care Urinary Incontinence

NURSING DIAGNOSIS: Urinary Incontinence: Reflex

DEFINITION: Involuntary loss of urine at somewhat predictable intervals when a specific bladder volume is reached.

Outcome	Major Interventions	Suggested Interventions	Optional Interventions
Neurological Status: Autonomic			
DEFINITION: Ability of the autonomic nervous system to coordinate visceral and homeostatic function	Urinary Bladder Training Urinary Catheterization: Intermittent	Dysreflexia Management Fluid Management Teaching: Procedure/ Treatment Urinary Elimination Management Urinary Retention Care	Tube Care: Urinary Urinary Catheterization Urinary Incontinence Care
Tissue Integrity: Skin & Mucous Membranes			
DEFINITION: Structural intactness and normal physiological function of skin and mucous membranes	Perineal Care Urinary Incontinence Care	Bathing Self-Care Assistance: Toileting	Teaching: Toilet Training

Continued

Outcome	Major Interventions	Suggested Interventions	Optional Interventions
Urinary Continence			
DEFINITION: Control of elimination of urine from the bladder	Urinary Bladder Training Urinary Catheterization: Intermittent	Pelvic Muscle Exercise Tube Care: Urinary Urinary Catheterization Urinary Elimination Management Urinary Habit Training Urinary Incontinence Care Urinary Retention Care	Fluid Management Fluid Monitoring Self-Care Assistance: Toileting Teaching: Procedure/ Treatment
Urinary Elimination			
DEFINITION: Collection and discharge of urine	Urinary Elimination Management	Pelvic Muscle Exercise Self-Care Assistance: Toileting Urinary Bladder Training Urinary Catheterization: Intermittent	Fluid Management Tube Care: Urinary Urinary Catheterization Urinary Incontinence Care Urinary Retention Care

NURSING DIAGNOSIS: Urinary Incontinence: Stress

DEFINITION: Loss of less than 50 mL of urine occurring with increased abdominal pressure.

Outcome	Major Interventions	Suggested Interventions	Optional Interventions
Urinary Continence DEFINITION: Control of elimination of urine from the bladder	Pelvic Muscle Exercise Urinary Incontinence Care	Biofeedback Medication Management Pessary Management Teaching: Individual Urinary Elimination Management Urinary Habit Training Weight Management	Environmental Management Perineal Care Postpartal Care Self-Care Assistance: Toileting Teaching: Prescribed Medication
Urinary Elimination DEFINITION: Collection and discharge of urine	Urinary Elimination Management	Medication Administration Pelvic Muscle Exercise Teaching: Individual Teaching: Prescribed Medication Urinary Habit Training Urinary Incontinence Care	Self-Care Assistance: Toileting

NURSING DIAGNOSIS: Urinary Incontinence: Total

DEFINITION: Continuous and unpredictable loss of urine.

Outcome	Major Interventions	Suggested Interventions	Optional Interventions

Tissue Integrity: Skin & Mucous Membranes
DEFINITION: Structural intactness and normal physiological function of skin and mucous membranes
	Skin Surveillance
	Urinary
	  Incontinence Care
		Bathing
		Perineal Care
		Skin Care:
		  Topical
		  Treatments
			Medication
			  Administration:
			  Skin
			Self-Care Assistance:
			  Toileting

Urinary Continence
DEFINITION: Control of elimination of urine from the bladder
	Urinary
	  Incontinence Care
		Environmental
		  Management
		Self-Care
		  Assistance:
		  Toileting
		Tube Care: Urinary
		Urinary
		  Catheterization
			Fluid Management
			Fluid Monitoring
			Teaching:
			  Procedure/
			  Treatment

Urinary Elimination
DEFINITION: Collection and discharge of urine
	Urinary Elimination
	  Management
		Self-Care
		  Assistance:
		  Toileting
		Urinary
		  Catheterization
		Urinary
		  Incontinence Care
			Fluid Management
			Tube Care: Urinary

NURSING DIAGNOSIS: Urinary Incontinence: Urge

DEFINITION: Involuntary passage of urine occurring soon after a strong sense of urgency to void.

Outcome	Major Interventions	Suggested Interventions	Optional Interventions
Self-Care: Toileting			
DEFINITION: Ability to toilet self independently with or without assistive device	Self-Care Assistance: Toileting	Environmental Management Fluid Management Urinary Elimination Management	Perineal Care Urinary Incontinence Care
Urinary Continence			
DEFINITION: Control of elimination of urine from the bladder	Urinary Habit Training Urinary Incontinence Care	Environmental Management Fluid Management Fluid Monitoring Medication Management Urinary Elimination Management	Bathing Perineal Care Self-Care Assistance: Toileting Teaching: Prescribed Medication Teaching: Toilet Training Tube Care: Urinary Urinary Catheterization Urinary Catheterization: Intermittent
Urinary Elimination			
DEFINITION: Collection and discharge of urine	Urinary Elimination Management Urinary Habit Training	Medication Administration Self-Care Assistance: Toileting Urinary Incontinence Care	Fluid Management Pelvic Muscle Exercise

NURSING DIAGNOSIS: Urinary Retention

DEFINITION: Incomplete emptying of the bladder.

Outcome	Major Interventions	Suggested Interventions	Optional Interventions
Urinary Continence			
DEFINITION: Control of elimination of urine from the bladder	Urinary Catheterization Urinary Retention Care	Bladder Irrigation Fluid Management Fluid Monitoring Medication Administration Medication Management Tube Care: Urinary Urinary Catheterization: Intermittent Urinary Elimination Management Urinary Incontinence Care	Anxiety Reduction Exercise Promotion Exercise Therapy: Ambulation Exercise Therapy: Muscle Control Perineal Care Postpartal Care Simple Relaxation Therapy
Urinary Elimination			
DEFINITION: Collection and discharge of urine	Urinary Elimination Management Urinary Retention Care	Fluid Management Fluid Monitoring Medication Administration Medication Management Specimen Management Urinary Catheterization: Intermittent	Exercise Promotion Self-Care Assistance: Toileting Tube Care: Urinary Urinary Catheterization

NURSING DIAGNOSIS: Ventilation, Impaired Spontaneous

DEFINITION: Decreased energy reserves result in an individual's inability to maintain breathing adequate to support life.

Outcome	Major Interventions	Suggested Interventions	Optional Interventions
Allergic Response: Systemic			
DEFINITION: Severity of systemic hypersensitive immune response to a specific environmental (exogenous) antigen	Airway Management Emergency Care Medication Administration: Intramuscular [IM] Medication Administration: Intravenous [IV]	Airway Suctioning Allergy Management Anxiety Reduction Fluid Management Intravenous [IV] Insertion Intravenous [IV] Therapy Oxygen Therapy	Aspiration Precautions Calming Technique Positioning Resuscitation Resuscitation: Neonate Vital Signs Monitoring
Mechanical Ventilation Response: Adult			
DEFINITION: Alveolar exchange and tissue perfusion are supported by mechanical ventilation	Aspiration Precautions Mechanical Ventilation Oxygen Therapy	Airway Management Airway Suctioning Anxiety Reduction Calming Technique Emotional Support Environmental Management: Comfort Environmental Management: Safety Infection Protection Oral Health Maintenance Respiratory Monitoring Skin Surveillance Vital Signs Monitoring	Bed Rest Care Chest Physiotherapy Energy Management Fluid Management Infection Control Mechanical Ventilatory Weaning Patient Rights Protection Physical Restraint Pressure Management Surveillance: Safety

Continued

Outcome	Major Interventions	Suggested Interventions	Optional Interventions
Respiratory Status: Gas Exchange DEFINITION: Alveolar exchange of carbon dioxide and oxygen to maintain arterial blood gas concentrations	Oxygen Therapy Respiratory Monitoring Ventilation Assistance	Acid-Base Management Acid-Base Management: Respiratory Acidosis Acid-Base Management: Respiratory Alkalosis Acid-Base Monitoring Airway Insertion and Stabilization Airway Management Airway Suctioning Anxiety Reduction Chest Physiotherapy Energy Management Positioning	Aspiration Precautions Cough Enhancement Fluid/Electrolyte Management Fluid Management Fluid Monitoring Infection Control Infection Protection Intravenous (IV) Insertion Intravenous (IV) Therapy Laboratory Data Interpretation

Outcome	Major Interventions	Suggested Interventions	Optional Interventions
Respiratory Status: Ventilation			
DEFINITION: Movement of air in and out of the lungs	Airway Management Artificial Airway Management Respiratory Monitoring Ventilation Assistance	Acid-Base Monitoring Airway Insertion and Stabilization Airway Suctioning Anxiety Reduction Aspiration Precautions Calming Technique Chest Physiotherapy Emotional Support Energy Management Fluid Management Oxygen Therapy Positioning Resuscitation: Neonate Vital Signs Monitoring	Coping Enhancement Emergency Care Endotracheal Extubation Phlebotomy: Arterial Blood Sample Security Enhancement Surveillance Technology Management Tube Care: Chest

Continued

Outcome	Major Interventions	Suggested Interventions	Optional Interventions
Vital Signs			
DEFINITION: Extent to which temperature, pulse, respiration, and blood pressure are within normal range	Respiratory Monitoring Vital Signs Monitoring	Acid-Base Management Airway Management Anxiety Reduction Environmental Management Fluid/Electrolyte Management Fluid Management Intravenous (IV) Insertion Intravenous (IV) Therapy Medication Administration Medication Management Ventilation Assistance	Emergency Care Infection Control Infection Protection Oxygen Therapy Pain Management Resuscitation

NURSING DIAGNOSIS: Ventilatory Weaning Response, Dysfunctional

DEFINITION: Inability to adjust to lowered levels of mechanical ventilator support that interrupts and prolongs the weaning process.

Outcome	Major Interventions	Suggested Interventions	Optional Interventions
Anxiety Level			
DEFINITION: Severity of manifested apprehension, tension, or uneasiness arising from an unidentifiable source	Anxiety Reduction Preparatory Sensory Information	Calming Technique Coping Enhancement Distraction Medication Administration Music Therapy Presence Security Enhancement Simple Guided Imagery Simple Relaxation Therapy	Biofeedback Emotional Support Environmental Management: Comfort

Continued

Outcome	Major Interventions	Suggested Interventions	Optional Interventions
Mechanical Ventilation Weaning Response: Adult			
DEFINITION: Respiratory and psychological adjustment to progressive removal of mechanical ventilation	Mechanical Ventilation Mechanical Ventilatory Weaning Ventilation Assistance	Acid-Base Management Airway Management Anxiety Reduction Artificial Airway Management Aspiration Precautions Calming Technique Distraction Environmental Management: Comfort Environmental Management: Safety Preparatory Sensation Information	Emotional Support Energy Management Music Therapy Phlebotomy: Arterial Blood Sample Presence Sleep Enhancement Surveillance

Outcome	Major Interventions	Suggested Interventions	Optional Interventions
Respiratory Status: Gas Exchange			
DEFINITION: Alveolar exchange of carbon dioxide and oxygen to maintain arterial blood gas concentrations	Respiratory Monitoring Ventilation Assistance	Acid-Base Management: Respiratory Acidosis Acid-Base Management: Respiratory Alkalosis Acid-Base Monitoring Airway Management Anxiety Reduction Artificial Airway Management Aspiration Precautions Oxygen Therapy Positioning	Airway Insertion and Stabilization Airway Suctioning Chest Physiotherapy Cough Enhancement Energy Management Laboratory Data Interpretation Phlebotomy: Arterial Blood Sample
Respiratory Status: Ventilation			
DEFINITION: Movement of air in and out of the lungs	Mechanical Ventilation Mechanical Ventilatory Weaning Respiratory Monitoring	Airway Insertion and Stabilization Airway Management Airway Suctioning Artificial Airway Management Aspiration Precautions Energy Management Environmental Management: Safety Positioning Ventilation Assistance	Acid-Base Monitoring Anxiety Reduction Calming Technique Cough Enhancement Emotional Support Oxygen Therapy Presence Simple Relaxation Therapy

Continued

Outcome	Major Interventions	Suggested Interventions	Optional Interventions
Vital Signs			
DEFINITION: Extent to which temperature, pulse, respiration, and blood pressure are within normal range	Respiratory Monitoring Vital Signs Monitoring	Airway Management Anxiety Reduction Environmental Management Medication Administration Medication Management Ventilation Assistance	Environmental Management: Comfort Music Therapy Oxygen Therapy Pain Management Resuscitation Simple Relaxation Therapy

NURSING DIAGNOSIS: Walking, Impaired

DEFINITION: Limitation of independent movement within the environment on foot.

Outcome	Major Interventions	Suggested Interventions	Optional Interventions
Ambulation			
DEFINITION: Ability to walk from place to place independently with or without assistive device	Exercise Therapy: Ambulation	Body Mechanics Promotion Energy Management Exercise Promotion Exercise Promotion: Strength Training Exercise Promotion: Stretching Exercise Therapy: Balance Exercise Therapy: Joint Mobility Exercise Therapy: Muscle Control Teaching: Prescribed Activity/Exercise Transport	Environmental Management Environmental Management: Safety Fall Prevention Lower Extremity Monitoring Medication Management Pain Management Positioning Weight Reduction Assistance
Balance			
DEFINITION: Ability to maintain body equilibrium	Exercise Therapy Ambulation Exercise Therapy: Balance	Environmental Management: Safety Exercise Promotion: Strength Training Exercise Therapy: Muscle Control Fall Prevention Teaching: Prescribed Activity/Exercise	Energy Management Exercise Therapy: Joint Mobility

Continued

Outcome	Major Interventions	Suggested Interventions	Optional Interventions
Coordinated Movement			
DEFINITION: Ability of muscles to work together voluntarily for purposeful movement	Exercise Therapy: Muscle Control	Body Mechanics Promotion Exercise Promotion: Strength Training Exercise Therapy: Ambulation Exercise Therapy: Balance	Exercise Promotion Exercise Promotion: Stretching Pain Management
Endurance			
DEFINITION: Capacity to sustain activity	Energy Management	Exercise Promotion Nutrition Management Sleep Enhancement Teaching: Prescribed Activity/Exercise	Environmental Management Exercise Therapy: Ambulation Exercise Therapy: Balance Exercise Therapy: Joint Mobility Exercise Therapy: Muscle Control Mutual Goal Setting Weight Management
Joint Movement: Ankle, Hip, Knee			
DEFINITION: Active range of motion of _____ (specify joint) with self-initiated movement	Exercise Therapy: Joint Mobility	Exercise Promotion Exercise Promotion: Strength Training Exercise Promotion: Stretching Exercise Therapy: Ambulation	Energy Management Fall Prevention Pain Management

Outcome	Major Interventions	Suggested Interventions	Optional Interventions
Mobility			
DEFINITION: Ability to move purposefully in own environment independently with or without assistive device	Exercise Therapy: Ambulation	Body Mechanics Promotion Energy Management Exercise Promotion: Strength Training Exercise Therapy: Balance Exercise Therapy: Joint Mobility Exercise Therapy: Muscle Control	Analgesic Administration Environmental Management: Safety Exercise Promotion Exercise Promotion: Stretching Pain Management Positioning Teaching: Prescribed Activity/Exercise

W

W

NURSING DIAGNOSIS: Wandering

DEFINITION: Meandering, aimless, or repetitive locomotion that exposes the individual to harm; frequently incongruent with boundaries, limits, or obstacles.

Outcome	Major Interventions	Suggested Interventions	Optional Interventions
Anxiety Level			
DEFINITION: Severity of manifested apprehension, tension, or uneasiness arising from an unidentifiable source	Anxiety Reduction Dementia Management	Behavior Management: Overactivity/ Inattention Calming Technique Elopement Precautions Medication Management Pain Management	Area Restriction Environmental Management: Safety Patient Rights Protection Surveillance: Safety
Fall Prevention Behavior			
DEFINITION: Personal or family caregiver actions to minimize risk factors that might precipitate falls in the personal environment	Dementia Management Fall Prevention	Area Restriction Elopement Precautions Environmental Management: Safety Surveillance: Safety	Behavior Management Medication Management
Safe Home Environment			
DEFINITION: Physical arrangements to minimize environmental factors that might cause physical harm or injury in the home	Elopement Precautions Environmental Management: Safety Surveillance: Safety	Fall Prevention Limit Setting Medication Management	Family Involvement Promotion Pain Management Reality Orientation Respite Care Self-Care Assistance Teaching: Toddler Safety

"Risk for" Diagnoses Linked to NOC and NIC

NURSING DIAGNOSIS: Activity Intolerance, Risk for

DEFINITION: At risk for experiencing insufficient physiological or psychological energy to endure or complete required or desired daily activities.

Outcome	Major Interventions	Suggested Interventions	Optional Interventions
Activity Tolerance DEFINITION: Physiologic response to energy-consuming movements with daily activities	Energy Management Exercise Promotion Exercise Promotion: Strength Training	Activity Therapy Exercise Therapy: Ambulation Exercise Therapy: Joint Mobility Exercise Therapy: Muscle Control Nutrition Management Pain Management Security Enhancement Sleep Enhancement Smoking Cessation Assistance Vital Signs Monitoring	Dementia Management Emotional Support Hope Instillation Medication Management Oxygen Therapy Self-Esteem Enhancement Teaching: Prescribed Activity/Exercise Weight Reduction Assistance

Continued

Outcome	Major Interventions	Suggested Interventions	Optional Interventions
Endurance DEFINITION: Capacity to sustain activity	Energy Management Exercise Promotion: Strength Training	Activity Therapy Emotional Support Exercise Promotion Exercise Promotion: Stretching Health Screening Nutrition Management Oxygen Therapy Pain Management Risk Identification Sleep Enhancement Smoking Cessation Assistance Teaching: Prescribed Activity/Exercise Teaching: Prescribed Diet Vital Signs Monitoring	Cardiac Care: Rehabilitative Counseling Dementia Management Eating Disorders Management Exercise Therapy: Ambulation Exercise Therapy: Balance Exercise Therapy: Joint Mobility Exercise Therapy: Muscle Control Mood Management Mutual Goal Setting Support System Enhancement Weight Management

Outcome	Major Interventions	Suggested Interventions	Optional Interventions
Energy Conservation DEFINITION: Personal actions to manage energy for initiating and sustaining activity	Energy Management	Body Mechanics Promotion Environmental Management Environmental Management: Comfort Exercise Promotion Nutrition Management Nutritional Monitoring Pain Management Self-Care Assistance: IADL Sleep Enhancement Teaching: Prescribed Activity/Exercise	Exercise Therapy: Ambulation Exercise Therapy: Balance Exercise Therapy: Joint Mobility Exercise Therapy: Muscle Control Mood Management Oxygen Therapy Simple Relaxation Therapy Smoking Cessation Assistance Weight Management

For interventions and outcomes related to specific risk factors, refer to the following diagnoses: Breathing Pattern, Ineffective; Cardiac Output, Decreased; Failure to Thrive, Adult; Fatigue; Gas Exchange, Impaired; Health Maintenance, Ineffective.

NURSING DIAGNOSIS: Aspiration, Risk for

DEFINITION: At risk for entry of gastrointestinal secretions, oropharyngeal secretions, solids, or fluids, into tracheobronchial passages.

Outcome	Major Interventions	Suggested Interventions	Optional Interventions
Aspiration Prevention DEFINITION: Personal actions to prevent the passage of fluid and solid particles into the lung	Aspiration Precautions Swallowing Therapy Vomiting Management	Airway Suctioning Amnioinfusion Artificial Airway Management Gastrointestinal Intubation Positioning Postanesthesia Care Respiratory Monitoring Resuscitation: Neonate Sedation Management Surveillance Teaching: Infant Safety Teaching: Toddler Safety	Enteral Tube Feeding Feeding Medication Administration: Enteral Neurologic Monitoring Vital Signs Monitoring
Respiratory Status: Ventilation DEFINITION: Movement of air in and out of the lungs	Airway Management Aspiration Precautions Respiratory Monitoring	Airway Suctioning Mechanical Ventilation Positioning	Anxiety Reduction Chest Physiotherapy Cough Enhancement Mechanical Ventilatory Weaning

Outcome	Major Interventions	Suggested Interventions	Optional Interventions
Swallowing Status DEFINITION: Safe passage of fluids and/or solids from the mouth to the stomach	Aspiration Precautions Swallowing Therapy	Enteral Tube Feeding Feeding Oral Health Maintenance Positioning Self-Care Assistance: Feeding Surveillance	Airway Management Airway Suctioning Vomiting Management

For interventions and outcomes related to specific risk factors, refer to the following diagnoses: Confusion, Acute; Confusion, Chronic; Infant Feeding Pattern, Ineffective; Physical Mobility, Impaired; Self-Care Deficit: Feeding; Swallowing, Impaired.

NURSING DIAGNOSIS: Autonomic Dysreflexia, Risk for

DEFINITION: At risk for life-threatening, uninhibited response of the sympathetic nervous system, post spinal shock, in an individual with spinal cord injury or lesion at T6 or above (has been demonstrated in patients with injuries at T7 and T8).

Outcome	Major Interventions	Suggested Interventions	Optional Interventions
Neurological Status: Autonomic			
DEFINITION: Ability of the autonomic nervous system to coordinate visceral and homeostatic function	Dysreflexia Management Neurologic Monitoring Vital Signs Monitoring	Bowel Management Emergency Care Fever Treatment Fluid Management Fluid Monitoring Infection Control Medication Administration Medication Management Positioning Shock Management Skin Surveillance Temperature Regulation Urinary Retention Care	Anxiety Reduction Heat Exposure Treatment Infection Protection Intravenous (IV) Therapy Respiratory Monitoring Surveillance: Safety Urinary Catheterization Urinary Catheterization: Intermittent Urinary Elimination Management
Symptom Severity			
DEFINITION: Severity of perceived adverse changes in physical, emotional, and social functioning	Dysreflexia Management	Anxiety Reduction Medication Administration Pain Management Peripheral Sensation Management Positioning Pressure Management Temperature Regulation	Energy Management Flatulence Reduction Lower Extremity Monitoring Medication Management

Outcome	Major Interventions	Suggested Interventions	Optional Interventions
Vital Signs DEFINITION: Extent to which temperature, pulse, respiration, and blood pressure are within normal range	Dysreflexia Management Vital Signs Monitoring	Dysrhythmia Management Emergency Care Environmental Management Fever Treatment Fluid Management Heat Exposure Treatment Hemodynamic Regulation Medication Administration Medication Management Pain Management Shock Management Shock Prevention Temperature Regulation	Airway Management Anxiety Reduction Exercise Promotion Infection Protection Intravenous (IV) Insertion Intravenous (IV) Therapy Medication Prescribing Nutrition Management Respiratory Monitoring

For interventions and outcomes related to specific risk factors, refer to the following diagnoses: Body Temperature, Risk for Imbalanced; Constipation; Hyperthermia; Infection, Risk for; Knowledge, Deficient (Specify); Pain, Acute; Sexual Dysfunction; Skin Integrity, Impaired; Thermoregulation, Ineffective; Urinary Retention.

NURSING DIAGNOSIS: Body Temperature, Risk for Imbalanced

DEFINITION: At risk for failure to maintain body temperature within normal range.

Outcome	Major Interventions	Suggested Interventions	Optional Interventions
Thermoregulation			
DEFINITION: Balance among heat production, gain, and heat loss	Temperature Regulation Temperature Regulation: Intraoperative Vital Signs Monitoring	Cerebral Edema Management Environmental Management Fever Treatment Fluid Management Fluid Monitoring Heat Exposure Treatment Malignant Hyperthermia Precautions Medication Administration Postanesthesia Care	Bathing Emergency Care Energy Management Environmental Management: Comfort Fluid Monitoring Heat/Cold Application Hemodynamic Regulation
Thermoregulation: Newborn			
DEFINITION: Balance among heat production, heat gain, and heat loss during the first 28 days of life	Newborn Care Temperature Regulation Vital Signs Monitoring	Environmental Management Fluid Management Newborn Monitoring	Environmental Management: Comfort Fever Treatment Heat Exposure Treatment Parent Education: Infant Phototherapy: Neonate Resuscitation: Neonate

For interventions and outcomes related to the specific risk factors, refer to the following diagnoses: Fluid Volume Deficient; Infant Behavior, Disorganized; Infection, Risk for; Protection, Ineffective; Skin Integrity, Impaired; Surgical Recovery, Delayed.

NURSING DIAGNOSIS: Caregiver Role Strain, Risk for

DEFINITION: Caregiver is vulnerable for felt difficulty in performing the family caregiver role.

Outcome	Major Interventions	Suggested Interventions	Optional Interventions
Caregiver Emotional Health	Caregiver Support	Active Listening	Counseling
DEFINITION: Emotional well-being of a family care provider while caring for a family member	Emotional Support Respite Care	Anger Control Assistance Anticipatory Guidance Coping Enhancement Decision-Making Support Family Involvement Promotion Grief Work Facilitation Guilt Work Facilitation Hope Instillation Socialization Enhancement Spiritual Support	Family Integrity Promotion Family Mobilization Family Process Maintenance Family Support Referral Simple Relaxation Therapy Support Group Support System Enhancement

Continued

Outcome	Major Interventions	Suggested Interventions	Optional Interventions
Caregiver Home Care Readiness			
DEFINITION: Extent of preparedness of a caregiver to assume responsibility for the health care of a family member in the home	Caregiver Support Family Involvement Promotion Parenting Promotion	Anticipatory Guidance Anxiety Reduction Coping Enhancement Decision-Making Support Discharge Planning Emotional Support Environmental Management: Home Preparation Family Mobilization Family Process Maintenance Family Support Health System Guidance Home Maintenance Assistance Normalization Promotion Parent Education: Adolescent Parent Education: Childrearing Family Parent Education: Infant Referral Respite Care Support System Enhancement	Financial Resource Assistance Insurance Authorization Teaching: Disease Process Teaching: Infant Nutrition Teaching: Infant Safety Teaching: Infant Stimulation Teaching: Prescribed Activity/Exercise Teaching: Prescribed Diet Teaching: Prescribed Medication Teaching: Procedure/ Treatment Teaching: Psychomotor Skill Teaching: Toddler Nutrition Teaching: Toddler Safety Teaching: Toilet Training

Outcome	Major Interventions	Suggested Interventions	Optional Interventions
Caregiver Physical Health			
DEFINITION: Physical well-being of a family care provider while caring for a family member	Energy Management Health Screening Respite Care	Coping Enhancement Family Mobilization Infection Protection Nutrition Management Risk Identification Sleep Enhancement Weight Management	Body Mechanics Promotion Caregiver Support Exercise Promotion Family Involvement Promotion Family Support Health System Guidance Medication Management Referral
Caregiver Stressors			
DEFINITION: Severity of biopsychosocial pressure on a family care provider caring for another over an extended period of time	Caregiver Support Coping Enhancement	Decision-Making Support Emotional Support Family Involvement Promotion Family Mobilization Family Support Home Maintenance Assistance Meditation Facilitation Normalization Promotion Recreation Therapy Respite Care Simple Relaxation Therapy Support Group Support System Enhancement	Active Listening Anticipatory Guidance Counseling Energy Management Family Integrity Promotion Family Process Maintenance Family Therapy Financial Resource Assistance Guilt Work Facilitation Referral Spiritual Support

Continued

Outcome	Major Interventions	Suggested Interventions	Optional Interventions
Caregiving Endurance Potential			
DEFINITION: Factors that promote family care provider continuance over an extended period of time	Caregiver Support Coping Enhancement	Decision-Making Support Energy Management Exercise Promotion Family Involvement Promotion Parenting Promotion Respite Care Spiritual Support Support Group Support System Enhancement	Assertiveness Training Emotional Support Family Mobilization Family Support Recreation Therapy Role Enhancement Simple Relaxation Therapy

Outcome	Major Interventions	Suggested Interventions	Optional Interventions
Parenting Performance DEFINITION: Parental actions to provide a child a nurturing and constructive physical, emotional, and social environment	Parent Education: Childrearing Family Parent Education: Infant Parenting Promotion	Abuse Protection Support: Child Anticipatory Guidance Coping Enhancement Counseling Family Integrity Promotion Family Mobilization Family Process Maintenance Family Support Parent Education: Adolescent Respite Care Risk Identification Role Enhancement Support System Enhancement	Emotional Support Family Therapy Health System Guidance Home Maintenance Assistance Self-Esteem Enhancement Socialization Enhancement Support Group

For interventions and outcomes related to specific risk factors, refer to the following diagnoses: Decisional Conflict (Specify); Diversional Activity, Deficient; Family Therapeutic Regimen Management, Ineffective; Family Processes, Interrupted; Fatigue; Grieving, Dysfunctional; Home Maintenance, Impaired; Hopelessness; Knowledge, Deficient (Specify); Parenteral Role Conflict; Powerlessness; Role Performance, Ineffective; Sleep Deprivation; Social Interaction, Impaired; Social Isolation; Sudden Infant Death Syndrome, Risk for.

NURSING DIAGNOSIS: Constipation, Risk for

DEFINITION: At risk for a decrease in normal frequency of defecation accompanied by difficult or incomplete passage of stool and/or passage of excessively hard, dry stool.

Outcome	Major Interventions	Suggested Interventions	Optional Interventions
Bowel Elimination			
DEFINITION: Formation and evacuation of stool	Constipation/ Impaction Management	Bowel Management	Exercise Therapy: Ambulation
		Bowel Training	Flatulence Reduction
		Diet Staging	Medication Administration: Oral
		Exercise Promotion	Ostomy Care
		Fluid Management	Pain Management
		Fluid Monitoring	Rectal Prolapse Management
		Medication Management	
		Medication Prescribing	
		Nutrition Management	
		Nutritional Monitoring	
Self-Care: Toileting			
DEFINITION: Ability to toilet self independently with or without assistive device	Self-Care Assistance: Toileting	Constipation/ Impaction Management	Anxiety Reduction
		Bowel Management	Exercise Promotion
		Bowel Training	Perineal Care
		Exercise Therapy: Ambulation	Simple Relaxation Therapy
		Exercise Therapy: Joint Mobility	

For interventions and outcomes related to specific risk factors, refer to the following diagnoses: Confusion, Chronic; Denial, Ineffective; Fluid Volume, Deficient; Health Maintenance, Ineffective; Mobility: Physical, Impaired; Nutrition: Imbalanced, Less Than Body Requirements; Self-Care Deficit: Feeding; Self-Care Deficit: Toileting; Sorrow: Chronic.

NURSING DIAGNOSIS: Development, Risk for Delayed

DEFINITION: At risk for delay of 25% or more in one or more of the areas of social or self-regulatory behavior, or cognitive, language, gross or fine motor skills.

Outcome	Major Interventions	Suggested Interventions	Optional Interventions
Child Development: 1 Month			
DEFINITION: Milestones of physical, cognitive, and psychosocial progression by 1 month of age	Attachment Promotion Newborn Care	Anticipatory Guidance Bottle Feeding Breastfeeding Assistance Environmental Management: Attachment Process Family Integrity Promotion: Childbearing Family Genetic Counseling Lactation Counseling Nonnutritive Sucking Teaching: Infant Safety Teaching: Infant Stimulation	Abuse Protection Support: Child Circumcision Care Family Involvement Promotion Home Maintenance Assistance Sibling Support Tube Care: Umbilical Line

Continued

Outcome	Major Interventions	Suggested Interventions	Optional Interventions
Child Development: 2 Months			
DEFINITION: Milestones of physical, cognitive, and psychosocial progression by 2 months of age	Infant Care Parent Education: Infant Teaching: Infant Safety	Anticipatory Guidance Bottle Feeding Breastfeeding Assistance Environmental Management: Attachment Process Family Integrity Promotion: Childbearing Family Immunization/ Vaccination Management	Abuse Protection Support: Child Caregiver Support Home Maintenance Assistance Nonnutritive Sucking Parent Education: Childrearing Family Sibling Support
Child Development: 4 Months			
DEFINITION: Milestones of physical, cognitive, and psychosocial progression by 4 months of age	Infant Care Parent Education: Infant	Anticipatory Guidance Bottle Feeding Family Integrity Promotion: Childbearing Family Family Involvement Promotion Family Process Maintenance Health Screening Parent Education: Childrearing Family Teaching: Infant Nutrition Teaching: Infant Safety	Abuse Protection Support: Child Caregiver Support Environmental Management: Attachment Process Family Support Immunization/ Vaccination Management Sibling Support

Outcome	Major Interventions	Suggested Interventions	Optional Interventions
Child Development: 6 Months			
DEFINITION: Milestones of physical, cognitive, and psychosocial progression by 6 months of age	Infant Care Teaching: Infant Nutrition	Anticipatory Guidance Bottle Feeding Family Integrity Promotion: Childbearing Family Family Involvement Promotion Family Process Maintenance Health Screening Nutrition Management Surveillance: Safety	Abuse Protection Support: Child Caregiver Support Environmental Management: Safety Family Support Immunization/ Vaccination Management Respite Care Sibling Support

Continued

Outcome	Major Interventions	Suggested Interventions	Optional Interventions
Child Development: 12 Months DEFINITION: Milestones of physical, cognitive, and psychosocial progression by 12 months of age	Infant Care Parent Education: Infant	Anticipatory Guidance Developmental Enhancement: Child Environmental Management: Safety Family Integrity Promotion: Childbearing Family Health Screening Immunization/Vaccination Management Nutrition Management Nutritional Monitoring Security Enhancement Socialization Enhancement Surveillance: Safety Teaching: Toilet Training	Abuse Protection Support: Child Caregiver Support Family Support Health System Guidance Nutritional Counseling Respite Care Sibling Support Sleep Enhancement Support System Enhancement Sustenance Support

Outcome	Major Interventions	Suggested Interventions	Optional Interventions
Child Development: 2 Years			
DEFINITION: Milestones of physical, cognitive, and psychosocial progression by 2 years of age	Developmental Enhancement: Child Environmental Management: Safety Risk Identification	Anticipatory Guidance Bowel Training Caregiver Support Family Integrity Promotion Family Involvement Promotion Health Screening Nutrition Management Parenting Promotion Security Enhancement Sleep Enhancement Socialization Surveillance: Safety Teaching: Toddler Nutrition Teaching: Toddler Safety Teaching: Toilet Training	Abuse Protection Support: Child Behavior Management Family Process Maintenance Family Support Family Therapy Health System Guidance Nutritional Counseling Nutritional Monitoring Sibling Support Support System Enhancement Sustenance Support Urinary Habit Training

Continued

Outcome	Major Interventions	Suggested Interventions	Optional Interventions
Child Development: 3 Years			
DEFINITION: Milestones of physical, cognitive, and psychosocial progression by 3 years of age	Developmental Enhancement: Child Environmental Management: Safety Health Screening Risk Identification	Anticipatory Guidance Behavior Management Bowel Management Bowel Training Family Integrity Promotion Family Involvement Promotion Nutrition Management Parenting Promotion Security Enhancement Socialization Enhancement Urinary Habit Training	Abuse Protection Support: Child Bowel Incontinence Care: Encopresis Family Process Maintenance Family Support Family Therapy Health System Guidance Nutritional Monitoring Sibling Support Sleep Enhancement Surveillance: Safety Therapeutic Play Urinary Incontinence Care: Enuresis

Outcome	Major Interventions	Suggested Interventions	Optional Interventions
Child Development: 4 Years			
DEFINITION: Milestones of physical, cognitive, and psychosocial progression by 4 years of age	Developmental Enhancement: Child Health Screening Risk Identification	Anticipatory Guidance Behavior Management Environmental Management: Safety Family Integrity Promotion Family Involvement Promotion Learning Facilitation Nutrition Management Security Enhancement Socialization Enhancement Support System Enhancement Urinary Habit Training	Abuse Protection Support: Child Behavior Management: Overactivity/ Inattention Behavior Modification Energy Management Family Process Maintenance Family Support Family Therapy Health System Guidance Sibling Support Sleep Enhancement Sustenance Support Therapeutic Play Urinary Incontinence Care: Enuresis

Continued

Outcome	Major Interventions	Suggested Interventions	Optional Interventions
Child Development: 5 Years			
DEFINITION: Milestones of physical, cognitive, and psychosocial progression by 5 years of age	Developmental Enhancement: Child Health Screening Risk Identification	Anticipatory Guidance Behavior Management Environmental Management: Safety Family Integrity Promotion Family Involvement Promotion Learning Facilitation Nutrition Management Nutritional Monitoring Parenting Promotion Security Enhancement Socialization Enhancement Support System Enhancement	Abuse Protection Support: Child Behavior Management: Overactivity/ Inattention Behavior Modification Counseling Energy Management Family Process Maintenance Family Support Family Therapy Health System Guidance Nutritional Counseling Sibling Support Sleep Enhancement Sustenance Support Therapeutic Play Urinary Habit Training Urinary Incontinence Care: Enuresis

Outcome	Major Interventions	Suggested Interventions	Optional Interventions
Child Development: Middle Childhood			
DEFINITION: Milestones of physical, cognitive, and psychosocial progression from 6 years through 11 years of age	Development Enhancement: Child Health Screening Risk Identification	Anticipatory Guidance Behavior Modification: Social Skills Body Image Enhancement Exercise Promotion Family Integrity Promotion Family Involvement Promotion Impulse Control Training Learning Facilitation Nutrition Management Nutritional Monitoring Parenting Promotion Self-Awareness Enhancement Self-Esteem Enhancement Self-Modification Assistance Self-Responsibility Facilitation Socialization Enhancement Spiritual Support Substance Use Prevention Teaching: Individual Teaching: Safe Sex Teaching: Sexuality	Abuse Protection Support: Child Behavior Management Behavior Modification Counseling Eating Disorders Management Family Process Maintenance Family Support Family Therapy Fire-Setting Precautions Health System Guidance Sibling Support Sustenance Support Therapeutic Play Weight Management

Continued

Outcome	Major Interventions	Suggested Interventions	Optional Interventions
Child Development: Adolescence			
DEFINITION: Milestones of physical, cognitive, and psychosocial progression from 12 years through 17 years of age	Developmental Enhancement: Adolescent Parent Education: Adolescent Risk Identification	Anticipatory Guidance Body Image Enhancement Exercise Promotion Health Screening Health System Guidance Impulse Control Training Learning Readiness Enhancement Mutual Goal Setting Nutrition Management Nutritional Counseling Self-Awareness Enhancement Self-Esteem Enhancement Self-Modification Assistance Self-Responsibility Facilitation Sleep Enhancement Socialization Enhancement Spiritual Support Substance Use Prevention Teaching: Individual Teaching: Safe Sex Teaching: Sexuality Values Clarification	Abuse Protection Support Behavior Management: Sexual Behavior Modification Counseling Decision-Making Support Eating Disorders Management Family Process Maintenance Family Support Family Therapy Sexual Counseling Support System Enhancement Weight Management

Outcome	Major Interventions	Suggested Interventions	Optional Interventions
Hyperactivity Level			
DEFINITION: Severity of patterns of inattention or impulsivity in a child from 1 year through 17 years of age	Behavior Management: Overactivity/ Inattention Developmental Enhancement: Child	Anticipatory Guidance Behavior Management Behavior Modification Energy Management Environmental Management Family Integrity Promotion Family Process Maintenance Family Support Family Therapy Impulse Control Training Risk Identification	Environmental Management: Safety Family Involvement Promotion Nutrition Management Parent Education: Childrearing Family Parenting Promotion Resiliency Promotion
Preterm Infant Organization			
DEFINITION: Extrauterine integration of physiologic and behavioral function by the infant born 24 to 37 (term) weeks' gestation	Developmental Care Environmental Management: Attachment Process	Anticipatory Guidance Attachment Promotion Bottle Feeding Counseling Family Integrity Promotion: Childbearing Family Kangaroo Care Newborn Care Newborn Monitoring Nonnutritive Sucking	Breastfeeding Assistance Caregiver Support Lactation Counseling Phototherapy: Neonate Resuscitation: Neonate Support Group Teaching: Individual Teaching: Infant Stimulation

Continued

Outcome	Major Interventions	Suggested Interventions	Optional Interventions
Social Interaction Skills DEFINITION: Personal behaviors that promote effective relationships	Behavior Modification: Social Skills Developmental Enhancement: Adolescent Developmental Enhancement: Child	Active Listening Assertiveness Training Complex Relationship Building Counseling Family Integrity Promotion Family Process Maintenance Recreation Therapy Role Enhancement Self-Awareness Enhancement Self-Esteem Enhancement Self-Responsibility Facilitation	Anger Control Assistance Anxiety Reduction Attachment Promotion Body Image Enhancement Coping Enhancement Family Therapy Impulse Control Training Sexual Counseling Support Group Therapy Group

For interventions and outcomes related to specific risk factors, refer to the following diagnoses: Body Image, Disturbed; Breastfeeding, Ineffective; Caregiver Role Strain; Family Coping, Compromised; Growth and Development, Delayed; Infant Feeding Pattern, Ineffective; Parent Infant/Child Attachment, Risk for Impaired; Parenting, Impaired; Parental Role Conflict; Social Isolation; Spiritual Distress.

NURSING DIAGNOSIS: Disuse Syndrome, Risk for

DEFINITION: At risk for deterioration of body systems as the result of prescribed or unavoidable musculoskeletal inactivity.

Outcome	Major Interventions	Suggested Interventions	Optional Interventions
Endurance			
DEFINITION: Capacity to sustain activity	Activity Therapy Energy Management	Exercise Promotion Exercise Promotion: Strength Training Nutrition Management Risk Identification Sleep Enhancement Teaching: Prescribed Activity/Exercise	Environmental Management Exercise Therapy: Ambulation Exercise Therapy: Balance Exercise Therapy: Joint Mobility Exercise Therapy: Muscle Control Pain Management

Continued

Outcome	Major Interventions	Suggested Interventions	Optional Interventions
Immobility Consequences: Physiological DEFINITION: Severity of compromise in physiological functioning due to impaired physical mobility	Energy Management	Bowel Management Circulatory Care: Venous Insufficiency Cough Enhancement Embolus Precautions Exercise Promotion: Stretching Exercise Therapy: Joint Mobility Exercise Therapy: Muscle Control Fluid Management Fluid Monitoring Infection Protection Medication Administration Medication Management Positioning Pressure Ulcer Prevention Simple Massage Skin Surveillance Urinary Elimination Management	Environmental Management Exercise Therapy: Ambulation Fall Prevention Positioning: Wheelchair Physical Restraint Surveillance

Outcome	Major Interventions	Suggested Interventions	Optional Interventions
Immobility Consequences: Psycho-Cognitive			
DEFINITION: Severity of compromise in psycho-cognitive functioning due to impaired physical mobility	Cognitive Stimulation Environmental Management	Coping Enhancement Emotional Support Medication Administration Medication Management Presence Simple Relaxation Therapy Sleep Enhancement	Animal-Assisted Therapy Counseling Environmental Management: Comfort Humor Mood Management Progressive Muscle Relaxation Reality Orientation
Mobility			
DEFINITION: Ability to move purposefully in own environment independently with or without assistive device	Exercise Therapy: Ambulation Exercise Therapy: Balance Exercise Therapy: Joint Mobility Exercise Therapy: Muscle Control	Activity Therapy Body Mechanics Promotion Energy Management Exercise Promotion Exercise Promotion: Strength Training Exercise Promotion: Stretching Fall Prevention	Analgesic Administration Environmental Management Pain Management Positioning Positioning: Wheelchair Teaching: Prescribed Activity/Exercise

For interventions and outcomes related to specific risk factors, refer to the following diagnoses: Confusion, Chronic; Fatigue; Pain, Chronic; Mobility: Physical, Impaired; Thought Processes, Disturbed; Walking, Impaired.

NURSING DIAGNOSIS: Falls, Risk for

DEFINITION: Increased susceptibility to falling that may cause physical harm.

Outcome	Major Interventions	Suggested Interventions	Optional Interventions
Balance			
DEFINITION: Ability to maintain body equilibrium	Exercise Therapy: Balance Fall Prevention	Environmental Management: Safety Self-Care Assistance: Toileting Self-Care Assistance: Transfer Surveillance: Safety	Positioning: Wheelchair Urinary Elimination Management Vital Signs Monitoring
Coordinated Movement			
DEFINITION: Ability of muscles to work together voluntarily for purposeful movement	Body Mechanics Promotion Exercise Therapy: Muscle Control Fall Prevention	Energy Management Exercise Promotion Exercise Promotion: Strength Training Exercise Promotion: Stretching Exercise Therapy: Ambulation Exercise Therapy: Joint Mobility Self-Care Assistance	Medication Management Pain Management Positioning

Outcome	Major Interventions	Suggested Interventions	Optional Interventions
Fall Prevention Behavior			
DEFINITION: Personal or family caregiver actions to minimize risk factors that might precipitate falls in the personal environment	Environmental Management: Safety Fall Prevention	Medication Management Positioning Positioning: Wheelchair Security Enhancement Seizure Precautions Surveillance: Safety	Home Maintenance Assistance Pain Management Self-Care Assistance Substance Use Treatment
Falls Occurrence			
DEFINITION: Number of falls in the past _____ (define period of time)	Fall Prevention Risk Identification	Area Restriction Dementia Management Dementia Management: Bathing Environmental Management: Safety Self-Care Assistance	Chemical Restraint Physical Restraint Positioning Positioning: Wheelchair Transport
Knowledge: Fall Prevention			
DEFINITION: Extent of understanding conveyed about prevention of falls	Teaching: Infant Safety Teaching: Toddler Safety	Parent Education: Infant Teaching: Individual Teaching: Prescribed Activity/Exercise Teaching: Prescribed Medication	Environmental Management: Safety

For interventions and outcomes related to specific risk factors, refer to the following diagnoses: Confusion, Chronic; Diarrhea; Environmental Interpretation Syndrome, Impaired; Failure to Thrive, Adult; Knowledge, Deficient; Mobility: Bed, Impaired; Mobility: Physical, Impaired; Mobility: Wheelchair, Impaired; Parenting, Impaired; Protection, Ineffective; Self-Care Deficit: Toileting; Sensory Perception, Disturbed; Transfer Ability, Impaired; Urinary Incontinence: Functional; Urinary Incontinence: Stress; Urinary Incontinence: Urge; Urinary Incontinence: Urge, Risk for; Walking, Impaired; Wandering.

NURSING DIAGNOSIS: Fluid Volume, Risk for Deficient

DEFINITION: At risk for experiencing vascular, cellular, or intracellular dehydration.

Outcome	Major Interventions	Suggested Interventions	Optional Interventions
Electrolyte & Acid/Base Balance			
DEFINITION: Balance of the electrolytes and non-electrolytes in the intracellular and extracellular compartments of the body	Electrolyte Management Fluid/Electrolyte Management Fluid Management	Acid-Base Management Acid-Base Monitoring Dysrhythmia Management Electrolyte Monitoring Fluid Monitoring Hemodynamic Regulation Intravenous (IV) Insertion Intravenous (IV) Therapy Laboratory Data Interpretation Vital Signs Monitoring	Electrolyte Management: Hypercalcemia Electrolyte Management: Hyperkalemia Electrolyte Management: Hypermagnesemia Electrolyte Management: Hypernatremia Electrolyte Management: Hyperphosphatemia Electrolyte Management: Hypocalcemia Electrolyte Management: Hypokalemia Electrolyte Management: Hypomagnesemia Electrolyte Management: Hyponatremia Electrolyte Management: Hypophosphatemia

Outcome	Major Interventions	Suggested Interventions	Optional Interventions
Fluid Balance			
DEFINITION: Water balance in the intracellular and extracellular compartments of the body	Fluid Management Fluid Monitoring Hypovolemia Management Intravenous (IV) Therapy	Bedside Laboratory Testing Diarrhea Management Electrolyte Management Electrolyte Monitoring Fluid/Electrolyte Management Fluid Resuscitation Intravenous (IV) Insertion Laboratory Data Interpretation Nutrition Management Total Parenteral Nutrition (TPN) Administration Venous Access Device (VAD) Maintenance Vital Signs Monitoring	Autotransfusion Bleeding Precautions Bleeding Reduction Blood Products Administration Cardiac Care: Acute Hemodynamic Regulation Hemorrhage Control Nutritional Monitoring Peripherally Inserted Central (PIC) Catheter Care Shock Prevention Surveillance

Continued

Outcome	Major Interventions	Suggested Interventions	Optional Interventions
Hydration			
DEFINITION: Adequate water in the intracellular and extracellular compartments of the body	Fluid Management Hypovolemia Management	Bottle Feeding Diarrhea Management Electrolyte Management Electrolyte Monitoring Feeding Fever Treatment Fluid/Electrolyte Management Fluid Monitoring Heat Exposure Treatment Nutrition Management Nutritional Monitoring Vital Signs Monitoring	Bleeding Precautions Bleeding Reduction Bleeding Reduction: Gastrointestinal Shock Prevention Temperature Regulation
Nutritional Status: Food & Fluid Intake			
DEFINITION: Amount of food and fluid taken into the body over a 24-hour period	Fluid Monitoring Nutritional Monitoring	Enteral Tube Feeding Feeding Fluid Management Nutrition Management Self-Care Assistance: Feeding Total Parenteral Nutrition (TPN) Administration	Bottle Feeding Intravenous (IV) Therapy Lactation Counseling Oral Health Restoration Swallowing Therapy Teaching: Prescribed Diet

For interventions and outcomes related to specific risk factors, refer to the following diagnoses: Diarrhea; Failure to Thrive, Adult; Hyperthermia; Infant Feeding Pattern, Ineffective; Knowledge, Deficient; Mobility: Physical, Impaired; Nausea; Nutrition: Imbalanced, Less than Body Requirements; Self-Care Deficit: Feeding; Swallowing, Impaired.

NURSING DIAGNOSIS: Fluid Volume, Risk for Imbalanced

DEFINITION: At risk of a decrease, increase, or rapid shift from one to the other of intravascular, interstitial, and/or intracellular fluid. This refers to body fluid loss, gain, or both.

Outcome	Major Interventions	Suggested Interventions	Optional Interventions
Electrolyte & Acid/Base Balance			
DEFINITION: Balance of the electrolytes and non-electrolytes in the intracellular and extracellular compartments of the body	Electrolyte Management Fluid/Electrolyte Management Fluid Management	Acid-Base Management Acid-Base Monitoring Dysrhythmia Management Electrolyte Monitoring Fluid Monitoring Hemodialysis Therapy Hemodynamic Regulation Intravenous (IV) Insertion Intravenous (IV) Therapy Laboratory Data Interpretation Neurologic Monitoring Respiratory Monitoring Vital Signs Monitoring	Electrolyte Management: Hypercalcemia Electrolyte Management: Hyperkalemia Electrolyte Management: Hypermagnesemia Electrolyte Management: Hypernatremia Electrolyte Management: Hyperphosphatemia Electrolyte Management: Hypocalcemia Electrolyte Management: Hypokalemia Electrolyte Management: Hypomagnesemia Electrolyte Management: Hyponatremia Electrolyte Management: Hypophosphatemia

Continued

Outcome	Major Interventions	Suggested Interventions	Optional Interventions
Fluid Balance DEFINITION: Water balance in the intracellular and extracellular compartments of the body	Fluid Management Fluid Monitoring	Bedside Laboratory Testing Diarrhea Management Electrolyte Management Electrolyte Monitoring Fluid/Electrolyte Management Fluid Resuscitation Hypervolemia Management Hypovolemia Management Intravenous (IV) Insertion Intravenous (IV) Therapy Laboratory Data Interpretation Medication Administration Medication Management Medication Prescribing Nutrition Management Nutritional Monitoring Surveillance Total Parenteral Nutrition (TPN) Administration Urinary Elimination Management Vital Signs Monitoring	Bleeding Precautions Bleeding Reduction Bleeding Reduction: Gastrointestinal Blood Products Administration Hemodialysis Therapy Hemodynamic Regulation Hemorrhage Control Intracranial Pressure (ICP) Monitoring Invasive Hemodynamic Monitoring Peritoneal Dialysis Therapy Phlebotomy: Arterial Blood Sample Phlebotomy: Cannulated Vessel Phlebotomy: Venous Blood Sample Respiratory Monitoring Shock Prevention Venous Access Device (VAD) Maintenance

Outcome	Major Interventions	Suggested Interventions	Optional Interventions
Hydration			
DEFINITION: Adequate water in the intracellular and extracellular compartments of the body	Fluid Management Fluid Monitoring	Bottle Feeding Diarrhea Management Electrolyte Management Electrolyte Monitoring Feeding Fever Treatment Fluid/Electrolyte Management Fluid Resuscitation Heat Exposure Treatment Hypovolemia Management Intravenous (IV) Insertion Intravenous (IV) Therapy Nutrition Management Nutritional Monitoring Shock Management: Volume Urinary Elimination Management Vital Signs Monitoring	Bleeding Precautions Bleeding Reduction Hemorrhage Control Temperature Regulation

For interventions and outcomes related to specific risk factors, refer to the following diagnoses: Diarrhea; Failure to Thrive, Adult; Fluid Balance, Readiness for Enhanced; Fluid Volume, Deficient; Fluid Volume, Excess; Hyperthermia; Infant Feeding Pattern, Ineffective; Knowledge, Deficient; Mobility: Physical, Impaired; Nausea; Nutrition: Imbalanced, Less than Body Requirements; Nutrition: Imbalanced, More than Body Requirements; Self-Care Deficit: Feeding; Swallowing, Impaired; Urinary Elimination, Impaired.

NURSING DIAGNOSIS: Grieving, Dysfunctional, Risk for

DEFINITION: At risk for extended, unsuccessful use of intellectual and emotional responses and behaviors by an individual, family, or community following a death or perception of loss.

Outcome	Major Interventions	Suggested Interventions	Optional Interventions
Coping			
DEFINITION: Personal actions to manage stressors that tax an individual's resources	Coping Enhancement Grief Work Facilitation Grief Work Facilitation: Perinatal Death	Anxiety Reduction Counseling Decision-Making Support Emotional Support Family Support Family Therapy Hope Instillation Support Group Support System Enhancement Therapy Group	Animal-Assisted Therapy Mood Management Simple Relaxation Therapy Spiritual Support Truth Telling
Family Coping			
DEFINITION: Family actions to manage stressors that tax family resources	Coping Enhancement Family Therapy	Counseling Family Integrity Promotion Family Integrity Promotion: Childbearing Family Family Process Maintenance Grief Work Facilitation: Perinatal Death	Normalization Promotion Sibling Support Support Group Support System Enhancement

Outcome	Major Interventions	Suggested Interventions	Optional Interventions
Grief Resolution			
DEFINITION: Adjustment to actual or impending loss	Grief Work Facilitation Grief Work Facilitation: Perinatal Death	Active Listening Coping Enhancement Counseling Family Integrity Promotion: Childbearing Family Family Therapy Spiritual Support Support Group Support System Enhancement	Anger Control Assistance Anxiety Reduction Crisis Intervention Family Process Maintenance Family Support Mood Management Normalization Promotion

For interventions and outcomes related to specific risk factors, refer to the following diagnoses: Anxiety; Coping, Ineffective; Thought Processes, Disturbed; Parenting, Impaired.

NURSING DIAGNOSIS: Growth, Risk for Disproportionate

DEFINITION: At risk for growth above the 97th percentile or below the 3rd percentile for age, crossing two percentile channels; disproportionate growth.

Outcome	Major Interventions	Suggested Interventions	Optional Interventions
Child Development: 6 Months			
DEFINITION: Milestones of physical, cognitive, and psychosocial progression by 6 months of age	Infant Care Teaching: Infant Nutrition	Attachment Promotion Bottle Feeding Kangaroo Care Lactation Counseling Parent Education: Infant Risk Identification Sleep Enhancement	Abuse Protection Support: Child Caregiver Support Health System Guidance Nutritional Monitoring Surveillance Sustenance Support
Child Development: 12 Months			
DEFINITION: Milestones of physical, cognitive, and psychosocial progression by 12 months of age	Infant Care Teaching: Infant Nutrition	Bottle Feeding Lactation Counseling Nutrition Management Nutritional Monitoring Parent Education: Infant Risk Identification Sleep Enhancement	Abuse Protection Support: Child Attachment Promotion Caregiver Support Health System Guidance Respite Care Sibling Support Surveillance Sustenance Support

Outcome	Major Interventions	Suggested Interventions	Optional Interventions
Child Development: 2 Years DEFINITION: Milestones of physical, cognitive, and psychosocial progression by 2 years of age	Health Screening Teaching: Toddler Nutrition	Nutrition Management Nutritional Counseling Nutritional Monitoring Parent Education: Childrearing Family Risk Identification Sleep Enhancement	Abuse Protection Support: Child Family Therapy Health System Guidance Support System Enhancement Surveillance Sustenance Support
Child Development: 3 Years DEFINITION: Milestones of physical, cognitive, and psychosocial progression by 3 years of age	Health Screening Nutritional Monitoring Teaching: Toddler Nutrition	Nutrition Management Nutritional Counseling Parent Education: Childrearing Family Risk Identification Support System Enhancement	Abuse Protection Support: Child Energy Management Family Therapy Health System Guidance Sleep Enhancement Sustenance Support
Child Development: 4 Years DEFINITION: Milestones of physical, cognitive, and psychosocial progression by 4 years of age	Health Screening Nutritional Monitoring Teaching: Toddler Nutrition	Nutrition Management Nutritional Counseling Parent Education: Childrearing Family Risk Identification Support System Enhancement Weight Management	Abuse Protection Support: Child Behavior Management Behavior Modification Energy Management Health System Guidance Sleep Enhancement Sustenance Support

Continued

G

Outcome	Major Interventions	Suggested Interventions	Optional Interventions
Child Development: 5 Years			
DEFINITION: Milestones of physical, cognitive, and psychosocial progression by 5 years of age	Nutrition Management Nutritional Monitoring	Health Screening Nutritional Counseling Parent Education: Childrearing Family Risk Identification Weight Management	Abuse Protection Support: Child Behavior Management Behavior Modification Energy Management Health System Guidance Sleep Enhancement Sustenance Support
Child Development: Middle Childhood			
DEFINITION: Milestones of physical, cognitive, and psychosocial progression from 6 years through 11 years of age	Nutrition Management Nutritional Monitoring Weight Management	Behavior Modification Counseling Eating Disorders Management Exercise Promotion Health Screening Learning Facilitation Nutritional Counseling Patient Contracting Substance Use Prevention Teaching: Prescribed Diet	Abuse Protection Support: Child Behavior Management Coping Enhancement Family Support Family Therapy Health System Guidance Parent Education: Childrearing Family Self-Modification Assistance Self-Responsibility Facilitation Weight Gain Assistance Weight Reduction Assistance

Outcome	Major Interventions	Suggested Interventions	Optional Interventions
Child Development: Adolescence			
DEFINITION: Milestones of physical, cognitive, and psychosocial progression from 12 years through 17 years of age	Nutrition Management Weight Management	Behavior Modification Counseling Eating Disorders Management Exercise Promotion Health Screening Mutual Goal Setting Nutrition Therapy Nutritional Counseling Nutritional Monitoring Patient Contracting Substance Use Prevention Teaching: Prescribed Diet	Family Support Family Therapy Health System Guidance Parent Education: Adolescent Self-Modification Assistance Self-Responsibility Facilitation Weight Gain Assistance Weight Reduction Assistance

Continued

Outcome	Major Interventions	Suggested Interventions	Optional Interventions
Growth DEFINITION: Normal increase in bone size and body weight during growth years	Nutrition Management Nutritional Monitoring Weight Management	Bottle Feeding Breastfeeding Assistance Counseling Developmental Enhancement: Child Eating Disorders Management Energy Management Health Education Health Screening Lactation Counseling Nutrition Therapy Nutritional Counseling Prenatal Care Teaching: Infant Nutrition Teaching: Prescribed Diet Teaching: Toddler Nutrition Weight Gain Assistance Weight Reduction Assistance	Abuse Protection Support: Child Enteral Tube Feeding Family Therapy High-Risk Pregnancy Care Parent Education: Adolescent Parent Education: Childrearing Family Parent Education: Infant Preconception Counseling Referral Substance Use Prevention Substance Use Treatment Support System Enhancement Sustenance Support Swallowing Therapy Total Parenteral Nutrition (TPN) Administration

For interventions and outcomes related to specific risk factors, refer to the following diagnoses: Breastfeeding, Ineffective; Diarrhea; Health Maintenance, Ineffective; Infant Feeding Pattern, Ineffective; Infection, Risk for; Nutrition: Imbalanced, More than Body Requirements; Oral Mucous Membrane, Impaired; Parenting, Impaired, Swallowing, Impaired; Violence: Other-Directed, Risk for.

NURSING DIAGNOSIS: Infant Behavior, Risk for Disorganized

DEFINITION: Risk for alteration in integrating and modulation of the physiological and behavioral systems of functioning (i.e., autonomic, motor, state, organizational, self-regulatory, and attentional-interactional systems).

Outcome	Major Interventions	Suggested Interventions	Optional Interventions
Child Development: 1 Month			
DEFINITION: Milestones of physical, cognitive, and psychosocial progression by 1 month of age	Newborn Care Parent Education: Infant Risk Identification	Attachment Promotion Bottle Feeding Breastfeeding Assistance Environmental Management: Comfort Family Involvement Promotion Lactation Counseling Nonnutritive Sucking Sleep Enhancement	Abuse Protection Support: Child Caregiver Support Respiratory Monitoring Teaching: Infant Safety Teaching: Infant Stimulation
Child Development: 2 Months			
DEFINITION: Milestones of physical, cognitive, and psychosocial progression by 2 months of age	Infant Care Parent Education: Infant Risk Identification	Attachment Promotion Bottle Feeding Breastfeeding Assistance Family Integrity Promotion: Childbearing Family Family Involvement Promotion Family Support Lactation Counseling Nonnutritive Sucking Sleep Enhancement	Abuse Protection Support: Child Caregiver Support Environmental Management: Comfort Health System Guidance Nutritional Monitoring Support System Enhancement Surveillance

Continued

Outcome	Major Interventions	Suggested Interventions	Optional Interventions
Child Development: 4 Months			
DEFINITION: Milestones of physical, cognitive, and psychosocial progression by 4 months of age	Infant Care Parent Education: Infant Risk Identification	Bottle Feeding Family Integrity Promotion: Childbearing Family Family Process Maintenance Family Support Health Screening Lactation Counseling Security Enhancement Sleep Enhancement	Abuse Protection Support: Child Attachment Promotion Caregiver Support Health System Guidance Nonnutritive Sucking Nutrition Management Nutritional Monitoring Sibling Support Support System Enhancement Surveillance
Preterm Infant Organization			
DEFINITION: Extrauterine integration of physiologic and behavioral function by the infant born 24 to 37 (term) weeks' gestation	Developmental Care Environmental Management: Attachment Process Newborn Care Positioning	Environmental Management Infant Care Kangaroo Care Neurologic Monitoring Nonnutritive Sucking Pain Management Respiratory Monitoring Surveillance Vital Signs Monitoring	Bottle Feeding Breastfeeding Assistance Lactation Counseling Nutritional Monitoring Teaching: Infant Safety Temperature Regulation

For interventions and outcomes related to specific risk factors, refer to the following diagnoses: Growth and Development, Delayed; Pain, Acute; Protection, Ineffective; Sensory Perception, Disturbed.

NURSING DIAGNOSIS: Infection, Risk for

DEFINITION: At increased risk for being invaded by pathogenic organisms.

Outcome	Major Interventions	Suggested Interventions	Optional Interventions
Community Risk Control: Communicable Disease			
DEFINITION: Community actions to eliminate or reduce the spread of infectious agents that threaten public health	Communicable Disease Management Surveillance: Community	Bioterrorism Preparedness Environmental Risk Protection Health Education Health Screening Immunization/ Vaccination Management	Case Management Infection Control Infection Protection
Immune Status			
DEFINITION: Natural and acquired appropriately targeted resistance to internal and external antigens	Health Screening Immunization/ Vaccination Management	Allergy Management Health Education Health System Guidance Infection Protection Laboratory Data Interpretation Medication Administration Parent Education: Infant Risk Identification Surveillance	Newborn Care Teaching: Disease Process Teaching: Prescribed Medication

Continued

Outcome	Major Interventions	Suggested Interventions	Optional Interventions
Infection Severity			
DEFINITION: Severity of infection and associated symptoms	Immunization/ Vaccination Management Infection Control Infection Protection	Bedside Laboratory Testing Bladder Irrigation Environmental Management Health Screening High-Risk Pregnancy Care Incision Site Care Infection Control: Intraoperative Labor Induction Laboratory Data Interpretation Medication Administration Medication Management Medication Prescribing Perineal Care Respiratory Monitoring Skin Surveillance Urinary Catheterization Urinary Retention Care Vital Signs Monitoring Wound Care Wound Care: Closed Drainage	Airway Management Allergy Management Amputation Care Artificial Airway Management Aspiration Precautions Asthma Management Bathing Birthing Cesarean Section Care Cough Enhancement Intrapartal Care Intrapartal Care: High-Risk Delivery Nutrition Management Oral Health Maintenance Postpartal Care Pregnancy Termination Care Pressure Ulcer Care Tube Care Tube Care: Chest Tube Care: Gastrointestinal Tube Care: Umbilical Line Tube Care: Urinary Tube Care: Ventriculostomy/ Lumbar Drain

Outcome	Major Interventions	Suggested Interventions	Optional Interventions
Infection Severity: Newborn			
DEFINITION: Severity of infection and associated symptoms during the first 28 days of life	Infection Control Infection Protection	Circumcision Care Environmental Management Fever Treatment Fluid Management Medication Administration Newborn Care Newborn Monitoring Respiratory Monitoring Skin Surveillance Vital Signs Monitoring	Aspiration Precautions Hypothermia Treatment Temperature Regulation
Risk Control: Sexually Transmitted Diseases (STD)			
DEFINITION: Personal actions to prevent, eliminate, or reduce behaviors associated with sexually transmitted diseases	Infection Protection Teaching: Safe Sex Teaching: Sexuality	Anticipatory Guidance Behavior Management: Sexual Environmental Management: Community Health Education Health Screening Health System Guidance Patient Contracting Risk Identification Self-Responsibility Facilitation Sexual Counseling	Fertility Preservation Impulse Control Training Support Group

Continued

Outcome	Major Interventions	Suggested Interventions	Optional Interventions
Wound Healing: Primary Intention			
DEFINITION: Extent of regeneration of cells and tissue following intentional closure	Incision Site Care Wound Care	Circulatory Precautions Fluid/Electrolyte Management Infection Control: Intraoperative Infection Protection Medication Administration Medication Administration: Skin Nutrition Management Skin Care: Topical Treatments Skin Surveillance Suturing Teaching: Prescribed Medication Teaching: Procedure/ Treatment Wound Care: Closed Drainage	Bathing Bed Rest Care Cesarean Section Care Hyperglycemia Management

Outcome	Major Interventions	Suggested Interventions	Optional Interventions
Wound Healing: Secondary Intention			
DEFINITION: Extent of regeneration of cells and tissue in an open wound	Circulatory Care: Arterial Insufficiency Infection Control Wound Care	Circulatory Precautions Fluid/Electrolyte Management Infection Protection Medication Administration Medication Administration: Skin Nutrition Therapy Skin Care: Topical Treatments Skin Surveillance Teaching: Disease Process Teaching: Prescribed Medication Teaching: Procedure/ Treatment Wound Care: Closed Drainage Wound Irrigation	Bathing Hyperglycemia Management Leech Therapy Nutrition Management Positioning Pressure Ulcer Care Total Parenteral Nutrition (TPN) Administration

For interventions and outcomes related to specific risk factors, refer to the following diagnoses: Dentition, Impaired; Failure to Thrive, Adult; Health Maintenance, Ineffective; Individual Management of Therapeutic Regimen, Ineffective; Knowledge, Deficient; Nutrition: Imbalanced, Less than Body Requirements; Oral Mucous Membrane, Impaired; Protection, Ineffective; Surgical Recovery, Delayed; Tissue Integrity, Impaired.

NURSING DIAGNOSIS: Injury, Risk for

DEFINITION: At risk of injury as a result of environmental conditions interacting with the individual's adaptive and defensive resources.

Outcome	Major Interventions	Suggested Interventions	Optional Interventions
Falls Occurrence			
DEFINITION: Number of falls in the past _____ (define period of time)	Fall Prevention Surveillance: Safety	Environmental Management: Safety Home Maintenance Assistance Incident Reporting Risk Identification Security Enhancement	Area Restriction Delusion Management Dementia Management Physical Restraint Seizure Precautions Teaching: Prescribed Activity/Exercise
Fetal Status: Intrapartum			
DEFINITION: Extent to which fetal signs are within normal limits from onset of labor to delivery	Electronic Fetal Monitoring: Intrapartum	Intrapartal Care Intrapartal Care: High-Risk Delivery Labor Induction Resuscitation: Fetus	Birthing High-Risk Pregnancy Care Labor Suppression
Maternal Status: Intrapartum			
DEFINITION: Extent to which maternal well-being is within normal limits from onset of labor to delivery	Labor Induction Intrapartal Care: High-Risk Delivery	Bleeding Precautions Bleeding Reduction Environmental Management Infection Protection Intrapartal Care Labor Suppression Medication Administration Medication Management	High-Risk Pregnancy Care Neurologic Monitoring Seizure Management Surgical Precautions Surgical Preparation Ultrasonography: Limited Obstetric

Outcome	Major Interventions	Suggested Interventions	Optional Interventions
Personal Safety Behavior			
DEFINITION: Personal actions of an adult to control behaviors that cause physical injury	Environmental Management: Safety Health Education	Allergy Management Anger Control Assistance Artificial Airway Management Asthma Management Bleeding Precautions Environmental Management: Violence Prevention Impulse Control Training Latex Precautions Risk Identification Sport-Injury Prevention: Youth Substance Use Prevention Surveillance: Safety Teaching: Safe Sex	Abuse Protection Support Behavior Management: Overactivity/ Inattention Behavior Management: Self-Harm Behavior Management: Sexual Environmental Management: Worker Safety First Aid Physical Restraint Security Enhancement

Continued

Outcome	Major Interventions	Suggested Interventions	Optional Interventions
Physical Injury Severity			
DEFINITION: Severity of injuries from accidents and trauma	Fall Prevention Surveillance: Safety	Emergency Care Environmental Management: Safety Environmental Management: Violence Prevention Environmental Management: Worker Safety Incident Reporting Malignant Hyperthermia Precautions Security Enhancement	Delusion Management Dementia Management Electroconvulsive Therapy (ECT) Management Elopement Precautions Hallucination Management Laser Precautions Physical Restraint Pneumatic Tourniquet Precautions Positioning: Intraoperative Postanesthesia Care Seizure Management Seizure Precautions Sports-Injury Prevention: Youth

Outcome	Major Interventions	Suggested Interventions	Optional Interventions
Risk Control			
DEFINITION: Personal actions to prevent, eliminate, or reduce modifiable health threats	Health Education Risk Identification	Environmental Management Environmental Management: Violence Prevention Environmental Management: Worker Safety Health Screening Health System Guidance Learning Facilitation Learning Readiness Enhancement Mutual Goal Setting Patient Contracting Self-Responsibility Facilitation Support System Enhancement Teaching: Disease Process	Allergy Management Asthma Management Bleeding Precautions Family Involvement Promotion Immunization/ Vaccination Management Infection Control Laser Precautions Latex Precautions Surgical Precautions Surgical Preparation Surveillance: Late Pregnancy Surveillance: Remote Electronic
Safe Home Environment			
DEFINITION: Physical arrangements to minimize environmental factors that might cause physical harm or injury in the home	Environmental Management: Safety Surveillance: Safety	Abuse Protection Support: Child Abuse Protection Support: Domestic Partner Abuse Protection Support: Elder Fall Prevention Fire-Setting Precautions Home Maintenance Assistance Risk Identification	Delusion Management Dementia Management Incident Reporting Seizure Precautions Teaching: Infant Safety Teaching: Toddler Safety

Continued

Outcome	Major Interventions	Suggested Interventions	Optional Interventions
Sensory Function Status			
DEFINITION: Extent to which an individual correctly perceives skin stimulation, sounds, proprioception, taste and smell, and visual images	Communication Enhancement: Hearing Communication Enhancement: Visual Environmental Management: Safety	Body Mechanics Promotion Dementia Management Environmental Management Exercise Therapy: Balance Fall Prevention Hallucination Management Lower Extremity Monitoring Peripheral Sensation Management	Neurologic Monitoring Reality Orientation Surveillance: Safety Vital Signs Monitoring

For interventions and outcomes related to specific risk factors, refer to the following diagnoses: Breathing Pattern, Ineffective; Community Coping, Ineffective; Confusion, Chronic; Coping, Ineffective; Latex Allergy Response; Nutrition: Imbalanced, Less than Body Requirements; Post-Trauma Syndrome; Protection, Ineffective; Thermoregulation, Ineffective; Tissue Perfusion, Ineffective; Tissue Integrity, Impaired.

NURSING DIAGNOSIS: Latex Allergy Response, Risk for

DEFINITION: At risk for allergic response to natural latex rubber products.

Outcome	Major Interventions	Suggested Interventions	Optional Interventions
Allergic Response: Localized			
DEFINITION: Severity of localized hypersensitive immune response to a specific environmental (exogenous) antigen	Latex Precautions	Allergy Management Environmental Management Environmental Risk Protection Risk Identification Surveillance Teaching: Individual	Environmental Management: Worker Safety Health Care Information Exchange Health System Guidance Skin Surveillance Surveillance
Tissue Integrity: Skin & Mucous Membranes			
DEFINITION: Structural intactness and normal physiological function of skin and mucous membranes	Latex Precautions Skin Surveillance	Allergy Management Pruritus Management Skin Care: Topical Treatments	Infection Protection Medication Administration: Oral Medication Administration: Skin

For interventions and outcomes related to specific risk factors, refer to the following diagnoses: Protection, Ineffective; Skin Integrity, Impaired; Tissue Integrity, Impaired.

NURSING DIAGNOSIS: Loneliness, Risk for

DEFINITION: At risk of experiencing vague dysphoria.

Outcome	Major Interventions	Suggested Interventions	Optional Interventions

Loneliness Severity
 	
DEFINITION:
Severity of
emotional, social,
or existential
isolation response
	Socialization
	  Enhancement
	Spiritual Support
	Visitation
	  Facilitation
		Activity Therapy
		Animal-Assisted
		  Therapy
		Behavior
		  Modification:
		  Social Skills
		Complex
		  Relationship
		  Building
		Coping
		  Enhancement
		Counseling
		Emotional Support
		Environmental
		  Management
		Family Integrity
		  Promotion
		Family Involvement
		  Promotion
		Family Mobilization
		Hope Instillation
		Mood Management
		Presence
		Recreation Therapy
		Role Enhancement
		Self-Awareness
		  Enhancement
		Self-Esteem
		  Enhancement
		Support Group
		Support System
		  Enhancement
		Therapeutic Play
		Therapy Group
		Touch
			Art Therapy
			Communication
			  Enhancement:
			  Hearing Deficit
			Communication
			  Enhancement: Speech
			  Deficit
			Communication
			  Enhancement: Visual
			  Deficit
			Family Therapy
			Grief Work Facilitation
			Reminiscence Therapy

Outcome	Major Interventions	Suggested Interventions	Optional Interventions
Social Involvement			
DEFINITION: Social interactions with persons, groups, or organizations	Socialization Enhancement	Activity Therapy Anxiety Reduction Art Therapy Assertiveness Training Complex Relationship Building Energy Management Recreation Therapy Relocation Stress Reduction Role Enhancement Self-Awareness Enhancement Self-Esteem Enhancement Self-Responsibility Facilitation Therapeutic Play Visitation Facilitation	Animal-Assisted Therapy Behavior Management Body Image Enhancement Counseling Culture Brokerage Developmental Enhancement: Child Family Mobilization Family Therapy Milieu Therapy Mood Management Presence Support Group Support System Enhancement

For interventions and outcomes related to specific risk factors, refer to the following diagnoses: Diversional Activity, Deficient; Social Interaction, Impaired; Social Isolation; Sorrow: Chronic; Spiritual Distress.

NURSING DIAGNOSIS: Nutrition: Imbalanced, Risk for More than Body Requirements

DEFINITION: At risk of experiencing an intake of nutrients that exceeds metabolic needs.

Outcome	Major Interventions	Suggested Interventions	Optional Interventions
Nutritional Status: Food & Fluid Intake DEFINITION: Amount of food and fluid taken into the body over a 24-hour period	Nutrition Management Nutritional Monitoring	Behavior Modification Fluid Management Fluid Monitoring Teaching: Prescribed Diet Weight Management Weight Reduction Assistance	Eating Disorders Management Mutual Goal Setting Patient Contracting Self-Responsibility Facilitation Teaching Infant Nutrition Teaching: Toddler Nutrition
Nutritional Status: Nutrient Intake DEFINITION: Adequacy of usual pattern of nutrient intake	Nutrition Management	Behavior Modification Nutrition Therapy Nutritional Counseling Nutritional Monitoring Teaching: Infant Nutrition Teaching: Prescribed Diet Teaching: Toddler Nutrition	Teaching: Individual Weight Management Weight Reduction Assistance

Outcome	Major Interventions	Suggested Interventions	Optional Interventions
Weight Control			
DEFINITION: Personal actions to achieve and maintain optimum body weight	Nutrition Management Weight Management	Behavior Modification Exercise Promotion Nutritional Counseling Nutritional Monitoring Patient Contracting Self-Responsibility Facilitation	Mutual Goal Setting Teaching: Individual Teaching: Prescribed Diet Weight Reduction Assistance

For interventions and outcomes related to specific risk factors, refer to the following diagnoses: Anxiety; Body Image, Disturbed; Coping, Ineffective; Diversional Activity, Deficient; Health Maintenance, Ineffective; Mobility: Physical, Impaired; Self-Esteem, Chronic Low; Sorrow: Chronic; Walking, Impaired.

NURSING DIAGNOSIS: Parent/Infant/Child Attachment, Risk for Impaired

DEFINITION: Disruption of the interactive process between parent/significant other, child, and infant that fosters the development of a protective and nurturing reciprocal relationship.

Outcome	Major Interventions	Suggested Interventions	Optional Interventions
Parent-Infant Attachment			
DEFINITION: Parent and infant behaviors that demonstrate an enduring affectionate bond	Attachment Promotion Environmental Management: Attachment Process Parent Education: Infant	Anticipatory Guidance Anxiety Reduction Breastfeeding Assistance Coping Enhancement Infant Care Kangaroo Care Lactation Counseling Risk Identification: Childbearing Family Role Enhancement	Emotional Support Family Integrity Promotion Family Involvement Promotion Family Process Maintenance

Continued

Outcome	Major Interventions	Suggested Interventions	Optional Interventions
Parenting Performance			
DEFINITION: Parental actions to provide a child a nurturing and constructive physical, emotional, and social environment	Parent Education: Infant Parenting Promotion	Abuse Protection Support: Child Anticipatory Guidance Coping Enhancement Environmental Management Family Integrity Promotion: Childbearing Family Family Involvement Promotion Family Process Maintenance Family Support Respite Care Role Enhancement Self-Awareness Enhancement Self-Esteem Enhancement Self-Responsibility Facilitation Socialization Enhancement Support System Enhancement	Breastfeeding Assistance Developmental Enhancement: Child Emotional Support Family Integrity Promotion Family Therapy Sibling Support Substance Use Prevention Substance Use Treatment Support Group Therapy Group

Outcome	Major Interventions	Suggested Interventions	Optional Interventions
Role Performance			
DEFINITION: Congruence of an individual's role behavior with role expectations	Parenting Promotion Role Enhancement	Anticipatory Guidance Attachment Promotion Caregiver Support Coping Enhancement Emotional Support Self-Awareness Enhancement Self-Responsibility Facilitation Values Clarification	Childbirth Preparation Family Integrity Promotion: Childbearing Family Kangaroo Care Parent Education: Childrearing Family Parent Education: Infant Self-Esteem Enhancement Support Group Support System Enhancement

For interventions and outcomes related to specific risk factors, refer to the following diagnoses: Breastfeeding, Ineffective; Breastfeeding, Interrupted; Caregiver Role Strain; Coping, Ineffective; Family Coping, Compromised; Family Processes, Interrupted; Coping, Ineffective; Infant Behavior, Disorganized; Knowledge, Deficient; Parental Role Conflict; Parenting, Impaired; Role Performance, Ineffective; Self-Esteem: Situational Low.

NURSING DIAGNOSIS: Parenting, Risk for Impaired

DEFINITION: Risk for inability of the primary caretaker to create, maintain, or regain an environment that promotes the optimum growth and development of the child.

Outcome	Major Interventions	Suggested Interventions	Optional Interventions
Parenting: Adolescent Physical Safety			
DEFINITION: Parental actions to prevent physical injury in an adolescent from 12 years through 17 years of age	Parent Education: Adolescent	Abuse Protection Support: Child Parenting Promotion Sports-Injury Prevention: Youth Vehicle Safety Promotion	Developmental Enhancement: Adolescent Environmental Management: Safety Health Education
Parenting: Early/Middle Childhood Physical Safety			
DEFINITION: Parental actions to avoid physical injury of a child from 3 years through 11 years of age	Parent Education: Childrearing Family	Abuse Protection Support: Child Environmental Management: Safety Parenting Promotion Sports-Injury Prevention: Youth	Developmental Enhancement: Child Fire Setting Precautions Health Education Surveillance: Safety Vehicle Safety Promotion

Continued

Outcome	Major Interventions	Suggested Interventions	Optional Interventions
Parenting: Infant/Toddler Physical Safety			
DEFINITION: Parental actions to avoid physical injury of a child from birth through 2 years of age	Teaching: Infant Safety Teaching: Toddler Safety	Abuse Protection Support: Child Environmental Management: Safety Parent Education: Infant Parenting Promotion Vehicle Safety Promotion	Infant Care Fall Prevention Immunization/ Vaccination Management Infection Protection Surveillance: Safety
Parenting Performance			
DEFINITION: Parental actions to provide a child a nurturing and constructive physical, emotional, and social environment	Developmental Enhancement: Adolescent Developmental Enhancement: Child Family Integrity Promotion: Childbearing Family Parenting Promotion	Abuse Protection Support: Child Anticipatory Guidance Attachment Promotion Caregiver Support Coping Enhancement Parent Education: Adolescent Parent Education: Childrearing Family Parent Education: Infant Resiliency Promotion Role Enhancement Self-Esteem Enhancement Sibling Support Support System Enhancement	Breastfeeding Assistance Childbirth Preparation Emotional Support Family Integrity Promotion Family Involvement Promotion Family Process Maintenance Family Support Financial Resource Assistance Health Education Health System Guidance Home Maintenance Assistance Infant Care Newborn Care Postpartal Care Respite Care Security Enhancement Support Group

Outcome	Major Interventions	Suggested Interventions	Optional Interventions
Parenting: Psychosocial Safety			
DEFINITION: Parental actions to protect a child from social contacts that might cause harm or injury	Abuse Protection Support: Child Family Integrity Promotion Childbearing Family	Anticipatory Guidance Developmental Enhancement: Adolescent Developmental Enhancement: Child Family Integrity Promotion Health Screening Parent Education: Adolescent Parent Education: Childrearing Family Risk Identification Risk Identification: Childbearing Family Socialization Enhancement Surveillance: Safety	Counseling Emotional Support Family Support Self-Esteem Enhancement Self-Modification Assistance Self-Responsibility Facilitation Substance Use Prevention Support Group Teaching: Individual

Continued

Outcome	Major Interventions	Suggested Interventions	Optional Interventions
Role Performance			
DEFINITION: Congruence of an individual's role behavior with role expectations	Parenting Promotion Role Enhancement	Anticipatory Guidance Caregiver Support Coping Enhancement Emotional Support Resiliency Promotion Self-Awareness Enhancement Support System Enhancement Values Clarification	Attachment Promotion Childbirth Preparation Decision-Making Support Energy Management Family Integrity Promotion Family Therapy Health Education Parent Education: Adolescent Parent Education: Childrearing Family Parent Education: Infant Self-Esteem Enhancement Support Group

For interventions and outcomes related to specific risk factors, refer to the following diagnoses: Breastfeeding, Ineffective; Breastfeeding, Interrupted; Caregiver Role Strain; Coping, Ineffective; Family Coping: Compromised; Family Processes, Interrupted; Infant Behavior, Disorganized; Knowledge, Deficient; Parental Role Conflict; Parenting, Impaired; Role Performance, Ineffective; Self-Esteem: Situational Low.

NURSING DIAGNOSIS: Perioperative Positioning Injury, Risk for

DEFINITION: At risk for injury as a result of the environmental conditions found in the perioperative setting.

Outcome	Major Interventions	Suggested Interventions	Optional Interventions
Circulation Status			
DEFINITION: Unobstructed, unidirectional blood flow at an appropriate pressure through large vessels of the systemic and pulmonary circuits	Circulatory Care: Arterial Insufficiency Circulatory Care: Venous Insufficiency Positioning: Intraoperative	Bleeding Reduction: Wound Circulatory Care: Mechanical Assist Device Circulatory Precautions Embolus Care: Peripheral Embolus Precautions Hemodynamic Regulation Hypovolemia Management Shock Prevention	Blood Products Administration Cerebral Perfusion Promotion Fluid Resuscitation Intravenous (IV) Insertion Intravenous (IV) Therapy Invasive Hemodynamic Monitoring Surgical Precautions
Neurological Status: Spinal Sensory/Motor Function			
DEFINITION: Ability of the spinal nerves to convey sensory and motor impulses	Positioning: Intraoperative	Fluid Management Fluid Monitoring Neurologic Monitoring Peripheral Sensation Management Surgical Precautions Surveillance	Seizure Management Seizure Precautions Vital Signs Monitoring

Continued

Outcome	Major Interventions	Suggested Interventions	Optional Interventions
Tissue Perfusion: Peripheral			
DEFINITION: Adequacy of blood flow through the small vessels of the extremities to maintain tissue function	Positioning: Intraoperative Pressure Management	Bleeding Reduction Circulatory Care: Arterial Insufficiency Circulatory Care: Mechanical Assist Device Circulatory Care: Venous Insufficiency Circulatory Precautions Embolus Care: Peripheral Embolus Precautions Hypovolemia Management Skin Surveillance	Fluid Management Surgical Precautions Temperature Regulation: Intraoperative

For interventions and outcomes related to specific risk factors, refer to the following diagnoses: Failure to Thrive, Adult; Fluid Volume Excess; Mobility: Bed, Impaired; Nutrition: Imbalanced, Less than Body Requirements; Sensory/Perception, Disturbed; Thought Processes, Disturbed; Tissue Perfusion, Ineffective.

NURSING DIAGNOSIS: Peripheral Neurovascular Dysfunction, Risk for

DEFINITION: At risk for disruption in circulation, sensation, or motion of an extremity.

Outcome	Major Interventions	Suggested Interventions	Optional Interventions
Coordinated Movement DEFINITION: Ability of muscles to work together voluntarily for purposeful movement	Exercise Promotion: Strength Training Exercise Therapy: Joint Mobility Exercise Therapy: Muscle Control	Exercise Promotion Progressive Muscle Relaxation Simple Massage Simple Relaxation Therapy	Bed Rest Care Heat/Cold Application Pain Management Teaching: Prescribed Activity/Exercise
Neurological Status: Spinal Sensory/ Motor Function DEFINITION: Ability of the spinal nerves to convey sensory and motor impulses	Peripheral Sensation Management Positioning: Neurologic	Embolus Care: Peripheral Embolus Precautions Environmental Management: Safety Lower Extremity Monitoring Neurologic Monitoring Pneumatic Tourniquet Precautions Pressure Management Pressure Ulcer Prevention Skin Surveillance Traction/ Immobilization Care Vital Signs Monitoring	Exercise Promotion: Stretching Exercise Therapy: Joint Mobility Exercise Therapy: Muscle Control Positioning Risk Identification Skin Care: Topical Treatments Splinting

Continued

Outcome	Major Interventions	Suggested Interventions	Optional Interventions
Tissue Perfusion: Peripheral			
DEFINITION: Adequacy of blood flow through the small vessels of the extremities to maintain tissue function	Circulatory Care: Arterial Insufficiency Circulatory Care: Venous Insufficiency Circulatory Precautions	Bleeding Reduction Cardiac Care Cardiac Precautions Circulatory Care: Mechanical Assist Device Embolus Care: Peripheral Fluid Management Pneumatic Tourniquet Precautions Pressure Management	Cast Care: Maintenance Cast Care: Wet Cutaneous Stimulation Heat/Cold Application Positioning Positioning: Wheelchair Skin Surveillance

For interventions and outcomes related to specific risk factors, refer to the following diagnoses: Mobility: Bed, Impaired; Mobility: Physical, Impaired; Perioperative Positioning Injury, Risk for; Protection, Ineffective; Surgical Recovery, Delayed; Tissue Perfusion, Ineffective; Trauma, Risk for; Unilateral Neglect.

NURSING DIAGNOSIS: Poisoning, Risk for

DEFINITION: Accentuated risk of accidental exposure to, or ingestion of, drugs or dangerous products in doses sufficient to cause poisoning.

Outcome	Major Interventions	Suggested Interventions	Optional Interventions
Safe Home Environment			
DEFINITION: Physical arrangements to minimize environmental factors that might cause physical harm or injury in the home	Environmental Management: Safety Surveillance: Safety	Environmental Management: Worker Safety Home Maintenance Assistance Risk Identification Teaching: Infant Safety Teaching: Toddler Safety	Dementia Management Environmental Risk Protection Parent Education: Childrearing Family Parent Education: Infant
Personal Safety Behavior			
DEFINITION: Personal actions of an adult to control behaviors that cause physical injury	Environmental Management: Safety Health Education	Home Maintenance Assistance Medication Management Risk Identification Substance Use Prevention Surveillance: Safety	Environmental Management: Worker Security Enhancement Surveillance
Physical Injury Severity			
DEFINITION: Severity of injuries from accidents and trauma	Environmental Safety	Emergency Care Environmental Management: Worker Safety First Aid Risk Identification Surveillance: Safety	Dementia Management Hallucination Management Vital Signs Monitoring

For interventions and outcomes related to specific risk factors, refer to the following diagnoses: Confusion, Acute; Confusion, Chronic; Home Maintenance, Impaired; Memory, Impaired; Parenting, Impaired.

NURSING DIAGNOSIS: Post-Trauma Syndrome, Risk for

DEFINITION: At risk for sustained maladaptive response to a traumatic, overwhelming event.

Outcome	Major Interventions	Suggested Interventions	Optional Interventions
Abuse Recovery Status			
DEFINITION: Extent of healing following physical or psychological abuse that may include sexual or financial exploitation	Abuse Protection Support Coping Enhancement Crisis Intervention	Abuse Protection Support: Child Abuse Protection Support: Elder Active Listening Anger Control Assistance Anxiety Reduction Assertiveness Training Counseling Emotional Support Forgiveness Facilitation Guilt Work Facilitation Hope Instillation Mood Management Presence Rape-Trauma Treatment Self-Esteem Enhancement Sexual Counseling Support Group Support System Enhancement	Activity Therapy Animal-Assisted Therapy Behavior Management: Self-Harm Behavior Management: Sexual Complex Relationship Building Decision-Making Support Eating Disorders Management Family Involvement Promotion Health System Guidance Self-Awareness Enhancement Simple Relaxation Therapy Socialization Spiritual Support Substance Use Prevention Suicide Prevention Therapy Group

Outcome	Major Interventions	Suggested Interventions	Optional Interventions
Aggression Self-Control			
DEFINITION: Self-restraint of assaultive, combative, or destructive behaviors toward others	Anger-Control Assistance Impulse Control Training	Behavior Modification Cognitive Restructuring Counseling Emotional Support Exercise Promotion Grief Work Facilitation Guilt Work Facilitation Mood Management Patient Contracting Self-Awareness Enhancement Self-Modification Assistance Self-Responsibility Facilitation Support Group Therapy Group	Crisis Intervention Environmental Management: Violence Prevention Medication Management Spiritual Support Substance Use Prevention Support System Enhancement Therapeutic Play

Continued

Outcome	Major Interventions	Suggested Interventions	Optional Interventions
Coping			
DEFINITION: Personal actions to manage stressors that tax an individual's resources	Coping Enhancement Counseling Crisis Intervention	Active Listening Animal-Assisted Therapy Anxiety Reduction Decision-Making Support Emotional Support Exercise Promotion Guilt Work Facilitation Hope Instillation Hypnosis Meditation Facilitation Presence Simple Relaxation Therapy Spiritual Support Support Group Support System Enhancement	Behavior Modification Environmental Management Family Therapy Mood Management Normalization Promotion Progressive Muscle Relaxation Rape-Trauma Treatment Religious Addiction Prevention Relocation Stress Reduction Reminiscence Therapy Sibling Support Therapy Group Truth Telling
Depression Self-Control			
DEFINITION: Personal actions to minimize melancholy and maintain interest in life events	Mood Management	Activity Therapy Behavior Management Behavior Management: Self-Harm Exercise Promotion Medication Management Nutrition Management Self-Modification Assistance Sleep Enhancement	Grief Work Facilitation Guilt Work Facilitation Substance Use Prevention

For interventions and outcomes related to specific risk factors, refer to the following diagnoses: Grieving, Dysfunctional; Hopelessness; Powerlessness; Relocation Stress Syndrome; Self-Esteem: Situational Low; Social Interaction, Impaired; Social Isolation; Sorrow: Chronic; Spiritual Distress.

NURSING DIAGNOSIS: Powerlessness, Risk for

DEFINITION: At risk for perceived lack of control over a situation and/or one's ability to significantly affect on outcome.

Outcome	Major Interventions	Suggested Interventions	Optional Interventions
Health Beliefs: Perceived Ability to Perform DEFINITION: Personal conviction that one can carry out a given health behavior	Self-Esteem Enhancement Self-Responsibility Facilitation	Assertiveness Training Anxiety Reduction Cognitive Restructuring Decision-Making Support Health System Guidance Teaching: Individual	Complex Relationship Building Emotional Support Learning Facilitation Mutual Goal Setting
Health Beliefs: Perceived Control DEFINITION: Personal conviction that one can influence a health outcome	Self-Awareness Enhancement Self-Esteem Enhancement	Assertiveness Training Behavior Modification Complex Relationship Building Decision-Making Support Mutual Goal Setting Self-Modification Assistance Self-Responsibility Facilitation	Anxiety Reduction Emotional Support Environmental Management Relocation Stress Reduction

Continued

Outcome	Major Interventions	Suggested Interventions	Optional Interventions
Personal Autonomy			
DEFINITION: Personal actions of a competent individual to exercise governance in life decisions	Decision-Making Support Self-Esteem Enhancement	Assertiveness Training Emotional Support Health System Guidance Learning Facilitation Self-Responsibility Facilitation Values Clarification	Cognitive Restructuring Crisis Intervention Presence Teaching: Individual

For interventions and outcomes related to specific risk factors, refer to the following diagnoses: Body Image, Disturbed; Confusion, Chronic; Coping, Ineffective; Death Anxiety; Family Processes, Dysfunctional: Alcoholism.

NURSING DIAGNOSIS: Religiosity, Impaired, Risk for

DEFINITION: At risk for impaired ability to exercise reliance on religious beliefs and/or participate in rituals of a particular faith tradition.

Outcome	Major Interventions	Suggested Interventions	Optional Interventions
Spiritual Health DEFINITION: Connectedness with self, others, higher power, all life, nature, and the universe that transcends and empowers the self	Emotional Support Spiritual Support	Coping Enhancement Counseling Hope Instillation Mood Management Security Enhancement Spiritual Growth Facilitation Support System Enhancement	Culture Brokerage Guilt Work Facilitation Pain Management Presence Resiliency Promotion

For interventions and outcomes related to specific risk factors, refer to the following diagnoses: Coping, Ineffective; Hopelessness; Loneliness, Risk for; Mobility: Physical, Impaired; Pain, Acute; Pain, Chronic; Social Isolation; Sorrow, Chronic.

Continued

NURSING DIAGNOSIS: Relocation Stress Syndrome, Risk for

DEFINITION: At risk for physiological and/or psychosocial disturbance following transfer from one environment to another.

Outcome	Major Interventions	Suggested Interventions	Optional Interventions
Discharge Readiness: Supported Living			
DEFINITION: Readiness of a patient to relocate from a health care institution to a lower level of supported living	Anxiety Reduction Discharge Planning Relocation Stress Reduction	Anger Control Assistance Emotional Support Family Involvement Promotion Family Mobilization Mutual Goal Setting Patient Rights Protection	Active Listening Coping Enhancement Family Support Presence Spiritual Support Visitation Facilitation
Personal Health Status			
DEFINITION: Overall physical, psychological, social, and spiritual functioning of an adult 18 years or older	Relocation Stress Reduction	Anger Control Assistance Anxiety Reduction Coping Enhancement Energy Management Exercise Promotion Hope Instillation Nutrition Management Nutritional Monitoring Self-Responsibility Facilitation Socialization Enhancement Spiritual Support	Activity Therapy Animal-Assisted Therapy Emotional Support Nutrition Therapy Patient Rights Protection Security Enhancement Sleep Enhancement

Outcome	Major Interventions	Suggested Interventions	Optional Interventions
Psychosocial Adjustment: Life Change			
DEFINITION: Adaptive psychosocial response of an individual to a significant life change	Coping Enhancement Relocation Stress Reduction	Active Listening Anticipatory Guidance Discharge Planning Emotional Support Family Involvement Promotion Patient Rights Protection Security Enhancement Socialization Enhancement Spiritual Support Support System Enhancement Visitation Facilitation	Anger Control Assistance Counseling Dementia Management Grief Work Facilitation Hope Instillation Nutritional Monitoring Recreation Therapy Reminiscence Therapy Sleep Enhancement

For interventions and outcomes related to specific risk factors, refer to the following diagnoses: Adjustment, Impaired; Confusion, Chronic; Coping, Ineffective; Grieving, Anticipatory; Hopelessness; Memory, Impaired; Powerlessness; Social Interaction, Impaired; Spiritual Distress.

NURSING DIAGNOSIS: Self-Esteem: Situational Low, Risk for

DEFINITION: At risk for developing negative perception of self-worth in response to a current situation (specify).

Outcome	Major Interventions	Suggested Interventions	Optional Interventions
Abuse Recovery Status DEFINITION: Extent of healing following physical or psychological abuse that may include sexual or financial exploitation	Abuse Protection Support Self-Esteem Enhancement	Assertiveness Training Coping Enhancement Counseling Self-Awareness Enhancement Self-Modification Assistance Self-Responsibility Facilitation Support Group Therapy Group Trauma Therapy: Child	Anger Control Assistance Body Image Enhancement Developmental Enhancement: Adolescent Developmental Enhancement: Child Emotional Support Mood Management Mutual Goal Setting Substance Use Prevention
Neglect Recovery DEFINITION: Extent of healing following the cessation of substandard care	Counseling Self-Esteem Enhancement	Decision-Making Support Developmental Enhancement: Adolescent Developmental Enhancement: Child Emotional Support Hope Instillation Security Enhancement	Abuse Protection Support Spiritual Support Support System Enhancement Weight Management

Outcome	Major Interventions	Suggested Interventions	Optional Interventions
Self-Esteem			
DEFINITION: Personal judgment of self-worth	Self-Esteem Enhancement	Assertiveness Training Body Image Enhancement Counseling Emotional Support Mood Management Role Enhancement Substance Use Treatment Support Group Weight Management	Animal-Assisted Bowel Incontinence Care: Encopresis Developmental Enhancement: Adolescent Developmental Enhancement: Child Reproductive Technology Management Urinary Incontinence Care: Enuresis

For interventions and outcomes related to specific risk factors, refer to the following diagnoses: Body Image, Disturbed; Bowel Incontinence; Development, Risk for Delayed; Grieving, Dysfunctional; Growth and Development, Delayed; Post-Trauma Syndrome; Powerlessness; Rape-Trauma Syndrome; Role Performance, Ineffective; Urinary Incontinence: Total.

NURSING DIAGNOSIS: Self-Mutilation, Risk for

DEFINITION: At risk for deliberate self-injurious behavior causing tissue damage with the intent of causing nonfatal injury to attain relief of tension.

Outcome	Major Interventions	Suggested Interventions	Optional Interventions
Impulse Self-Control DEFINITION: Self-restraint of compulsive or impulsive behaviors	Behavior Management: Self-Harm Impulse Control Training	Anger Control Assistance Anxiety Reduction Behavior Management Behavior Modification Calming Technique Counseling Environmental Management: Safety Environmental Management: Violence Prevention Fire-Setting Precautions Limit Setting Milieu Therapy Mutual Goal Setting Patient Contracting Self-Modification Assistance Self-Responsibility Facilitation	Coping Enhancement Developmental Enhancement: Child Emotional Support Mood Management Risk Identification Security Enhancement Socialization Enhancement Support System Enhancement Surveillance: Safety Therapy Group

Outcome	Major Interventions	Suggested Interventions	Optional Interventions
Self-Mutilation Restraint			
DEFINITION: Personal actions to refrain from intentional self-inflicted injury (non-lethal)	Anger Control Assistance Behavior Management: Self-Harm Environmental Management: Safety	Anxiety Reduction Area Restriction Behavior Management Behavior Modification Calming Technique Cognitive Restructuring Coping Enhancement Counseling Emotional Support Environmental Management: Violence Prevention Impulse Control Training Limit Setting Mood Management Mutual Goal Setting Patient Contracting Physical Restraint Self-Awareness Enhancement Self-Esteem Enhancement Suicide Prevention Surveillance: Safety	Active Listening Activity Therapy Animal-Assisted Therapy Body Image Enhancement Family Therapy Hallucination Management Medication Administration Milieu Therapy Mutual Goal Setting Presence Security Enhancement Therapy Group

For interventions and outcomes related to specific risk factors, refer to the following diagnoses: Anxiety; Body Image Disturbed; Coping, Ineffective; Family Processes, Interrupted; Hopelessness; Personal Identity, Disturbed; Post-Trauma Syndrome; Rape-Trauma Syndrome; Self-Esteem: Chronic Low; Sorrow: Chronic; Spiritual Distress.

NURSING DIAGNOSIS: Skin Integrity, Risk for Impaired

DEFINITION: At risk for skin being adversely altered.

Outcome	Major Interventions	Suggested Interventions	Optional Interventions
Immobility Consequences: Physiological			
DEFINITION: Severity of compromise in physiological functioning due to impaired physical mobility	Bed Rest Care Pressure Management	Circulatory Precautions Embolus Care: Peripheral Embolus Precautions Exercise Promotion: Strength Training Exercise Promotion: Stretching Exercise Therapy: Joint Mobility Exercise Therapy: Muscle Control Positioning Pressure Ulcer Prevention Simple Massage Skin Surveillance Traction/ Immobilization Care	Bathing Foot Care Lower Extremity Monitoring Nail Care Perineal Care Positioning: Intraoperative Skin Care: Topical Treatments Surveillance Vital Signs Monitoring

Outcome	Major Interventions	Suggested Interventions	Optional Interventions
Tissue Integrity: Skin & Mucous Membranes			
DEFINITION: Structural intactness and normal physiological function of skin and mucous membranes	Pressure Management Pressure Ulcer Prevention Skin Surveillance	Amputation Care Bathing Bed Rest Care Bowel Incontinence Care Cast Care: Maintenance Chemotherapy Management Circulatory Precautions Foot Care Incision Site Care Infection Control Infection Protection Latex Precautions Medication Administration: Skin Medication Management Nutrition Management Ostomy Care Positioning Radiation Therapy Management Skin Care: Topical Treatments Traction/ Immobilization Care	Allergy Management Cutaneous Stimulation Diarrhea Management Fluid Management Lactation Counseling Nail Care Nutrition Therapy Perineal Care Positioning: Intraoperative Positioning: Wheelchair Prosthesis Care Self-Care Assistance: Bathing/Hygiene Self-Care Assistance: Toileting Urinary Incontinence Care Urinary Incontinence Care: Enuresis Wound Care

Continued

Outcome	Major Interventions	Suggested Interventions	Optional Interventions
Wound Healing: Primary Intention			
DEFINITION: Extent of regeneration of cells and tissue following intentional closure	Incision Site Care Wound Care	Amputation Care Circulatory Precautions Infection Control: Intraoperative Infection Protection Medication Administration Medication Administration: Skin Nutrition Management Skin Care: Topical Treatments Skin Surveillance Splinting Teaching: Prescribed Medication Teaching: Procedure/ Treatment Wound Care: Closed Drainage	Bathing Bed Rest Care Cesarean Section Care Exercise Therapy: Ambulation Hyperglycemia Management Perineal Care

For interventions and outcomes related to specific risk factors, refer to the following diagnoses: Diarrhea; Bowel Incontinence; Hyperthermia; Latex Allergy Response; Mobility: Physical, Impaired; Nutrition: Imbalanced, Less than Body Requirements; Sensory Perception, Disturbed; Tissue Perfusion, Ineffective; Urinary Incontinence: Total.

NURSING DIAGNOSIS: Spiritual Distress, Risk for

DEFINITION: At risk for an impaired ability to experience and integrate meaning and purpose in life through a person's connectedness with self, other persons, art, music, literature, and/or a power greater than oneself.

Outcome	Major Interventions	Suggested Interventions	Optional Interventions
Hope			
DEFINITION: Optimism that is personally satisfying and life-supporting	Hope Instillation Spiritual Support	Anxiety Reduction Coping Enhancement Emotional Support Forgiveness Facilitation Grief Work Facilitation Self-Awareness Enhancement Support Group Support System Enhancement Values Clarification	Animal-Assisted Therapy Counseling Family Support Mood Management Presence Socialization Enhancement Truth Telling
Spiritual Health			
DEFINITION: Connectedness with self, others, higher power, all life, nature, and the universe that transcends and empowers the self	Spiritual Growth Facilitation Spiritual Support	Emotional Support Forgiveness Facilitation Grief Work Facilitation Hope Instillation Meditation Facilitation Mood Management Religious Ritual Enhancement Resiliency Promotion Support Group Values Clarification	Abuse Protection Support: Religious Bibliotherapy Music Therapy Patient Rights Protection Referral Religious Addiction Prevention Reminiscence Therapy

Continued

Outcome	Major Interventions	Suggested Interventions	Optional Interventions
Suffering Severity DEFINITION: Severity of anguish associated with a distressing symptom, injury, or loss that has potential long-term effects	Hope Instillation Spiritual Growth Facilitation Spiritual Support	Active Listening Anticipatory Guidance Anxiety Reduction Coping Enhancement Emotional Support Grief Work Facilitation Presence Support Group Values Clarification	Animal-Assisted Therapy Decision-Making Support Forgiveness Facilitation Mood Management Reminiscence Therapy Truth Telling

For interventions and outcomes related to specific risk factors, refer to the following diagnoses: Anxiety; Death Anxiety; Grieving, Dysfunctional; Hopelessness; Loneliness, Risk for; Self-Esteem: Chronic Low; Social Interaction, Impaired; Sorrow: Chronic.

NURSING DIAGNOSIS: Sudden Infant Death Syndrome, Risk for

DEFINITION: Presence of risk factors for sudden death of an infant under 1 year of age.

Outcome	Major Interventions	Suggested Interventions	Optional Interventions
Parenting: Infant/Toddler Physical Safety DEFINITION: Parental actions to avoid physical injury of a child from birth through 2 years of age	Parent Education: Infant Teaching: Infant Safety	Anticipatory Guidance Childbirth Preparation Family Involvement Promotion Family Support Infant Care Newborn Care Resuscitation: Neonate	Caregiver Support Developmental Care Parenting Promotion Respiratory Monitoring Risk Identification: Childbearing Family
Preterm Infant Organization DEFINITION: Extrauterine integration of physiologic and behavioral function by the infant born 24 to 37 (term) weeks' gestation	Developmental Care Teaching: Infant Safety	Anticipatory Guidance Infant Care Kangaroo Care Newborn Care Parent Education: Infant Parenting Promotion Teaching: Infant Stimulation Temperature Regulation	Risk Identification: Childbearing Family Respiratory Monitoring Resuscitation: Neonate

For interventions and outcomes related to specific risk factors, refer to the following diagnoses: Breathing Pattern, Ineffective; Infant Behavior, Disorganized; Parenting, Impaired; Protection, Ineffective; Suffocation, Risk for; Thermoregulation, Ineffective; Ventilation, Impaired Spontaneous.

NURSING DIAGNOSIS: Suffocation, Risk for

DEFINITION: Accentuated risk of accidental suffocation (inadequate air available for inhalation).

Outcome	Major Interventions	Suggested Interventions	Optional Interventions
Aspiration Prevention DEFINITION: Personal actions to prevent the passage of fluid and solid particles into the lung	Aspiration Precautions Respiratory Monitoring	Airway Management Airway Suctioning Artificial Airway Management Environmental Management: Safety Positioning Teaching: Infant Safety Ventilation Assistance	Cough Enhancement Infant Care Parent Education: Infant Surveillance: Safety Swallowing Therapy Vital Signs Monitoring

Outcome	Major Interventions	Suggested Interventions	Optional Interventions
Asthma Self-Management			
DEFINITION: Personal actions to reverse inflammatory condition resulting in bronchial constriction of the airways	Airway Management Asthma Management	Cough Enhancement Emergency Care Environmental Management: Safety Medication Administration Medication Administration: Inhalation Medication Administration: Nasal Medication Administration: Oral Medication Management Respiratory Monitoring Teaching: Disease Process Teaching: Prescribed Medication Teaching: Procedure/ Treatment	Chest Physiotherapy Parent Education: Childrearing Family Surveillance Ventilation Assistance Vital Signs Monitoring

Continued

Outcome	Major Interventions	Suggested Interventions	Optional Interventions
Respiratory Status: Ventilation			
DEFINITION: Movement of air in and out of the lungs	Airway Management Respiratory Monitoring	Airway Insertion and Stabilization Airway Suctioning Artificial Airway Management Aspiration Precautions Positioning Surveillance Ventilation Assistance Vital Signs Monitoring	Chest Physiotherapy Cough Enhancement Infant Care Parent Education: Infant Teaching: Infant Safety

For interventions and outcomes related to specific risk factors, refer to the following diagnoses: Airway Clearance, Ineffective; Confusion, Chronic; Health Maintenance, Ineffective; Home Maintenance, Impaired; Infant Behavior, Disorganized; Infant Feeding Pattern, Ineffective; Knowledge, Deficient; Protection, Ineffective; Swallowing, Impaired; Ventilation, Impaired Spontaneous.

NURSING DIAGNOSIS: Suicide, Risk for

DEFINITION: At risk for self-inflicted, life-threatening injury.

Outcome	Major Interventions	Suggested Interventions	Optional Interventions
Mood Equilibrium DEFINITION: Appropriate adjustment of prevailing emotional tone in response to circumstances	Mood Management	Active Listening Coping Enhancement Counseling Delusion Management Grief Work Facilitation Guilt Work Facilitation Medication Management Suicide Prevention Support Group	Anxiety Reduction Calming Technique Emotional Support Exercise Promotion Presence

Continued

Outcome	Major Interventions	Suggested Interventions	Optional Interventions
Suicide Self-Restraint			
DEFINITION: Personal actions to refrain from gestures and attempts at killing self	Behavior Management: Self-Harm Suicide Prevention	Anger Control Assistance Area Restriction Behavior Modification Coping Enhancement Counseling Delusion Management Environmental Management: Safety Grief Work Facilitation Impulse Control Training Medication Management Mood Management Patient Contracting Surveillance: Safety Therapy Group	Anxiety Reduction Crisis Intervention Family Involvement Promotion Family Therapy Forgiveness Facilitation Hallucination Management Limit Setting Self-Esteem Enhancement Self-Responsibility Facilitation Substance Use Treatment

Outcome	Major Interventions	Suggested Interventions	Optional Interventions

Will to Live
 	
DEFINITION:
Desire,
determination,
and effort to
survive
	Hope Instillation
	Spiritual Support
	Suicide Prevention
		Coping
		  Enhancement
		Counseling
		Emotional Support
		Grief Work
		  Facilitation
		Mood Management
		Relocation Stress
		  Reduction
		Self-Awareness
		  Enhancement
		Self-Esteem
		  Enhancement
		Socialization
		  Enhancement
		Support Group
		Support System
		  Enhancement
		Values Clarification
			Behavior Management:
			  Self-Harm
			Crisis Intervention
			Family Involvement
			  Promotion
			Forgiveness Facilitation
			Guilt Work Facilitation
			Substance Use
			  Treatment

For interventions and outcomes related to specific risk factors, refer to the following diagnoses: Adjustment, Impaired; Anxiety; Coping, Ineffective; Family Processes, Dysfunctional: Alcoholism; Grieving, Dysfunctional; Hopelessness; Loneliness, Risk for; Relocation Stress Syndrome; Sorrow: Chronic; Thought Processes, Disturbed.

NURSING DIAGNOSIS: Trauma, Risk for

DEFINITION: Accentuated risk of accidental tissue injury (e.g., wound, burn, fracture).

Outcome	Major Interventions	Suggested Interventions	Optional Interventions
Personal Safety Behavior			
DEFINITION: Personal actions of an adult to control behaviors that cause physical injury	Environmental Management: Safety	Behavior Modification Health Education Risk Identification Seizure Precautions Sports-Injury Prevention: Youth Surveillance: Safety Teaching: Individual Teaching: Infant Safety Teaching: Toddler Safety Vehicle Safety Promotion	Behavior Management: Overactivity/ Inattention Embolus Precautions Environmental Management: Worker Safety Parent Education: Adolescent Parent Education: Childrearing Family Parent Education: Infant Physical Restraint Security Enhancement
Physical Injury Severity			
DEFINITION: Severity of injuries from accidents and trauma	Environmental Management: Safety	Environmental Management: Worker Safety Environmental Risk Protection Fall Prevention Home Maintenance Assistance Risk Identification Security Enhancement Surveillance: Safety Vital Signs Monitoring	Dementia Management Hallucination Management Seizure Precautions Sports-Injury Prevention: Youth

Outcome	Major Interventions	Suggested Interventions	Optional Interventions
Tissue Integrity: Skin & Mucous Membranes			
DEFINITION: Structural intactness and normal physiological function of skin and mucous membranes	Pressure Management Skin Surveillance	Bathing Chemotherapy Management Circulatory Precautions Infection Protection Medication Administration: Skin Nutrition Management Oral Health Maintenance Positioning Pressure Ulcer Prevention Radiation Therapy Management Self-Care Assistance: Bathing/Hygiene Self-Care Assistance: Toileting Self-Care Assistance: Transfer Simple Massage Skin Care: Topical Treatments	Bed Rest Care Eye Care Foot Care Laser Precautions Nail Care Perineal Care Peripheral Sensation Management Positioning: Wheelchair

For interventions and outcomes related to specific risk factors, refer to the following diagnoses: Community Coping, Ineffective; Fatigue; Home Maintenance, Impaired; Parenting, Impaired; Mobility: Physical, Impaired; Protection, Ineffective; Sleep Deprivation.

NURSING DIAGNOSIS: Urinary Incontinence: Urge, Risk for

DEFINITION: At risk for involuntary loss of urine associated with a sudden, strong sensation or urinary urgency.

Outcome	Major Interventions	Suggested Interventions	Optional Interventions
Urinary Continence			
DEFINITION: Control of elimination of urine from the bladder	Urinary Bladder Training Urinary Habit Training	Biofeedback Fluid Management Fluid Monitoring Medication Administration Medication Management Pelvic Muscle Exercise Self-Care Assistance: Toileting Urinary Elimination Management	Environmental Management Exercise Promotion Health Screening Pessary Management Prompted Voiding Tube Care: Urinary Urinary Catheterization Weight Management
Urinary Elimination			
DEFINITION: Collection and discharge of urine	Urinary Elimination Management	Fluid Management Fluid Monitoring Medication Administration Self-Care Assistance: Toileting Urinary Bladder Training	Pelvic Muscle Exercise Prompted Voiding Urinary Habit Training

For interventions and outcomes related to specific risk factors, refer to the following diagnoses: Growth and Development, Delayed; Therapeutic Regimen Management, Ineffective; Self-Care Deficit: Toileting.

NURSING DIAGNOSIS: Violence: Other-Directed, Risk for

DEFINITION: At risk for behaviors in which an individual demonstrates that he/she can be physically, emotionally, and/or sexually harmful to others.

Outcome	Major Interventions	Suggested Interventions	Optional Interventions
Abuse Cessation			
DEFINITION: Evidence that the victim is no longer hurt or exploited	Abuse Protection Support Behavior Management	Abuse Protection Support: Child Abuse Protection Support: Domestic Partner Abuse Protection Support: Elder Anger Control Assistance Coping Enhancement Counseling Environmental Management: Violence Prevention Risk Identification Self-Esteem Enhancement	Calming Technique Caregiver Support Emotional Support Family Involvement Promotion Family Support Guilt Work Facilitation Mood Management Parent Education: Childrearing Family Parent Education: Infant Role Enhancement Self-Awareness Enhancement Sexual Counseling Support Group

Continued

Outcome	Major Interventions	Suggested Interventions	Optional Interventions
Abusive Behavior Self-Restraint DEFINITION: Self-restraint of abusive and neglectful behaviors toward others	Anger Control Assistance Environmental Management: Violence Prevention	Abuse Protection Support Abuse Protection Support: Child Abuse Protection Support: Domestic Partner Abuse Protection Support: Elder Behavior Management Behavior Management: Sexual Behavior Modification Coping Enhancement Counseling Emotional Support Environmental Management: Safety Impulse Control Training Referral Risk Identification Self-Modification Assistance Self-Responsibility Facilitation Substance Use Treatment Substance Use Treatment: Alcohol Withdrawal Substance Use Treatment: Drug Withdrawal Surveillance	Medication Management Medication Prescribing Parent Education: Childrearing Family Self-Awareness Enhancement Self-Esteem Enhancement Support Group Support System Enhancement Teaching: Individual Values Clarification

Outcome	Major Interventions	Suggested Interventions	Optional Interventions
Aggression Self-Control			
DEFINITION: Self-restraint of assaultive, combative, or destructive behaviors toward others	Anger Control Assistance Environmental Management: Violence Prevention	Abuse Protection Support Area Restriction Assertiveness Training Behavior Management Behavior Modification Calming Technique Coping Enhancement Counseling Crisis Intervention Fire-Setting Precautions Impulse Control Training Limit Setting Medication Management Patient Contracting Physical Restraint Seclusion Surveillance: Safety	Animal-Assisted Therapy Art Therapy Behavior Management: Overactivity/ Inattention Behavior Modification: Social Skills Delusion Management Dementia Management Environmental Management Environmental Management: Safety Hallucination Management Self-Awareness Enhancement Self-Modification Assistance Self-Responsibility Facilitation Socialization Enhancement Therapeutic Play Triage: Emergency Center Triage: Telephone

Continued

Outcome	Major Interventions	Suggested Interventions	Optional Interventions
Impulse Self-Control DEFINITION: Self-restraint of compulsive or impulsive behaviors	Anger Control Assistance Impulse Control Training	Anxiety Reduction Behavior Management Behavior Modification Behavior Modification: Social Skills Environmental Management: Safety Environmental Management: Violence Prevention Fire-Setting Precautions Limit Setting Patient Contracting Physical Restraint Seclusion Self-Modification Assistance Self-Responsibility Facilitation	Coping Enhancement Emotional Support Mood Management Risk Identification Security Enhancement Substance Use Prevention Substance Use Treatment Support Group Support System Enhancement Surveillance: Safety Therapy Group

For interventions and outcomes related to specific risk factors, refer to the following diagnoses: Caregiver Role Strain; Coping, Ineffective; Family Coping, Disabled; Family Processes, Interrupted; Parenteral Role Conflict; Personal Identity, Disturbed; Self-Esteem: Chronic Low; Thought Processes, Disturbed.

NURSING DIAGNOSIS: Violence: Self-Directed, Risk for

DEFINITION: At risk for behaviors in which an individual demonstrates that he/she can be physically, emotionally, and/or sexually harmful to self.

Outcome	Major Interventions	Suggested Interventions	Optional Interventions
Impulse Self-Control DEFINITION: Self-restraint of compulsive or impulsive behaviors	Impulse Control Training	Anger Control Assistance Anxiety Reduction Area Restriction Behavior Management Behavior Management: Overactivity/ Inattention Behavior Management: Self-Harm Behavior Modification Environmental Management: Safety Environmental Management: Violence Prevention Limit Setting Patient Contracting Physical Restraint Self-Modification Assistance Self-Responsibility Facilitation	Behavior Modification: Social Skills Coping Enhancement Emotional Support Mood Management Risk Identification Security Enhancement Self-Awareness Enhancement Substance Use Prevention Substance Use Treatment Substance Use Treatment: Alcohol Withdrawal Substance Use Treatment: Drug Withdrawal Support Group Support System Enhancement Surveillance: Safety Therapy Group

Continued

Outcome	Major Interventions	Suggested Interventions	Optional Interventions
Self-Mutilation Restraint			
DEFINITION: Personal actions to refrain from intentional self-inflicted injury (non-lethal)	Behavior Management: Self-Harm Environmental Management: Violence Prevention	Anger Control Assistance Anxiety Reduction Area Restriction Behavior Modification Cognitive Restructuring Coping Enhancement Counseling Emotional Support Environmental Management: Safety Impulse Control Training Limit Setting Mood Management Patient Contracting Physical Restraint Security Enhancement Suicide Prevention Surveillance: Safety	Active Listening Crisis Intervention Delusion Management Family Involvement Promotion Hallucination Management Mutual Goal Setting Presence

Outcome	Major Interventions	Suggested Interventions	Optional Interventions
Suicide Self-Restraint DEFINITION: Personal actions to refrain from gestures and attempts at killing self	Behavior Management: Self-Harm Environmental Management: Violence Prevention Suicide Prevention	Area Restriction Cognitive Restructuring Coping Enhancement Counseling Delusion Management Elopement Precautions Emotional Support Environmental Management: Safety Hallucination Management Hope Instillation Impulse Control Training Mood Management Patient Contracting Physical Restraint Security Enhancement Substance Use Prevention Support Group Surveillance: Safety	Anger Control Assistance Anxiety Reduction Assertiveness Training Behavior Modification Crisis Intervention Family Involvement Promotion Family Support Grief Work Facilitation Guilt Work Facilitation Limit Setting Self-Esteem Enhancement Spiritual Support Substance Use Treatment Substance Use Treatment: Overdose

For interventions and outcomes related to specific risk factors, refer to the following diagnoses: Anxiety; Body Image, Disturbed; Coping, Ineffective; Family Processes, Interrupted; Hopelessness; Personal Identity, Disturbed; Post-Trauma Syndrome; Rape-Trauma Syndrome; Self-Esteem: Chronic Low; Sexual Dysfunction; Social Isolation; Sorrow: Chronic; Spiritual Distress.

PART III

APPENDIXES

NOC Outcome Labels and Definitions

330 Outcomes

2500	Abuse Cessation	Evidence that the victim is no longer hurt or exploited
2501	Abuse Protection	Protection of self or dependent others from abuse
2514	Abuse Recovery Status	Extent of healing following physical or psychological abuse that may include sexual or financial exploitation
2502	Abuse Recovery: Emotional	Extent of healing of psychological injuries due to abuse
2503	Abuse Recovery: Financial	Extent of control of monetary and legal matters following financial exploitation
2504	Abuse Recovery: Physical	Extent of healing of physical injuries due to abuse
2505	Abuse Recovery: Sexual	Extent of healing of physical and psychological injuries due to sexual abuse or exploitation
1400	Abusive Behavior Self-Restraint	Self-restraint of abusive and neglectful behaviors toward others
1300	Acceptance: Health Status	Reconciliation to significant change in health circumstances
0005	Activity Tolerance	Physiologic response to energy-consuming movements with daily activities
1308	Adaptation to Physical Disability	Adaptive response to a significant functional challenge due to a physical disability
1600	Adherence Behavior	Self-initiated actions to promote wellness, recovery, and rehabilitation
1401	Aggression Self-Control	Self-restraint of assaultive, combative, or destructive behaviors toward others

From Moorhead, S., Johnson, M., & Maas, M. (Eds.). (2004). *Nursing outcomes classification (NOC)* (3rd ed.). St. Louis: Mosby.

0705	Allergic Response: Localized	Severity of localized hypersensitive immune response to a specific environmental (exogenous) antigen
0706	Allergic Response: Systemic	Severity of systemic hypersensitive immune response to a specific environmental (exogenous) antigen
0200	Ambulation	Ability to walk from place to place independently with or without assistive device
0201	Ambulation: Wheelchair	Ability to move from place to place in a wheelchair
1211	Anxiety Level	Severity of manifested apprehension, tension, or uneasiness arising from an unidentifiable source
1402	Anxiety Self-Control	Personal actions to eliminate or reduce feelings of apprehension, tension, or uneasiness from an unidentifiable source
1014	Appetite	Desire to eat when ill or receiving treatment
1918	Aspiration Prevention	Personal actions to prevent the passage of fluid and solid particles into the lung
0704	Asthma Self-Management	Personal actions to reverse inflammatory condition resulting in bronchial constriction of the airways
0202	Balance	Ability to maintain body equilibrium
0409	Blood Coagulation	Extent to which blood clots within normal period of time
2300	Blood Glucose Level	Extent to which glucose levels in plasma and urine are maintained in normal range
0413	Blood Loss Severity	Severity of internal or external bleeding/hemorrhage
0700	Blood Transfusion Reaction	Severity of complications with blood transfusion reaction
1200	Body Image	Perception of own appearance and body functions
1616	Body Mechanics Performance	Personal actions to maintain proper body alignment and to prevent muscular skeletal strain
0203	Body Positioning: Self-Initiated	Ability to change own body position independently with or without assistive device
1104	Bone Healing	Extent of regeneration of cells and tissues following bone injury
0500	Bowel Continence	Control of passage of stool from the bowel
0501	Bowel Elimination	Formation and evacuation of stool

1000	Breastfeeding Establishment: Infant	Infant attachment to and sucking from the mother's breast for nourishment during the first 3 weeks of breastfeeding
1001	Breastfeeding Establishment: Maternal	Maternal establishment of proper attachment of an infant to and sucking from the breast for nourishment during the first 3 weeks of breastfeeding
1002	Breastfeeding Maintenance	Continuation of breastfeeding for nourishment of an infant/toddler
1003	Breastfeeding Weaning	Progressive discontinuation of breastfeeding
1617	Cardiac Disease Self-Management	Personal actions to manage heart disease and prevent disease progression
0400	Cardiac Pump Effectiveness	Adequacy of blood volume ejected from the left ventricle to support systemic perfusion pressure
2200	Caregiver Adaptation to Patient Institutionalization	Adaptive response of family caregiver when the care recipient is moved to an institution
2506	Caregiver Emotional Health	Emotional well-being of a family care provider while caring for a family member
2202	Caregiver Home Care Readiness	Extent of preparedness of a caregiver to assume responsibility for the health care of a family member in the home
2203	Caregiver Lifestyle Disruption	Severity of disturbances in the lifestyle of a family member due to caregiving
2204	Caregiver-Patient Relationship	Positive interactions and connections between the caregiver and care recipient
2205	Caregiver Performance: Direct Care	Provision by family care provider of appropriate personal and health care for a family member
2206	Caregiver Performance: Indirect Care	Arrangement and oversight by family care provider of appropriate care for a family member
2507	Caregiver Physical Health	Physical well-being of a family care provider while caring for a family member
2208	Caregiver Stressors	Severity of biopsychosocial pressure on a family care provider caring for another over an extended period of time
2508	Caregiver Well-Being	Extent of positive perception of primary care provider's health status and life circumstances
2210	Caregiving Endurance Potential	Factors that promote family care provider continuance over an extended period of time
1301	Child Adaptation to Hospitalization	Adaptive response of a child from 3 years through 17 years of age to hospitalization

NOC

0120	Child Development: 1 Month	Milestones of physical, cognitive, and psychosocial progression by 1 month of age
0100	Child Development: 2 Months	Milestones of physical, cognitive, and psychosocial progression by 2 months of age
0101	Child Development: 4 Months	Milestones of physical, cognitive, and psychosocial progression by 4 months of age
0102	Child Development: 6 Months	Milestones of physical, cognitive, and psychosocial progression by 6 months of age
0103	Child Development: 12 Months	Milestones of physical, cognitive, and psychosocial progression by 12 months of age
0104	Child Development: 2 Years	Milestones of physical, cognitive, and psychosocial progression by 2 years of age
0105	Child Development: 3 Years	Milestones of physical, cognitive, and psychosocial progression by 3 years of age
0106	Child Development: 4 Years	Milestones of physical, cognitive, and psychosocial progression by 4 years of age
0107	Child Development: 5 Years	Milestones of physical, cognitive, and psychosocial progression by 5 years of age
0108	Child Development: Middle Childhood	Milestones of physical, cognitive, and psychosocial progression from 6 years through 11 years of age
0109	Child Development: Adolescence	Milestones of physical, cognitive, and psychosocial progression from 12 years through 17 years of age
0401	Circulation Status	Unobstructed, unidirectional blood flow at an appropriate pressure through large vessels of the systemic and pulmonary circuits
3000	Client Satisfaction: Access to Care Resources	Extent of positive perception of access to nursing staff, supplies, and equipment needed for care
3001	Client Satisfaction: Caring	Extent of positive perception of nursing staff's concern for the client
3002	Client Satisfaction: Communication	Extent of positive perception of information exchanged between client and nursing staff
3003	Client Satisfaction: Continuity of Care	Extent of positive perception of coordination of care as the patient moves from one care setting to another
3004	Client Satisfaction: Cultural Needs Fulfillment	Extent of positive perception of integration of cultural beliefs, values and social structures into nursing care
3005	Client Satisfaction: Functional Assistance	Extent of positive perception of nursing assistance to achieve mobility and self-care as independently as health condition permits

NOC

3006	Client Satisfaction: Physical Care	Extent of positive perception of nursing care to maintain body functions and cleanliness
3007	Client Satisfaction: Physical Environment	Extent of positive perception of living environment, treatment environment, equipment and supplies in acute or long-term care settings
3008	Client Satisfaction: Protection of Rights	Extent of positive perception of protection of a client's legal and moral rights provided by nursing staff
3009	Client Satisfaction: Psychological Care	Extent of positive perception of nursing assistance to perform emotional and mental activities as independently as health condition permits
3010	Client Satisfaction: Safety	Extent of positive perception of procedures, information and nursing care to prevent harm or injury
3011	Client Satisfaction: Symptom Control	Extent of positive perception of nursing care to relieve symptoms of illness
3012	Client Satisfaction: Teaching	Extent of positive perception of instruction provided by nursing staff to improve knowledge, understanding and participation in care
3013	Client Satisfaction: Technical Aspects of Care	Extent of positive perception of nursing staff's knowledge and expertise used in providing care
0900	Cognition	Ability to execute complex mental processes
0901	Cognitive Orientation	Ability to identify person, place, and time accurately
2100	Comfort Level	Extent of positive perception of physical and psychological ease
2007	Comfortable Death	Physical and psychological ease with the impending end of life
0902	Communication	Reception, interpretation, and expression of spoken, written, and non-verbal messages
0903	Communication: Expressive	Expression of meaningful verbal and/or non-verbal messages
0904	Communication: Receptive	Reception and interpretation of verbal and/or non-verbal messages
2700	Community Competence	Capacity of a community to collectively problem solve to achieve community goals
2804	Community Disaster Readiness	Community preparedness to respond to a natural or man-made calamitous event
2701	Community Health Status	General state of well-being of a community or population

2800	Community Health Status: Immunity	Resistance of community members to the invasion and spread of an infectious agent that could threaten public health
2801	Community Risk Control: Chronic Disease	Community actions to reduce the risk of chronic diseases and related complications
2802	Community Risk Control: Communicable Disease	Community actions to eliminate or reduce the spread of infectious agents that threaten public health
2803	Community Risk Control: Lead Exposure	Community actions to reduce lead exposure and poisoning
2805	Community Risk Control: Violence	Community actions to eliminate or reduce intentional violent acts resulting in serious physical or psychological harm
2702	Community Violence Level	Incidence of violent acts compared with local, state, or national values
1601	Compliance Behavior	Personal actions to promote wellness, recovery, and rehabilitation based on professional advice
0905	Concentration	Ability to focus on a specific stimulus
0212	Coordinated Movement	Ability of muscles to work together voluntarily for purposeful movement
1302	Coping	Personal actions to manage stressors that tax an individual's resources
0906	Decision-Making	Ability to make judgments and choose between two or more alternatives
1208	Depression Level	Severity of melancholic mood and loss of interest in life events
1409	Depression Self-Control	Personal actions to minimize melancholy and maintain interest in life events
1619	Diabetes Self-Management	Personal actions to manage diabetes mellitus and prevent disease progression
1307	Dignified Life Closure	Personal actions to maintain control during approaching end of life
0311	Discharge Readiness: Independent Living	Readiness of a patient to relocate from a health care institution to living independently
0312	Discharge Readiness: Supported Living	Readiness of a patient to relocate from a health care institution to a lower level of supported living
1403	Distorted Thought Self-Control	Self-restraint of disruptions in perception, thought processes, and thought content
0600	Electrolyte & Acid/Base Balance	Balance of the electrolytes and non-electrolytes in the intracellular and extracellular compartments of the body
0001	Endurance	Capacity to sustain activity

0002	Energy Conservation	Personal actions to manage energy for initiating and sustaining activity
1909	Fall Prevention Behavior	Personal or family caregiver actions to minimize risk factors that might precipitate falls in the personal environment
1912	Falls Occurrence	Number of falls in the past _____ (define period of time)
2600	Family Coping	Family actions to manage stressors that tax family resources
2602	Family Functioning	Capacity of the family system to meet the needs of its members during developmental transitions
2606	Family Health Status	Overall health and social competence of family unit
2603	Family Integrity	Family members' behaviors that collectively demonstrate cohesion, strength, and emotional bonding
2604	Family Normalization	Capacity of the family system to maintain routines and develop strategies for optimal functioning when a member has a chronic illness or disability
2605	Family Participation in Professional Care	Family involvement in decision-making, delivery, and evaluation of care provided by health care personnel
2607	Family Physical Environment	Physical arrangements in the home that provide safety and stimulation to family members
2608	Family Resiliency	Capacity of the family system to successfully adapt and function competently following significant adversity or crises
2601	Family Social Climate	Supportive milieu as characterized by family member relationships and goals
2609	Family Support During Treatment	Family presence and emotional support for an individual undergoing treatment
1210	Fear Level	Severity of manifested apprehension, tension, or uneasiness arising from an identifiable source
1213	Fear Level: Child	Severity of manifested apprehension, tension, or uneasiness arising from an identifiable source in a child from 1 year through 17 years of age
1404	Fear Self-Control	Personal actions to eliminate or reduce disabling feelings of apprehension, tension, or uneasiness from an identifiable source

NOC

0111	Fetal Status: Antepartum	Extent to which fetal signs are within normal limits from conception to the onset of labor
0112	Fetal Status: Intrapartum	Extent to which fetal signs are within normal limits from onset of labor to delivery
0601	Fluid Balance	Water balance in the intracellular and extracellular compartments of the body
0603	Fluid Overload Severity	Severity of excess fluids in the intracellular and extracellular compartments of the body
1304	Grief Resolution	Adjustment to actual or impending loss
0110	Growth	Normal increase in bone size and body weight during growth years
1700	Health Beliefs	Personal convictions that influence health behaviors
1701	Health Beliefs: Perceived Ability to Perform	Personal conviction that one can carry out a given health behavior
1702	Health Beliefs: Perceived Control	Personal conviction that one can influence a health outcome
1703	Health Beliefs: Perceived Resources	Personal conviction that one has adequate means to carry out a health behavior
1704	Health Beliefs: Perceived Threat	Personal conviction that a threatening health problem is serious and has potential negative consequences for lifestyle
1705	Health Orientation	Personal commitment to health behaviors as lifestyle priorities
1602	Health Promoting Behavior	Personal actions to sustain or increase wellness
1603	Health Seeking Behavior	Personal actions to promote optimal wellness, recovery, and rehabilitation
1610	Hearing Compensation Behavior	Personal actions to identify, monitor, and compensate for hearing loss
1105	Hemodialysis Access	Functionality of a dialysis access site
1201	Hope	Optimism that is personally satisfying and life-supporting
0602	Hydration	Adequate water in the intracellular and extracellular compartments of the body
0915	Hyperactivity Level	Severity of patterns of inattention or impulsivity in a child from 1 year through 17 years of age
1202	Identity	Distinguishes between self and non-self and characterizes one's essence
0204	Immobility Consequences: Physiological	Severity of compromise in physiological functioning due to impaired physical mobility

0205	Immobility Consequences: Psycho-Cognitive	Severity of compromise in psycho-cognitive functioning due to impaired physical mobility
0707	Immune Hypersensitivity Response	Severity of inappropriate immune responses
0702	Immune Status	Natural and acquired appropriately targeted resistance to internal and external antigens
1900	Immunization Behavior	Personal actions to obtain immunization to prevent a communicable disease
1405	Impulse Self-Control	Self-restraint of compulsive or impulsive behaviors
0703	Infection Severity	Severity of infection and associated symptoms
0708	Infection Severity: Newborn	Severity of infection and associated symptoms during the first 28 days of life
0907	Information Processing	Ability to acquire, organize, and use information
0213	Joint Movement: Ankle	Active range of motion of the ankle with self-initiated movement
0214	Joint Movement: Elbow	Active range of motion of the elbow with self-initiated movement
0215	Joint Movement: Fingers	Active range of motion of the fingers with self-initiated movement
0216	Joint Movement: Hip	Active range of motion of the hip with self-initiated movement
0217	Joint Movement: Knee	Active range of motion of the knee with self-initiated movement
0218	Joint Movement: Neck	Active range of motion of the neck with self-initiated movement
0207	Joint Movement: Passive	Joint movement with assistance
0219	Joint Movement: Shoulder	Active range of motion of the shoulder with self-initiated movement
0220	Joint Movement: Spine	Active range of motion of the spine with self-initiated movement
0221	Joint Movement: Wrist	Active range of motion of the wrist with self-initiated movement
0504	Kidney Function	Filtration of blood and elimination of metabolic waste products through the formation of urine
1827	Knowledge: Body Mechanics	Extent of understanding conveyed about proper body alignment, balance, and coordinated movement
1800	Knowledge: Breastfeeding	Extent of understanding conveyed about lactation and nourishment of an infant through breastfeeding
1830	Knowledge: Cardiac Disease Management	Extent of understanding conveyed about heart disease and the prevention of complications

NOC

1801	Knowledge: Child Physical Safety	Extent of understanding conveyed about safely caring for a child from 1 year through 17 years of age
1821	Knowledge: Conception Prevention	Extent of understanding conveyed about prevention of unintended pregnancy
1820	Knowledge: Diabetes Management	Extent of understanding conveyed about diabetes mellitus and the prevention of complications
1802	Knowledge: Diet	Extent of understanding conveyed about recommended diet
1803	Knowledge: Disease Process	Extent of understanding conveyed about a specific disease process
1804	Knowledge: Energy Conservation	Extent of understanding conveyed about energy conservation techniques
1828	Knowledge: Fall Prevention	Extent of understanding conveyed about prevention of falls
1816	Knowledge: Fertility Promotion	Extent of understanding conveyed about fertility testing and the conditions that affect conception
1805	Knowledge: Health Behavior	Extent of understanding conveyed about the promotion and protection of health
1823	Knowledge: Health Promotion	Extent of understanding conveyed about information needed to obtain and maintain optimal health
1806	Knowledge: Health Resources	Extent of understanding conveyed about relevant health care resources
1824	Knowledge: Illness Care	Extent of understanding conveyed about illness-related information needed to achieve and maintain optimal health
1819	Knowledge: Infant Care	Extent of understanding conveyed about caring for a baby from birth to 1st birthday
1807	Knowledge: Infection Control	Extent of understanding conveyed about prevention and control of infection
1817	Knowledge: Labor & Delivery	Extent of understanding conveyed about labor and vaginal delivery
1808	Knowledge: Medication	Extent of understanding conveyed about the safe use of medication
1829	Knowledge: Ostomy Care	Extent of understanding conveyed about maintenance of an ostomy for elimination
1826	Knowledge: Parenting	Extent of understanding conveyed about provision of a nurturing and constructive environment for a child from 1 year through 17 years of age
1809	Knowledge: Personal Safety	Extent of understanding conveyed about prevention of unintentional injuries

1818	Knowledge: Postpartum Maternal Health	Extent of understanding conveyed about maternal health following delivery
1822	Knowledge: Preconception Maternal Health	Extent of understanding conveyed about maternal health prior to conception to insure a healthy pregnancy
1810	Knowledge: Pregnancy	Extent of understanding conveyed about promotion of a healthy pregnancy and prevention of complications
1811	Knowledge: Prescribed Activity	Extent of understanding conveyed about prescribed activity and exercise
1815	Knowledge: Sexual Functioning	Extent of understanding conveyed about sexual development and responsible sexual practices
1812	Knowledge: Substance Use Control	Extent of understanding conveyed about controlling the use of drugs, tobacco, or alcohol
1814	Knowledge: Treatment Procedure(s)	Extent of understanding conveyed about procedure(s) required as part of a treatment regimen
1813	Knowledge: Treatment Regimen	Extent of understanding conveyed about a specific treatment regimen
1604	Leisure Participation	Use of relaxing, interesting, and enjoyable activities to promote well-being
1203	Loneliness Severity	Severity of emotional, social, or existential isolation response
2509	Maternal Status: Antepartum	Extent to which maternal well-being is within normal limits from conception to the onset of labor
2510	Maternal Status: Intrapartum	Extent to which maternal well-being is within normal limits from onset of labor to delivery
2511	Maternal Status: Postpartum	Extent to which maternal well-being is within normal limits from delivery of placenta to completion of involution
0411	Mechanical Ventilation Response: Adult	Alveolar exchange and tissue perfusion are supported by mechanical ventilation
0412	Mechanical Ventilation Weaning Response: Adult	Respiratory and psychological adjustment to progressive removal of mechanical ventilation
2301	Medication Response	Therapeutic and adverse effects of prescribed medication
0908	Memory	Ability to cognitively retrieve and report previously stored information
0208	Mobility	Ability to move purposefully in own environment independently with or without assistive device

NOC

1204	Mood Equilibrium	Appropriate adjustment of prevailing emotional tone in response to circumstances
1209	Motivation	Inner urge that moves or prompts an individual to positive action(s)
1618	Nausea & Vomiting Control	Personal actions to control nausea, retching, and vomiting symptoms
2106	Nausea & Vomiting: Disruptive Effects	Severity of observed or reported disruptive effects of nausea, retching, and vomiting on daily functioning
2107	Nausea & Vomiting Severity	Severity of nausea, retching, and vomiting symptoms
2513	Neglect Cessation	Evidence that the victim is no longer receiving substandard care
2512	Neglect Recovery	Extent of healing following the cessation of substandard care
0909	Neurological Status	Ability of the peripheral and central nervous system to receive, process, and respond to internal and external stimuli
0910	Neurological Status: Autonomic	Ability of the autonomic nervous system to coordinate visceral and homeostatic function
0911	Neurological Status: Central Motor Control	Ability of the central nervous system to coordinate skeletal muscle activity for body movement
0912	Neurological Status: Consciousness	Arousal, orientation, and attention to the environment
0913	Neurological Status: Cranial Sensory/Motor Function	Ability of the cranial nerves to convey sensory and motor impulses
0914	Neurological Status: Spinal Sensory/Motor Function	Ability of the spinal nerves to convey sensory and motor impulses
0118	Newborn Adaptation	Adaptive response to the extrauterine environment by a physiologically mature newborn during the first 28 days
1004	Nutritional Status	Extent to which nutrients are available to meet metabolic needs
1005	Nutritional Status: Biochemical Measures	Body fluid components and chemical indices of nutritional status
1007	Nutritional Status: Energy	Extent to which nutrients and oxygen provide cellular energy
1008	Nutritional Status: Food & Fluid Intake	Amount of food and fluid taken into the body over a 24-hour period
1009	Nutritional Status: Nutrient Intake	Adequacy of usual pattern of nutrient intake
1100	Oral Hygiene	Condition of the mouth, teeth, gums, and tongue

NOC

NOC

1615	Ostomy Self-Care	Personal actions to maintain ostomy for elimination
1306	Pain: Adverse Psychological Response	Severity of observed or reported adverse cognitive and emotional responses to physical pain
1605	Pain Control	Personal actions to control pain
2101	Pain: Disruptive Effects	Severity of observed or reported disruptive effects of chronic pain on daily functioning
2102	Pain Level	Severity of observed or reported pain
1500	Parent-Infant Attachment	Parent and infant behaviors that demonstrate an enduring affectionate bond
2902	Parenting: Adolescent Physical Safety	Parental actions to prevent physical injury in an adolescent from 12 years through 17 years of age
2901	Parenting: Early/Middle Childhood Physical Safety	Parental actions to avoid physical injury of a child from 3 years through 11 years of age
2900	Parenting: Infant/Toddler Physical Safety	Parental actions to avoid physical injury of a child from birth through 2 years of age
2211	Parenting Performance	Parental actions to provide a child a nurturing and constructive physical, emotional, and social environment
1901	Parenting: Psychosocial Safety	Parental actions to protect a child from social contacts that might cause harm or injury
1606	Participation in Health Care Decisions	Personal involvement in selecting and evaluating health care options to achieve desired outcome
1614	Personal Autonomy	Personal actions of a competent individual to exercise governance in life decisions
2006	Personal Health Status	Overall physical, psychological, social, and spiritual functioning of an adult 18 years or older
1911	Personal Safety Behavior	Personal actions of an adult to control behaviors that cause physical injury
2002	Personal Well-Being	Extent of positive perception of one's health status and life circumstances
0113	Physical Aging	Normal physical changes that occur with the natural aging process
2004	Physical Fitness	Performance of physical activities with vigor
1913	Physical Injury Severity	Severity of injuries from accidents and trauma
0114	Physical Maturation: Female	Normal physical changes in the female that occur with the transition from childhood to adulthood
0115	Physical Maturation: Male	Normal physical changes in the male that occur with the transition from childhood to adulthood

0116	Play Participation	Use of activities by a child from 1 year through 11 years of age to promote enjoyment, entertainment, and development
2303	Post Procedure Recovery Status	Extent to which an individual returns to baseline function following a procedure(s) requiring anesthesia or sedation
1607	Prenatal Health Behavior	Personal actions to promote a healthy pregnancy and a healthy newborn
0117	Preterm Infant Organization	Extrauterine integration of physiologic and behavioral function by the infant born 24 to 37 (term) weeks' gestation
0006	Psychomotor Energy	Personal drive and energy to maintain activities of daily living, nutrition, and personal safety
1305	Psychosocial Adjustment: Life Change	Adaptive psychosocial response of an individual to a significant life change
2000	Quality of Life	Extent of positive perception of current life circumstances
0410	Respiratory Status: Airway Patency	Open, clear tracheobronchial passages for air exchange
0402	Respiratory Status: Gas Exchange	Alveolar exchange of carbon dioxide and oxygen to maintain arterial blood gas concentrations
0403	Respiratory Status: Ventilation	Movement of air in and out of the lungs
0003	Rest	Quantity and pattern of diminished activity for mental and physical rejuvenation
1902	Risk Control	Personal actions to prevent, eliminate, or reduce modifiable health threats
1903	Risk Control: Alcohol Use	Personal actions to prevent, eliminate, or reduce alcohol use that poses a threat to health
1917	Risk Control: Cancer	Personal actions to detect or reduce the threat of cancer
1914	Risk Control: Cardiovascular Health	Personal actions to eliminate or reduce threats to cardiovascular health
1904	Risk Control: Drug Use	Personal actions to prevent, eliminate, or reduce drug use that poses a threat to health
1915	Risk Control: Hearing Impairment	Personal actions to prevent, eliminate, or reduce threats to hearing function
1905	Risk Control: Sexually Transmitted Diseases (STD)	Personal actions to prevent, eliminate, or reduce behaviors associated with sexually transmitted disease
1906	Risk Control: Tobacco Use	Personal actions to prevent, eliminate, or reduce tobacco use

1907	Risk Control: Unintended Pregnancy	Personal actions to prevent or reduce the possibility of unintended pregnancy
1916	Risk Control: Visual Impairment	Personal actions to prevent, eliminate, or reduce threats to visual function
1908	Risk Detection	Personal actions to identify personal health threats
1501	Role Performance	Congruence of an individual's role behavior with role expectations
1910	Safe Home Environment	Physical arrangements to minimize environmental factors that might cause physical harm or injury in the home
1620	Seizure Control	Personal actions to reduce or minimize the occurrence of seizure episodes
0313	Self-Care Status	Ability to perform basic personal care activities and household tasks
0300	Self-Care: Activities of Daily Living (ADL)	Ability to perform the most basic physical tasks and personal care activities independently with or without assistive device
0301	Self-Care: Bathing	Ability to cleanse own body independently with or without assistive device
0302	Self-Care: Dressing	Ability to dress self independently with or without assistive device
0303	Self-Care: Eating	Ability to prepare and ingest food and fluid independently with or without assistive device
0305	Self-Care: Hygiene	Ability to maintain own personal cleanliness and kempt appearance independently with or without assistive device
0306	Self-Care: Instrumental Activities of Daily Living (IADL)	Ability to perform activities needed to function in the home or community independently with or without assistive device
0307	Self-Care: Non-Parenteral Medication	Ability to administer oral and topical medications to meet therapeutic goals independently with or without assistive device
0308	Self-Care: Oral Hygiene	Ability to care for own mouth and teeth independently with or without assistive device
0309	Self-Care: Parenteral Medication	Ability to administer parenteral medications to meet therapeutic goals independently with or without assistive device
0310	Self-Care: Toileting	Ability to toilet self independently with or without assistive device

1613	Self-Direction of Care	Care recipient actions taken to direct others who assist with or perform physical tasks and personal health care
1205	Self-Esteem	Personal judgment of self-worth
1406	Self-Mutilation Restraint	Personal actions to refrain from intentional self-inflicted injury (non-lethal)
2405	Sensory Function Status	Extent to which an individual correctly perceives skin stimulation, sounds, proprioception, taste and smell, and visual images
2400	Sensory Function: Cutaneous	Extent to which stimulation of the skin is correctly sensed
2401	Sensory Function: Hearing	Extent to which sounds are correctly sensed
2402	Sensory Function: Proprioception	Extent to which the position and movement of the head and body are correctly sensed
2403	Sensory Function: Taste & Smell	Extent to which chemicals inhaled or dissolved in saliva are correctly sensed
2404	Sensory Function: Vision	Extent to which visual images are correctly sensed
0119	Sexual Functioning	Integration of physical, socioemotional, and intellectual aspects of sexual expression and performance
1207	Sexual Identity	Acknowledgment and acceptance of own sexual identity
0211	Skeletal Function	Ability of the bones to support the body and facilitate movement
0004	Sleep	Natural periodic suspension of consciousness during which the body is restored
1502	Social Interaction Skills	Personal behaviors that promote effective relationships
1503	Social Involvement	Social interactions with persons, groups, or organizations
1504	Social Support	Perceived availability and actual provision of reliable assistance from others
2001	Spiritual Health	Connectedness with self, others, higher power, all life, nature, and the universe that transcends and empowers the self
1212	Stress Level	Severity of manifested physical or mental tension resulting from factors that alter an existing equilibrium
2005	Student Health Status	Physical, cognitive/emotional, and social status of school age children that contribute to school attendance, participation in school activities, and ability to learn

NOC

1407	Substance Addiction Consequences	Severity of change in health status and social functioning due to substance addiction
2003	Suffering Severity	Severity of anguish associated with a distressing symptom, injury, or loss that has potential long-term effects
1408	Suicide Self-Restraint	Personal actions to refrain from gestures and attempts at killing self
1010	Swallowing Status	Safe passage of fluids and/or solids from the mouth to the stomach
1011	Swallowing Status: Esophageal Phase	Safe passage of fluids and/or solids from the pharynx to the stomach
1012	Swallowing Status: Oral Phase	Preparation, containment and posterior movement of fluids and/or solids in the mouth
1013	Swallowing Status: Pharyngeal Phase	Safe passage of fluids and/or solids from the mouth to the esophagus
1608	Symptom Control	Personal actions to minimize perceived adverse changes in physical and emotional functioning
2103	Symptom Severity	Severity of perceived adverse changes in physical, emotional, and social functioning
2104	Symptom Severity: Perimenopause	Severity of symptoms caused by declining hormonal levels
2105	Symptom Severity: Premenstrual Syndrome (PMS)	Severity of symptoms caused by cyclic hormonal fluctuations
2302	Systemic Toxin Clearance: Dialysis	Clearance of toxins from the body with peritoneal or hemodialysis
0800	Thermoregulation	Balance among heat production, heat gain, and heat loss
0801	Thermoregulation: Newborn	Balance among heat production, heat gain, and heat loss during the first 28 days of life
1101	Tissue Integrity: Skin & Mucous Membranes	Structural intactness and normal physiological function of skin and mucous membranes
0404	Tissue Perfusion: Abdominal Organs	Adequacy of blood flow through the small vessels of the abdominal viscera to maintain organ function
0405	Tissue Perfusion: Cardiac	Adequacy of blood flow through the coronary vasculature to maintain heart function
0406	Tissue Perfusion: Cerebral	Adequacy of blood flow through the cerebral vasculature to maintain brain function
0407	Tissue Perfusion: Peripheral	Adequacy of blood flow through the small vessels of the extremities to maintain tissue function

0408	Tissue Perfusion: Pulmonary	Adequacy of blood flow through pulmonary vasculature to perfuse alveoli/capillary unit
0210	Transfer Performance	Ability to change body location independently with or without assistive device
1609	Treatment Behavior: Illness or Injury	Personal actions to palliate or eliminate pathology
0502	Urinary Continence	Control of elimination of urine from the bladder
0503	Urinary Elimination	Collection and discharge of urine
1611	Vision Compensation Behavior	Personal actions to compensate for visual impairment
0802	Vital Signs	Extent to which temperature, pulse, respiration, and blood pressure are within normal range
1006	Weight: Body Mass	Extent to which body weight, muscle, and fat are congruent to height, frame, gender, and age
1612	Weight Control	Personal actions to achieve and maintain optimum body weight
1206	Will to Live	Desire, determination, and effort to survive
1102	Wound Healing: Primary Intention	Extent of regeneration of cells and tissue following intentional closure
1103	Wound Healing: Secondary Intention	Extent of regeneration of cells and tissue in an open wound

NIC Interventions Labels and Definitions

514 Interventions

6400	Abuse Protection Support	Identification of high-risk dependent relationships and actions to prevent further infliction of physical or emotional harm
6402	Abuse Protection Support: Child	Identification of high-risk, dependent child relationships and actions to prevent possible or further infliction of physical, sexual, or emotional harm or neglect of basic necessities of life
6403	Abuse Protection Support: Domestic Partner	Identification of high-risk, dependent domestic relationships and actions to prevent possible or further infliction of physical, sexual, or emotional harm or exploitation of a domestic partner
6404	Abuse Protection Support: Elder	Identification of high-risk, dependent elder relationships and actions to prevent possible or further infliction of physical, sexual, or emotional harm; neglect of basic necessities of life; or exploitation
6408	Abuse Protection Support: Religious	Identification of high risk, controlling religious relationships and actions to prevent infliction of physical, sexual, or emotional harm and/or exploitation
1910	Acid-Base Management	Promotion of acid-base balance and prevention of complications resulting from acid-base imbalance
1911	Acid-Base Management: Metabolic Acidosis	Promotion of acid-base balance and prevention of complications resulting from serum HCO_3 levels lower than desired

Dochterman, J.C., & Bulechek, G.M. (Eds.). (2004). *Nursing Interventions Classification (NIC)* (4th ed.). St Louis, MO: Mosby.

NIC

1912	Acid-Base Management: Metabolic Alkalosis	Promotion of acid-base balance and prevention of complications resulting from serum HCO_3 levels higher than desired
1913	Acid-Base Management: Respiratory Acidosis	Promotion of acid-base balance and prevention of complications resulting from serum PCO_2 levels higher than desired
1914	Acid-Base Management: Respiratory Alkalosis	Promotion of acid-base balance and prevention of complications resulting from serum PCO_2 levels lower than desired
1920	Acid-Base Monitoring	Collection and analysis of patient data to regulate acid-base balance
4920	Active Listening	Attending closely to and attaching significance to a patient's verbal and nonverbal messages
4310	Activity Therapy	Prescription of and assistance with specific physical, cognitive, social, and spiritual activities to increase the range, frequency, or duration of an individual's (or group's) activity
1320	Acupressure	Application of firm, sustained pressure to special points on the body to decrease pain, produce relaxation, and prevent or reduce nausea
7310	Admission Care	Facilitating entry of a patient into a health care facility
3120	Airway Insertion and Stabilization	Insertion or assistance with insertion and stabilization of an artificial airway
3140	Airway Management	Facilitation of patency of air passages
3160	Airway Suctioning	Removal of airway secretions by inserting a suction catheter into the patient's oral airway and/or trachea
6410	Allergy Management	Identification, treatment, and prevention of allergic responses to food, medications, insect bites, contrast material, blood, and other substances
6700	Amnioinfusion	Infusion of fluid into the uterus during labor to relieve umbilical cord compression or to dilute meconium-stained fluid
3420	Amputation Care	Promotion of physical and psychological healing before and after amputation of a body part
2210	Analgesic Administration	Use of pharmacologic agents to reduce or eliminate pain
2214	Analgesic Administration: Intraspinal	Administration of pharmacologic agents into the epidural or intrathecal space to reduce or eliminate pain

6412	Anaphylaxis Management	Promotion of adequate ventilation and tissue perfusion for an individual with a severe allergic (antigen-antibody) reaction
2840	Anesthesia Administration	Preparation for and administration of anesthetic agents and monitoring of patient responsiveness during administration
4640	Anger Control Assistance	Facilitation of the expression of anger in an adaptive, nonviolent manner
4320	Animal-Assisted Therapy	Purposeful use of animals to provide affection, attention, diversion, and relaxation
5210	Anticipatory Guidance	Preparation of patient for an anticipated developmental and/or situational crisis
5820	Anxiety Reduction	Minimizing apprehension, dread, foreboding, or uneasiness related to an unidentified source of anticipated danger
6420	Area Restriction	Limitation of patient mobility to a specified area for purposes of safety or behavior management
1330	Aromatherapy	Administration of essential oils through massage, topical ointments or lotions, baths, inhalation, douches, or compresses (hot or cold) to calm and sooth, provide pain relief, and enhance relaxation and comfort
4330	Art Therapy	Facilitation of communication through drawings or other art forms
3180	Artificial Airway Management	Maintenance of endotracheal and tracheostomy tubes and prevention of complications associated with their use
3200	Aspiration Precautions	Prevention or minimization of risk factors in the patient at risk for aspiration
4340	Assertiveness Training	Assistance with the effective expression of feelings, needs, and ideas while respecting the rights of others
3210	Asthma Management	Identification, treatment, and prevention of reactions to inflammation/constriction in the airway passages
6710	Attachment Promotion	Facilitation of the development of the parent-infant relationship
5840	Autogenic Training	Assisting with self-suggestions about feelings of heaviness and warmth for the purpose of inducing relaxation
2860	Autotransfusion	Collecting and reinfusing blood that has been lost intraoperatively or postoperatively from clean wounds

NIC

1610	Bathing	Cleaning of the body for the purposes of relaxation, cleanliness, and healing
0740	Bed Rest Care	Promotion of comfort and safety and prevention of complications for a patient unable to get out of bed
7610	Bedside Laboratory Testing	Performance of laboratory tests at the bedside or point of care
4350	Behavior Management	Helping a patient to manage negative behavior
4352	Behavior Management: Overactivity/Inattention	Provision of a therapeutic milieu that safely accommodates the patient's attention deficit and/or overactivity while promoting optimal function
4354	Behavior Management: Self-Harm	Assisting the patient to decrease or eliminate self-mutilating or self-abusive behaviors
4356	Behavior Management: Sexual	Delineation and prevention of socially unacceptable sexual behaviors
4360	Behavior Modification	Promotion of a behavior change
4362	Behavior Modification: Social Skills	Assisting the patient to develop or improve interpersonal social skills
4680	Bibliotherapy	Use of literature to enhance the expression of feelings and the gaining of insight
5860	Biofeedback	Assisting the patient to modify a body function using feedback from instrumentation
8810	Bioterrorism Preparedness	Preparing for an effective response to bioterrorism events or disaster
6720	Birthing	Delivery of a baby
0550	Bladder Irrigation	Instillation of a solution into the bladder to provide cleansing or medication
4010	Bleeding Precautions	Reduction of stimuli that may induce bleeding or hemorrhage in at-risk patients
4020	Bleeding Reduction	Limitation of the loss of blood volume during an episode of bleeding
4021	Bleeding Reduction: Antepartum Uterus	Limitation of the amount of blood loss from the pregnant uterus during third trimester of pregnancy
4022	Bleeding Reduction: Gastrointestinal	Limitation of the amount of blood loss from the upper and lower gastrointestinal tract and related complications
4024	Bleeding Reduction: Nasal	Limitation of the amount of blood loss from the nasal cavity
4026	Bleeding Reduction: Postpartum Uterus	Limitation of the amount of blood loss from the postpartum uterus

4028	Bleeding Reduction: Wound	Limitation of the blood loss from a wound that may be a result of trauma, incisions, or placement of a tube or catheter
4030	Blood Products Administration	Administration of blood or blood products and monitoring of patient's response
5220	Body Image Enhancement	Improving a patient's conscious and unconscious perceptions and attitudes toward his/her body
0140	Body Mechanics Promotion	Facilitating the use of posture and movement in daily activities to prevent fatigue and musculoskeletal strain or injury
1052	Bottle Feeding	Preparation and administration of fluids to an infant via a bottle
0410	Bowel Incontinence Care	Promotion of bowel continence and maintenance of perianal skin integrity
0412	Bowel Incontinence Care: Encopresis	Promotion of bowel continence in children
0420	Bowel Irrigation	Instillation of a substance into the lower gastrointestinal tract
0430	Bowel Management	Establishment and maintenance of a regular pattern of bowel elimination
0440	Bowel Training	Assisting the patient to train the bowel to evacuate at specific intervals
6522	Breast Examination	Inspection and palpation of the breasts and related areas
1054	Breastfeeding Assistance	Preparing a new mother to breastfeed her infant
5880	Calming Technique	Reducing anxiety in patient experiencing acute distress
4035	Capillary Blood Sample	Obtaining an arteriovenous sample from a peripheral body site, such as the heel, finger or other transcutaneous site
4040	Cardiac Care	Limitation of complications resulting from an imbalance between myocardial oxygen supply and demand for a patient with symptoms of impaired cardiac function
4044	Cardiac Care: Acute	Limitation of complications for a patient recently experiencing an episode of an imbalance between myocardial oxygen supply and demand resulting in impaired cardiac function
4046	Cardiac Care: Rehabilitative	Promotion of maximum functional activity level for a patient who has experienced an episode of impaired cardiac function that resulted from an imbalance between myocardial oxygen supply and demand

4050	Cardiac Precautions	Prevention of an acute episode of impaired cardiac function by minimizing myocardial oxygen consumption or increasing myocardial oxygen supply
7040	Caregiver Support	Provision of the necessary information, advocacy, and support to facilitate primary patient care by someone other than a health care professional
7320	Case Management	Coordinating care and advocating for specified individuals and patient populations across settings to reduce cost, reduce resource use, improve quality of health care, and achieve desired outcomes
0762	Cast Care: Maintenance	Care of a cast after the drying period
0764	Cast Care: Wet	Care of a new cast during the drying period
2540	Cerebral Edema Management	Limitation of secondary cerebral injury resulting from swelling of brain tissue
2550	Cerebral Perfusion Promotion	Promotion of adequate perfusion and limitation of complications for a patient experiencing or at risk for inadequate cerebral perfusion
6750	Cesarean Section Care	Preparation and support of patient delivering a baby by cesarean section
6430	Chemical Restraint	Administration, monitoring, and discontinuation of psychotropic agents used to control an individual's extreme behavior
2240	Chemotherapy Management	Assisting the patient and family to understand the action and minimize side effects of antineoplastic agents
3230	Chest Physiotherapy	Assisting the patient to move airway secretions from peripheral airways to more central airways for expectoration and/or suctioning
6760	Childbirth Preparation	Providing information and support to facilitate childbirth and to enhance the ability of an individual to develop and perform the role of parent
4062	Circulatory Care: Arterial Insufficiency	Promotion of arterial circulation
4064	Circulatory Care: Mechanical Assist Device	Temporary support of the circulation through the use of mechanical devices or pumps
4066	Circulatory Care: Venous Insufficiency	Promotion of venous circulation

4070	Circulatory Precautions	Protection of a localized area with limited perfusion
3000	Circumcision Care	Preprocedural and postprocedural support to males undergoing circumcision
6140	Code Management	Coordination of emergency measures to sustain life
4700	Cognitive Restructuring	Challenging a patient to alter distorted thought patterns and view self and the world more realistically
4720	Cognitive Stimulation	Promotion of awareness and comprehension of surroundings by utilization of planned stimuli
8820	Communicable Disease Management	Working with a community to decrease and manage the incidence and prevalence of contagious diseases in a specific population
4974	Communication Enhancement: Hearing Deficit	Assistance in accepting and learning alternate methods for living with diminished hearing
4976	Communication Enhancement: Speech Deficit	Assistance in accepting and learning alternate methods for living with impaired speech
4978	Communication Enhancement: Visual Deficit	Assistance in accepting and learning alternate methods for living with diminished vision
8840	Community Disaster Preparedness	Preparing for an effective response to a large-scale disaster
8500	Community Health Development	Assisting members of a community to identify a community's health concerns, mobilize resources, and implement solutions
5000	Complex Relationship Building	Establishing a therapeutic relationship with a patient who has difficulty interacting with others
5020	Conflict Mediation	Facilitation of constructive dialogue between opposing parties with a goal of resolving disputes in a mutually acceptable manner
0450	Constipation/Impaction Management	Prevention and alleviation of constipation/impaction
7910	Consultation	Using expert knowledge to work with those who seek help in problem solving to enable individuals, families, groups, or agencies to achieve identified goals
1620	Contact Lens Care	Prevention of eye injury and lens damage by proper use of contact lenses

7620	Controlled Substance Checking	Promoting appropriate use and maintaining security of controlled substances
5230	Coping Enhancement	Assisting a patient to adapt to perceived stressors, changes, or threats that interfere with meeting life demands and roles
7630	Cost Containment	Management and facilitation of efficient and effective use of resources
3250	Cough Enhancement	Promotion of deep inhalation by the patient with subsequent generation of high intrathoracic pressures and compression of underlying lung parenchyma for the forceful expulsion of air
5240	Counseling	Use of an interactive helping process focusing on the needs, problems, or feelings of the patient and significant others to enhance or support coping, problem solving, and interpersonal relationships
6160	Crisis Intervention	Use of short-term counseling to help the patient cope with a crisis and resume a state of functioning comparable to or better than the pre-crisis state
7640	Critical Path Development	Constructing and using a timed sequence of patient care activities to enhance desired patient outcomes in a cost-efficient manner
7330	Culture Brokerage	The deliberate use of culturally competent strategies to bridge or mediate between the patient's culture and the biomedical health care system
1340	Cutaneous Stimulation	Stimulation of the skin and underlying tissues for the purpose of decreasing undesirable signs and symptoms such as pain, muscle spasm, or inflammation
5250	Decision-Making Support	Providing information and support for a patient who is making a decision regarding health care
7650	Delegation	Transfer of responsibility for the performance of patient care while retaining accountability for the outcome
6440	Delirium Management	Provision of a safe and therapeutic environment for the patient who is experiencing an acute confusional state
6450	Delusion Management	Promoting the comfort, safety, and reality orientation of a patient experiencing false, fixed beliefs that have little or no basis in reality

6460	Dementia Management	Provision of a modified environment for the patient who is experiencing a chronic confusional state
6462	Dementia Management: Bathing	Reduction of aggressive behavior during cleaning of the body
7930	Deposition/Testimony	Provision of recorded sworn testimony for legal proceedings based upon knowledge of the case
8250	Developmental Care	Structuring the environment and providing care in response to the behavioral cues and states of the preterm infant
8272	Developmental Enhancement: Adolescent	Facilitating optimal physical, cognitive, social, and emotional growth of individuals during the transition from childhood to adulthood
8274	Developmental Enhancement: Child	Facilitating or teaching parents/caregivers to facilitate the optimal gross motor, fine motor, language, cognitive, social, and emotional growth of preschool and school-aged children
4240	Dialysis Access Maintenance	Preservation of vascular (arterial-venous) access sites
0460	Diarrhea Management	Management and alleviation of diarrhea
1020	Diet Staging	Instituting required diet restrictions with subsequent progression of diet as tolerated
7370	Discharge Planning	Preparation for moving a patient from one level of care to another within or outside the current health care agency
5900	Distraction	Purposeful focusing of attention away from undesirable sensations
7920	Documentation	Recording of pertinent patient data in a clinical record
1630	Dressing	Choosing, putting on, and removing clothes for a person who cannot do this for self
5260	Dying Care	Promotion of physical comfort and psychological peace in the final phase of life
2560	Dysreflexia Management	Prevention and elimination of stimuli that cause hyperactive reflexes and inappropriate autonomic responses in a patient with a cervical or high thoracic cord lesion
4090	Dysrhythmia Management	Preventing, recognizing, and facilitating treatment of abnormal cardiac rhythms
1640	Ear Care	Prevention or minimization of threats to ear or hearing

1030	Eating Disorders Management	Prevention and treatment of severe diet restriction and overexercising or binging and purging of food and fluids
2570	Electroconvulsive Therapy (ECT) Management	Assisting with the safe and efficient provision of electroconvulsive therapy in the treatment of psychiatric illness
2000	Electrolyte Management	Promotion of electrolyte balance and prevention of complications resulting from abnormal or undesired serum electrolyte levels
2001	Electrolyte Management: Hypercalcemia	Promotion of calcium balance and prevention of complications resulting from serum calcium levels higher than desired
2002	Electrolyte Management: Hyperkalemia	Promotion of potassium balance and prevention of complications resulting from serum potassium levels higher than desired
2003	Electrolyte Management: Hypermagnesemia	Promotion of magnesium balance and prevention of complications resulting from serum magnesium levels higher than desired
2004	Electrolyte Management: Hypernatremia	Promotion of sodium balance and prevention of complications resulting from serum sodium levels higher than desired
2005	Electrolyte Management: Hyperphosphatemia	Promotion of phosphate balance and prevention of complications resulting from serum phosphate levels higher than desired
2006	Electrolyte Management: Hypocalcemia	Promotion of calcium balance and prevention of complications resulting from serum calcium levels lower than desired
2007	Electrolyte Management: Hypokalemia	Promotion of potassium balance and prevention of complications resulting from serum potassium levels lower than desired
2008	Electrolyte Management: Hypomagnesemia	Promotion of magnesium balance and prevention of complications resulting from serum magnesium levels lower than desired
2009	Electrolyte Management: Hyponatremia	Promotion of sodium balance and prevention of complications resulting from serum sodium levels lower than desired
2010	Electrolyte Management: Hypophosphatemia	Promotion of phosphate balance and prevention of complications resulting from serum phosphate levels lower than desired
2020	Electrolyte Monitoring	Collection and analysis of patient data to regulate electrolyte balance

6771	Electronic Fetal Monitoring: Antepartum	Electronic evaluation of fetal heart rate response to movement, external stimuli, or uterine contractions during antepartal testing
6772	Electronic Fetal Monitoring: Intrapartum	Electronic evaluation of fetal heart rate response to uterine contractions during intrapartal care
6470	Elopement Precautions	Minimizing the risk of a patient leaving a treatment setting without authorization when departure presents a threat to the safety of patient or others
4104	Embolus Care: Peripheral	Limitation of complications for a patient experiencing, or at risk for, occlusion of peripheral circulation
4106	Embolus Care: Pulmonary	Limitation of complications for a patient experiencing, or at risk for, occlusion of pulmonary circulation
4110	Embolus Precautions	Reduction of the risk of an embolus in a patient with thrombi or at risk for thrombus formation
6200	Emergency Care	Providing life-saving measures in life-threatening situations
7660	Emergency Cart Checking	Systematic review of the contents of an emergency cart at established time intervals
5270	Emotional Support	Provision of reassurance, acceptance, and encouragement during times of stress
3270	Endotracheal Extubation	Purposeful removal of the endotracheal tube from the nasopharyngeal or oropharyngeal airway
0180	Energy Management	Regulating energy use to treat or prevent fatigue and optimize function
1056	Enteral Tube Feeding	Delivering nutrients and water through a gastrointestinal tube
6480	Environmental Management	Manipulation of the patient's surroundings for therapeutic benefit, sensory appeal, and psychological well-being
6481	Environmental Management: Attachment Process	Manipulation of the patient's surroundings to facilitate the development of the parent-infant relationship
6482	Environmental Management: Comfort	Manipulation of the patient's surroundings for promotion of optimal comfort
6484	Environmental Management: Community	Monitoring and influencing of the physical, social, cultural, economic, and political conditions that affect the health of groups and communities

6485	Environmental Management: Home Preparation	Preparing the home for safe and effective delivery of care
6486	Environmental Management: Safety	Monitoring and manipulation of the physical environment to promote safety
6487	Environmental Management: Violence Prevention	Monitoring and manipulation of the physical environment to decrease the potential for violent behavior directed toward self, others, or environment
6489	Environmental Management: Worker Safety	Monitoring and manipulation of the worksite environment to promote safety and health of workers
8880	Environmental Risk Protection	Preventing and detecting disease and injury in populations at risk from environmental hazards
7680	Examination Assistance	Providing assistance to the patient and another health care provider during a procedure or exam
0200	Exercise Promotion	Facilitation of regular physical activity to maintain or advance to a higher level of fitness and health
0201	Exercise Promotion: Strength Training	Facilitating regular resistive muscle training to maintain or increase muscle strength
0202	Exercise Promotion: Stretching	Facilitation of systematic slow-stretch-hold muscle exercises to induce relaxation, to prepare muscles/joints for more vigorous exercise, or to increase or maintain body flexibility
0221	Exercise Therapy: Ambulation	Promotion and assistance with walking to maintain or restore autonomic and voluntary body functions during treatment and recovery from illness or injury
0222	Exercise Therapy: Balance	Use of specific activities, postures, and movements to maintain, enhance, or restore balance
0224	Exercise Therapy: Joint Mobility	Use of active or passive body movement to maintain or restore joint flexibility
0226	Exercise Therapy: Muscle Control	Use of specific activity or exercise protocols to enhance or restore controlled body movement
1650	Eye Care	Prevention or minimization of threats to eye or visual integrity
6490	Fall Prevention	Instituting special precautions with patient at risk for injury from falling
7100	Family Integrity Promotion	Promotion of family cohesion and unity

7104	Family Integrity Promotion: Childbearing Family	Facilitation of the growth of individuals or families who are adding an infant to the family unit
7110	Family Involvement Promotion	Facilitating family participation in the emotional and physical care of the patient
7120	Family Mobilization	Utilization of family strengths to influence patient's health in a positive direction
6784	Family Planning: Contraception	Facilitation of pregnancy prevention by providing information about the physiology of reproduction and methods to control conception
6786	Family Planning: Infertility	Management, education, and support of the patient and significant other undergoing evaluation and treatment for infertility
6788	Family Planning: Unplanned Pregnancy	Facilitation of decision-making regarding pregnancy outcome
7170	Family Presence Facilitation	Facilitation of the family's presence in support of an individual undergoing resuscitation and/or invasive procedures
7130	Family Process Maintenance	Minimization of family process disruption effects
7140	Family Support	Promotion of family values, interests, and goals
7150	Family Therapy	Assisting family members to move their family toward a more productive way of living
1050	Feeding	Providing nutritional intake for patient who is unable to feed self
7160	Fertility Preservation	Providing information, counseling, and treatment that facilitate reproductive health and the ability to conceive
3740	Fever Treatment	Management of a patient with hyperpyrexia caused by nonenvironmental factors
7380	Financial Resource Assistance	Assisting an individual/family to secure and manage finances to meet health care needs
6500	Fire-Setting Precautions	Prevention of fire-setting behaviors
6240	First Aid	Providing initial care for a minor injury
8550	Fiscal Resource Management	Procuring and directing the use of financial resources to ensure the development and continuation of programs and services
0470	Flatulence Reduction	Prevention of flatus formation and facilitation of passage of excessive gas
2080	Fluid/Electrolyte Management	Regulation and prevention of complications from altered fluid and/or electrolyte levels

4120	Fluid Management	Promotion of fluid balance and prevention of complications resulting from abnormal or undesired fluid levels
4130	Fluid Monitoring	Collection and analysis of patient data to regulate fluid balance
4140	Fluid Resuscitation	Administering prescribed intravenous fluids rapidly
1660	Foot Care	Cleansing and inspecting the feet for the purposes of relaxation, cleanliness, and healthy skin
5280	Forgiveness Facilitation	Assisting an individual to forgive and/or experience forgiveness in relationship with self, others, and higher power
1080	Gastrointestinal Intubation	Insertion of a tube into the gastrointestinal tract
5242	Genetic Counseling	Use of an interactive helping process focusing on assisting an individual, family or group, manifesting or at risk for developing or transmitting a birth defect or genetic condition, to cope
5290	Grief Work Facilitation	Assistance with the resolution of a significant loss
5294	Grief Work Facilitation: Perinatal Death	Assistance with the resolution of a perinatal loss
5300	Guilt Work Facilitation	Helping another to cope with painful feelings of responsibility, actual or perceived
1670	Hair Care	Promotion of neat, clean, attractive hair
6510	Hallucination Management	Promoting the safety, comfort, and reality orientation of a patient experiencing hallucinations
7960	Health Care Information Exchange	Providing patient care information to other health professionals
5510	Health Education	Developing and providing instruction and learning experiences to facilitate voluntary adaptation of behavior conducive to health in individuals, families, groups, or communities
7970	Health Policy Monitoring	Surveillance and influence of government and organization regulations, rules, and standards that affect nursing systems and practices to ensure quality care of patients
6520	Health Screening	Detecting health risks or problems by means of history, examination, and other procedures

7400	Health System Guidance	Facilitating a patient's location and use of appropriate health services
1380	Heat/Cold Application	Stimulation of the skin and underlying tissues with heat or cold for the purpose of decreasing pain, muscle spasms, or inflammation
3780	Heat Exposure Treatment	Management of patient overcome by heat due to excessive environmental heat exposure
2100	Hemodialysis Therapy	Management of extracorporeal passage of the patient's blood through a dialyzer
4150	Hemodynamic Regulation	Optimization of heart rate, preload, afterload, and contractility
2110	Hemofiltration Therapy	Cleansing of acutely ill patient's blood via a hemofilter controlled by the patient's hydrostatic pressure
4160	Hemorrhage Control	Reduction or elimination of rapid and excessive blood loss
6800	High-Risk Pregnancy Care	Identification and management of a high-risk pregnancy to promote healthy outcomes for mother and baby
7180	Home Maintenance Assistance	Helping the patient/family to maintain the home as a clean, safe, and pleasant place to live
5310	Hope Instillation	Facilitation of the development of a positive outlook in a given situation
2280	Hormone Replacement Therapy	Facilitation of safe and effective use of hormone replacement therapy
5320	Humor	Facilitating the patient to perceive, appreciate, and express what is funny, amusing, or ludicrous in order to establish relationships, relieve tension, release anger, facilitate learning, or cope with painful feelings
2120	Hyperglycemia Management	Preventing and treating above normal blood glucose levels
4170	Hypervolemia Management	Reduction in extracellular and/or intracellular fluid volume and prevention of complications in a patient who is fluid overloaded
5920	Hypnosis	Assisting a patient to induce an altered state of consciousness to create an acute awareness and a directed focus experience
2130	Hypoglycemia Management	Preventing and treating low blood glucose levels

NIC

3800	Hypothermia Treatment	Rewarming and surveillance of a patient whose core body temperature is below 35°C
4180	Hypovolemia Management	Expansion of intravascular fluid volume in a patient who is volume depleted
6530	Immunization/Vaccination Management	Monitoring immunization status, facilitating access to immunizations, and providing immunizations to prevent communicable disease
4370	Impulse Control Training	Assisting the patient to mediate impulsive behavior through application of problem-solving strategies to social and interpersonal situations
7980	Incident Reporting	Written and verbal reporting of any event in the process of patient care that is inconsistent with desired patient outcomes or routine operations of the health care facility
3440	Incision Site Care	Cleansing, monitoring, and promotion of healing in a wound that is closed with sutures, clips, or staples
6820	Infant Care	Provision of developmentally appropriate family-centered care to the child under 1 year of age
6540	Infection Control	Minimizing the acquisition and transmission of infectious agents
6545	Infection Control: Intraoperative	Preventing nosocomial infection in the operating room
6550	Infection Protection	Prevention and early detection of infection in a patient at risk
7410	Insurance Authorization	Assisting the patient and provider to secure payment for health services or equipment from a third party
2590	Intracranial Pressure (ICP) Monitoring	Measurement and interpretation of patient data to regulate intracranial pressure
6830	Intrapartal Care	Monitoring and management of stages one and two of the birth process
6834	Intrapartal Care: High-Risk Delivery	Assisting with vaginal delivery of multiple or malpositioned fetuses
4190	Intravenous (IV) Insertion	Insertion of a needle into a peripheral vein for the purpose of administering fluids, blood, or medications
4200	Intravenous (IV) Therapy	Administration and monitoring of intravenous fluids and medications
4210	Invasive Hemodynamic Monitoring	Measurement and interpretation of invasive hemodynamic parameters to determine cardiovascular function and regulate therapy as appropriate

NIC

6840	Kangaroo Care	Promoting closeness between parent and physiologically stable preterm infant by preparing the parent and providing the environment for skin-to-skin contact
6850	Labor Induction	Initiation or augmentation of labor by mechanical or pharmacological methods
6860	Labor Suppression	Controlling uterine contractions prior to 37 weeks of gestation to prevent preterm birth
7690	Laboratory Data Interpretation	Critical analysis of patient laboratory data in order to assist with clinical decision making
5244	Lactation Counseling	Use of an interactive helping process to assist in maintenance of successful breastfeeding
6870	Lactation Suppression	Facilitating the cessation of milk production and minimizing breast engorgement after giving birth
6560	Laser Precautions	Limiting the risk of laser-related injury to the patient
6570	Latex Precautions	Reducing the risk of systemic reaction to latex
5520	Learning Facilitation	Promoting the ability to process and comprehend information
5540	Learning Readiness Enhancement	Improving the ability and willingness to receive information
3460	Leech Therapy	Application of medicinal leeches to help drain replanted or transplanted tissue engorged with venous blood
4380	Limit Setting	Establishing the parameters of desirable and acceptable patient behavior
3480	Lower Extremity Monitoring	Collection, analysis, and use of patient data to categorize risk and prevent injury to the lower extremities
3840	Malignant Hyperthermia Precautions	Prevention or reduction of hypermetabolic response to pharmacological agents used during surgery
3300	Mechanical Ventilation	Use of an artificial device to assist a patient to breathe
3310	Mechanical Ventilatory Weaning	Assisting the patient to breathe without the aid of a mechanical ventilator
2300	Medication Administration	Preparing, giving, and evaluating the effectiveness of prescription and nonprescription drugs
2308	Medication Administration: Ear	Preparing and instilling otic medications
2301	Medication Administration: Enteral	Delivering medications through a tube inserted into the gastrointestinal system

NIC

2310	Medication Administration: Eye	Preparing and instilling ophthalmic medications
2311	Medication Administration: Inhalation	Preparing and administering inhaled medications
2302	Medication Administration: Interpleural	Administration of medication through an interpleural catheter for reduction of pain
2312	Medication Administration: Intradermal	Preparing and giving medications via the intradermal route
2313	Medication Administration: Intramuscular (IM)	Preparing and giving medications via the intramuscular route
2303	Medication Administration: Intraosseous	Insertion of a needle through the bone cortex into the medullary cavity for the purpose of short-term, emergency administration of fluid, blood, or medication
2319	Medication Administration: Intraspinal	Administration and monitoring of medication via an established epidural or intrathecal route
2314	Medication Administration: Intravenous (IV)	Preparing and giving medications via the intravenous route
2320	Medication Administration: Nasal	Preparing and giving medications via nasal passages
2304	Medication Administration: Oral	Preparing and giving medications by mouth
2315	Medication Administration: Rectal	Preparing and inserting rectal suppositories
2316	Medication Administration: Skin	Preparing and applying medications to the skin
2317	Medication Administration: Subcutaneous	Preparing and giving medications via the subcutaneous route
2318	Medication Administration: Vaginal	Preparing and inserting vaginal medications
2307	Medication Administration: Ventricular Reservoir	Administration and monitoring of medication through an indwelling catheter into the lateral ventricle of the brain
2380	Medication Management	Facilitation of safe and effective use of prescription and over-the-counter drugs
2390	Medication Prescribing	Prescribing medication for a health problem
5960	Meditation Facilitation	Facilitating a person to alter his/her level of awareness by focusing specifically on an image or thought
4760	Memory Training	Facilitation of memory
4390	Milieu Therapy	Use of people, resources, and events in the patient's immediate environment to promote optimal psychosocial functioning
5330	Mood Management	Providing for safety, stabilization, recovery, and maintenance of a patient who is experiencing dysfunctionally depressed or elevated mood

8020	Multidisciplinary Care Conference	Planning and evaluating patient care with health professionals from other disciplines
4400	Music Therapy	Using music to help achieve a specific change in behavior, feeling, or physiology
4410	Mutual Goal Setting	Collaborating with patient to identify and prioritize care goals, then developing a plan for achieving those goals
1680	Nail Care	Promotion of clean, neat, attractive nails and prevention of skin lesions related to improper care of nails
1450	Nausea Management	Prevention and alleviation of nausea
2620	Neurologic Monitoring	Collection and analysis of patient data to prevent or minimize neurologic complications
6880	Newborn Care	Management of neonate during the transition to extrauterine life and subsequent period of stabilization
6890	Newborn Monitoring	Measurement and interpretation of physiological status of the neonate the first 24 hours after delivery
6900	Nonnutritive Sucking	Provision of sucking opportunities for the infant
7200	Normalization Promotion	Assisting parents and other family members of children with chronic illnesses or disabilities in providing normal life experiences for their children and families
1100	Nutrition Management	Assisting with or providing a balanced dietary intake of foods and fluids
1120	Nutrition Therapy	Administration of food and fluids to support metabolic processes of a patient who is malnourished or at high risk for becoming malnourished
5246	Nutritional Counseling	Use of an interactive helping process focusing on the need for diet modification
1160	Nutritional Monitoring	Collection and analysis of patient data to prevent or minimize malnourishment
1710	Oral Health Maintenance	Maintenance and promotion of oral hygiene and dental health for the patient at risk for developing oral or dental lesions
1720	Oral Health Promotion	Promotion of oral hygiene and dental care for a patient with normal oral and dental health
1730	Oral Health Restoration	Promotion of healing for a patient who has an oral mucosa or dental lesion

NIC

8060	Order Transcription	Transferring information from order sheets to the nursing patient care planning and documentation system
6260	Organ Procurement	Guiding families through the donation process to ensure timely retrieval of vital organs and tissue for transplant
0480	Ostomy Care	Maintenance of elimination through a stoma and care of surrounding tissue
3320	Oxygen Therapy	Administration of oxygen and monitoring of its effectiveness
1400	Pain Management	Alleviation of pain or a reduction in pain to a level of comfort that is acceptable to the patient
5562	Parent Education: Adolescent	Assisting parents to understand and help their adolescent children
5566	Parent Education: Childrearing Family	Assisting parents to understand and promote the physical, psychological, and social growth and development of their toddler, preschool, or school-aged child/children
5568	Parent Education: Infant	Instruction on nurturing and physical care needed during the first year of life
8300	Parenting Promotion	Providing parenting information, support, and coordination of comprehensive services to high-risk families
7440	Pass Facilitation	Arranging a leave for a patient from a health care facility
4420	Patient Contracting	Negotiating an agreement with an individual that reinforces a specific behavior change
2400	Patient-Controlled Analgesia (PCA) Assistance	Facilitating patient control of analgesic administration and regulation
7460	Patient Rights Protection	Protection of health care rights of a patient, especially a minor, incapacitated, or incompetent patient unable to make decisions
7700	Peer Review	Systematic evaluation of a peer's performance compared with professional standards of practice
0560	Pelvic Muscle Exercise	Strengthening and training the levator ani and urogenital muscles through voluntary, repetitive contraction to decrease stress, urge, or mixed types of urinary incontinence
1750	Perineal Care	Maintenance of perineal skin integrity and relief of perineal discomfort

2660	Peripheral Sensation Management	Prevention or minimization of injury or discomfort in the patient with altered sensation
4220	Peripherally Inserted Central (PIC) Catheter Care	Insertion and maintenance of a peripherally inserted catheter either midline or centrally located
2150	Peritoneal Dialysis Therapy	Administration and monitoring of dialysis solution into and out of the peritoneal cavity
0630	Pessary Management	Placement and monitoring of a vaginal device for treating stress urinary incontinence, uterine retroversion, genital prolapse, or incompetent cervix
4232	Phlebotomy: Arterial Blood Sample	Obtaining a blood sample from an uncannulated artery to assess oxygen and carbon dioxide levels and acid-base balance
4234	Phlebotomy: Blood Unit Acquisition	Procuring blood and blood products from donors
4235	Phlebotomy: Cannulated Vessel	Aspirating a blood sample through an indwelling vascular catheter for laboratory tests
4238	Phlebotomy: Venous Blood Sample	Removal of a sample of venous blood from an uncannulated vein
6926	Phototherapy: Mood/Sleep Regulation	Administration of doses of bright light in order to elevate mood and/or normalize the body's internal clock
6924	Phototherapy: Neonate	Use of light therapy to reduce bilirubin levels in newborn infants
6580	Physical Restraint	Application, monitoring, and removal of mechanical restraining devices or manual restraints used to limit physical mobility of a patient
7710	Physician Support	Collaborating with physicians to provide quality patient care
6590	Pneumatic Tourniquet Precautions	Applying a pneumatic tourniquet, while minimizing the potential for patient injury from use of the device
0840	Positioning	Deliberative placement of the patient or a body part to promote physiological and/or psychological well-being
0842	Positioning: Intraoperative	Moving the patient or body part to promote surgical exposure while reducing the risk of discomfort and complications
0844	Positioning: Neurologic	Achievement of optimal, appropriate body alignment for the patient experiencing or at risk for spinal cord injury or vertebral irritability

NIC

0846	Positioning: Wheelchair	Placement of a patient in a properly selected wheelchair to enhance comfort, promote skin integrity, and foster independence
2870	Postanesthesia Care	Monitoring and management of the patient who has recently undergone general or regional anesthesia
1770	Postmortem Care	Providing physical care of the body of an expired patient and support for the family viewing the body
6930	Postpartal Care	Monitoring and management of the patient who has recently given birth
7722	Preceptor: Employee	Assisting and supporting a new or transferred employee through a planned orientation to a specific clinical area
7726	Preceptor: Student	Assisting and supporting learning experiences for a student
5247	Preconception Counseling	Screening and providing information and support to individuals of childbearing age before pregnancy to promote health and reduce risks
6950	Pregnancy Termination Care	Management of the physical and psychological needs of the woman undergoing a spontaneous or elective abortion
1440	Premenstrual Syndrome (PMS) Management	Alleviation of/attention to physical and/or behavioral symptoms occurring during the luteal phase of the menstrual cycle
6960	Prenatal Care	Monitoring and management of patient during pregnancy to prevent complications of pregnancy and promote a healthy outcome for both mother and infant
2880	Preoperative Coordination	Facilitating preadmission diagnostic testing and preparation of the surgical patient
5580	Preparatory Sensory Information	Describing in concrete and objective terms the typical sensory experiences and events associated with an upcoming stressful health care procedure/treatment
5340	Presence	Being with another, both physically and psychologically, during times of need
3500	Pressure Management	Minimizing pressure to body parts
3520	Pressure Ulcer Care	Facilitation of healing in pressure ulcers
3540	Pressure Ulcer Prevention	Prevention of pressure ulcers for an individual at high risk for developing them
7760	Product Evaluation	Determining the effectiveness of new products or equipment

8700	Program Development	Planning, implementing, and evaluating a coordinated set of activities designed to enhance wellness, or to prevent, reduce, or eliminate one or more health problems for a group or community
1460	Progressive Muscle Relaxation	Facilitating the tensing and releasing of successive muscle groups while attending to the resulting differences in sensation
0640	Prompted Voiding	Promotion of urinary continence through the use of timed verbal toileting reminders and positive social feedback for successful toileting
1780	Prosthesis Care	Care of a removable appliance worn by a patient and the prevention of complications associated with its use
3550	Pruritus Management	Preventing and treating itching
7800	Quality Monitoring	Systematic collection and analysis of an organization's quality indicators for the purpose of improving patient care
6600	Radiation Therapy Management	Assisting the patient to understand and minimize the side effects of radiation treatments
6300	Rape-Trauma Treatment	Provision of emotional and physical support immediately following a reported rape
4820	Reality Orientation	Promotion of patient's awareness of personal identity, time, and environment
5360	Recreation Therapy	Purposeful use of recreation to promote relaxation and enhancement of social skills
0490	Rectal Prolapse Management	Prevention and/or manual reduction of rectal prolapse
8100	Referral	Arrangement for services by another care provider or agency
5422	Religious Addiction Prevention	Prevention of a self-imposed controlling religious lifestyle
5424	Religious Ritual Enhancement	Facilitating participation in religious practices
5350	Relocation Stress Reduction	Assisting the individual to prepare for and cope with movement from one environment to another
4860	Reminiscence Therapy	Using the recall of past events, feelings, and thoughts to facilitate pleasure, quality of life, or adaptation to present circumstances
7886	Reproductive Technology Management	Assisting a patient through the steps of complex infertility treatment
8120	Research Data Collection	Collecting research data

8340	Resiliency Promotion	Assisting individuals, families, and communities in development, use, and strengthening of protective factors to be used in coping with environmental and societal stressors
3350	Respiratory Monitoring	Collection and analysis of patient data to ensure airway patency and adequate gas exchange
7260	Respite Care	Provision of short-term care to provide relief for family caregiver
6320	Resuscitation	Administering emergency measures to sustain life
6972	Resuscitation: Fetus	Administering emergency measures to improve placental perfusion or correct fetal acid-base status
6974	Resuscitation: Neonate	Administering emergency measures to support newborn adaptation to extrauterine life
6610	Risk Identification	Analysis of potential risk factors, determination of health risks, and prioritization of risk reduction strategies for an individual or group
6612	Risk Identification: Childbearing Family	Identification of an individual or family likely to experience difficulties in parenting and prioritization of strategies to prevent parenting problems
6614	Risk Identification: Genetic	Identification and analysis of potential genetic risk factors in an individual, family, or group
5370	Role Enhancement	Assisting a patient, significant other, and/or family to improve relationships by clarifying and supplementing specific role behaviors
6630	Seclusion	Solitary containment in a fully protective environment with close surveillance by nursing staff for purposes of safety or behavior management
5380	Security Enhancement	Intensifying a patient's sense of physical and psychological safety
2260	Sedation Management	Administration of sedatives, monitoring of the patient's response, and provision of necessary physiological support during a diagnostic or therapeutic procedure
2680	Seizure Management	Care of a patient during a seizure and the postictal state
2690	Seizure Precautions	Prevention or minimization of potential injuries sustained by a patient with a known seizure disorder

5390	Self-Awareness Enhancement	Assisting a patient to explore and understand his/her thoughts, feelings, motivations, and behaviors
1800	Self-Care Assistance	Assisting another to perform activities of daily living
1801	Self-Care Assistance: Bathing/Hygiene	Assisting patient to perform personal hygiene
1802	Self-Care Assistance: Dressing/Grooming	Assisting patient with clothes and makeup
1803	Self-Care Assistance: Feeding	Assisting a person to eat
1805	Self-Care Assistance: IADL	Assisting and instructing a person to perform instrumental activities of daily living (IADL) needed to function in the home or community
1804	Self-Care Assistance: Toileting	Assisting another with elimination
1806	Self-Care Assistance: Transfer	Assisting a person to change body location
5400	Self-Esteem Enhancement	Assisting a patient to increase his/her personal judgment of self worth
5922	Self-Hypnosis Facilitation	Teaching and monitoring the use of a self-initiated hypnotic state for therapeutic benefit
4470	Self-Modification Assistance	Reinforcement of self-directed change initiated by the patient to achieve personally important goals
4480	Self-Responsibility Facilitation	Encouraging a patient to assume more responsibility for own behavior
5248	Sexual Counseling	Use of an interactive helping process focusing on the need to make adjustments in sexual practice or to enhance coping with a sexual event/disorder
8140	Shift Report	Exchanging essential patient care information with other nursing staff at change of shift
4250	Shock Management	Facilitation of the delivery of oxygen and nutrients to systemic tissue with removal of cellular waste products in a patient with severely altered tissue perfusion
4254	Shock Management: Cardiac	Promotion of adequate tissue perfusion for a patient with severely compromised pumping function of the heart
4256	Shock Management: Vasogenic	Promotion of adequate tissue perfusion for a patient with severe loss of vascular tone
4258	Shock Management: Volume	Promotion of adequate tissue perfusion for a patient with severely compromised intravascular volume

NIC

4260	Shock Prevention	Detecting and treating a patient at risk for impending shock
7280	Sibling Support	Assisting a sibling to cope with a brother or sister's illness/chronic condition/disability
6000	Simple Guided Imagery	Purposeful use of imagination to achieve relaxation and/or direct attention away from undesirable sensations
1480	Simple Massage	Stimulation of the skin and underlying tissues with varying degrees of hand pressure to decrease pain, produce relaxation, and/or improve circulation
6040	Simple Relaxation Therapy	Use of techniques to encourage and elicit relaxation for the purpose of decreasing undesirable signs and symptoms such as pain, muscle tension, or anxiety
3582	Skin Care: Donor Site	Prevention of wound complications and promotion of healing at the donor site
3583	Skin Care: Graft Site	Prevention of wound complications and promotion of graft site healing
3584	Skin Care: Topical Treatments	Application of topical substances or manipulation of devices to promote skin integrity and minimize skin breakdown
3590	Skin Surveillance	Collection and analysis of patient data to maintain skin and mucous membrane integrity
1850	Sleep Enhancement	Facilitation of regular sleep/wake cycles
4490	Smoking Cessation Assistance	Helping another to stop smoking
5100	Socialization Enhancement	Facilitation of another person's ability to interact with others
7820	Specimen Management	Obtaining, preparing, and preserving a specimen for a laboratory test
5426	Spiritual Growth Facilitation	Facilitation of growth in patient's capacity to identify, connect with, and call upon the source of meaning, purpose, comfort, strength, and hope in his/her life
5420	Spiritual Support	Assisting the patient to feel balance and connection with a greater power
0910	Splinting	Stabilization, immobilization, and/or protection of an injured body part with a supportive appliance
6648	Sports-Injury Prevention: Youth	Reduce the risk of sports-related injury in young athletes
7850	Staff Development	Developing, maintaining, and monitoring competence of staff
7830	Staff Supervision	Facilitating the delivery of high-quality patient care by others

2720	Subarachnoid Hemorrhage Precautions	Reduction of internal and external stimuli or stressors to minimize risk of rebleeding prior to aneurysm surgery
4500	Substance Use Prevention	Prevention of an alcoholic or drug use lifestyle
4510	Substance Use Treatment	Supportive care of patient/family members with physical and psychosocial problems associated with the use of alcohol or drugs
4512	Substance Use Treatment: Alcohol Withdrawal	Care of the patient experiencing sudden cessation of alcohol consumption
4514	Substance Use Treatment: Drug Withdrawal	Care of a patient experiencing drug detoxification
4516	Substance Use Treatment: Overdose	Monitoring, treatment, and emotional support of a patient who has ingested prescription or over-the-counter drugs beyond the therapeutic range
6340	Suicide Prevention	Reducing risk of self-inflicted harm with intent to end life
7840	Supply Management	Ensuring acquisition and maintenance of appropriate items for providing patient care
5430	Support Group	Use of a group environment to provide emotional support and health-related information for members
5440	Support System Enhancement	Facilitation of support to patient by family, friends, and community
2900	Surgical Assistance	Assisting the surgeon/dentist with operative procedures and care of the surgical patient
2920	Surgical Precautions	Minimizing the potential for iatrogenic injury to the patient related to a surgical procedure
2930	Surgical Preparation	Providing care to a patient immediately prior to surgery and verifying required procedures/tests and documentation in the clinical record
6650	Surveillance	Purposeful and ongoing acquisition, interpretation, and synthesis of patient data for clinical decision making
6652	Surveillance: Community	Purposeful and ongoing acquisition, interpretation, and synthesis of data for decision making in the community
6656	Surveillance: Late Pregnancy	Purposeful and ongoing acquisition, interpretation, and synthesis of maternal-fetal data for treatment, observation, or admission

NIC

6658	Surveillance: Remote Electronic	Purposeful and ongoing acquisition of patient data via electronic modalities (telephone, video, conference, e-mail) from distant locations, as well as interpretation and synthesis of patient data for clinical decision making with individuals or populations
6654	Surveillance: Safety	Purposeful and ongoing collection and analysis of information about the patient and the environment for use in promoting and maintaining patient safety
7500	Sustenance Support	Helping a needy individual/family to locate food, clothing, or shelter
3620	Suturing	Approximating edges of a wound using sterile suture material and a needle
1860	Swallowing Therapy	Facilitating swallowing and preventing complications of impaired swallowing
5602	Teaching: Disease Process	Assisting the patient to understand information related to a specific disease process
5603	Teaching: Foot Care	Preparing a patient at risk and/or significant other to provide preventive foot care
5604	Teaching: Group	Development, implementation, and evaluation of a patient teaching program for a group of individuals experiencing the same health condition
5606	Teaching: Individual	Planning, implementation, and evaluation of a teaching program designed to address a patient's particular needs
5626	Teaching: Infant Nutrition	Instruction on nutrition and feeding practices during the first year of life
5628	Teaching: Infant Safety	Instruction on safety during first year of life
5605	Teaching: Infant Stimulation	Teaching parents and caregivers to provide developmentally appropriate sensory activities to promote development and movement during the first year of life
5610	Teaching: Preoperative	Assisting a patient to understand and mentally prepare for surgery and the postoperative recovery period
5612	Teaching: Prescribed Activity/Exercise	Preparing a patient to achieve and/or maintain a prescribed level of activity
5614	Teaching: Prescribed Diet	Preparing a patient to correctly follow a prescribed diet
5616	Teaching: Prescribed Medication	Preparing a patient to safely take prescribed medications and monitor for their effects

5618	Teaching: Procedure/Treatment	Preparing a patient to understand and mentally prepare for a prescribed procedure or treatment
5620	Teaching: Psychomotor Skill	Preparing a patient to perform a psychomotor skill
5622	Teaching: Safe Sex	Providing instruction concerning sexual protection during sexual activity
5624	Teaching: Sexuality	Assisting individuals to understand physical and psychosocial dimensions of sexual growth and development
5630	Teaching: Toddler Nutrition	Instruction on nutrition and feeding practices during the second and third years of life
5632	Teaching: Toddler Safety	Instruction on safety during the second and third years of life
5634	Teaching: Toilet Training	Instruction on determining the child's readiness and strategies to assist the child to learn independent toileting skills
7880	Technology Management	Use of technical equipment and devices to monitor patient condition or sustain life
8180	Telephone Consultation	Eliciting patient's concerns, listening, and providing support, information, or teaching in response to patient's stated concerns, over the telephone
8190	Telephone Follow-up	Providing results of testing or evaluating patient's response and determining potential for problems as a result of previous treatment, examination, or testing, over the telephone
3900	Temperature Regulation	Attaining and/or maintaining body temperature within a normal range
3902	Temperature Regulation: Intraoperative	Attaining and/or maintaining desired intraoperative body temperature
4092	Temporary Pacemaker Management	Temporary support of cardiac pumping through the insertion and use of temporary pacemakers
4430	Therapeutic Play	Purposeful and directive use of toys and other materials to assist children in communicating their perception and knowledge of their world and to help in gaining mastery of their environment
5465	Therapeutic Touch	Attuning to the universal healing field, seeking to act as an instrument for healing influence, and using the natural sensitivity of the hands to gently focus and direct the intervention process

NIC

5450	Therapy Group	Application of psychotherapeutic techniques to a group, including the utilization of interactions between members of the group
1200	Total Parenteral Nutrition (TPN) Administration	Preparation and delivery of nutrients intravenously and monitoring of patient responsiveness
5460	Touch	Providing comfort and communication through purposeful tactile contact
0940	Traction/Immobilization Care	Management of a patient who has traction and/or a stabilizing device to immobilize and stabilize a body part
1540	Transcutaneous Electrical Nerve Stimulation (TENS)	Stimulation of skin and underlying tissues with controlled, low-voltage electrical vibration via electrodes
0960	Transport	Moving a patient from one location to another
5410	Trauma Therapy: Child	Use of an interactive helping process to resolve a trauma experienced by a child
6362	Triage: Disaster	Establishing priorities of patient care for urgent treatment while allocating scarce resources
6364	Triage: Emergency Center	Establishing priorities and initiating treatment for patients in an emergency center
6366	Triage: Telephone	Determining the nature and urgency of a problem(s) and providing directions for the level of care required, over the telephone
5470	Truth Telling	Use of whole truth, partial truth, or decision delay to promote the patient's self-determination and well-being
1870	Tube Care	Management of a patient with an external drainage device exiting the body
1872	Tube Care: Chest	Management of a patient with an external water-seal drainage device exiting the chest cavity
1874	Tube Care: Gastrointestinal	Management of a patient with a gastrointestinal tube
1875	Tube Care: Umbilical Line	Management of a newborn with an umbilical catheter
1876	Tube Care: Urinary	Management of a patient with urinary drainage equipment
1878	Tube Care: Ventriculostomy/ Lumbar Drain	Management of a patient with an external cerebrospinal fluid drainage system
6982	Ultrasonography: Limited Obstetric	Performance of ultrasound exams to determine ovarian, uterine, or fetal status

2760	Unilateral Neglect Management	Protecting and safely reintegrating the affected part of the body while helping the patient adapt to disturbed perceptual abilities
0570	Urinary Bladder Training	Improving bladder function for those with urge incontinence by increasing the bladder's ability to hold urine and the patient's ability to suppress urination
0580	Urinary Catheterization	Insertion of a catheter into the bladder for temporary or permanent drainage of urine
0582	Urinary Catheterization: Intermittent	Regular periodic use of a catheter to empty the bladder
0590	Urinary Elimination Management	Maintenance of an optimum urinary elimination pattern
0600	Urinary Habit Training	Establishing a predictable pattern of bladder emptying to prevent incontinence for persons with limited cognitive ability who have urge, stress, or functional incontinence
0610	Urinary Incontinence Care	Assistance in promoting continence and maintaining perineal skin integrity
0612	Urinary Incontinence Care: Enuresis	Promotion of urinary continence in children
0620	Urinary Retention Care	Assistance in relieving bladder distention
5480	Values Clarification	Assisting another to clarify her/his own values in order to facilitate effective decision making
9050	Vehicle Safety Promotion	Assisting individuals, families, and communities to increase awareness of measures to reduce unintentional injuries in motorized and nonmotorized vehicle
2440	Venous Access Device (VAD) Maintenance	Management of the patient with prolonged venous access via tunneled and nontunneled (percutaneous) catheters, and implanted ports
3390	Ventilation Assistance	Promotion of an optimal spontaneous breathing pattern that maximizes oxygen and carbon dioxide exchange in the lungs
7560	Visitation Facilitation	Promoting beneficial visits by family and friends
6680	Vital Signs Monitoring	Collection and analysis of cardiovascular, respiratory, and body temperature data to determine and prevent complications
1570	Vomiting Management	Prevention and alleviation of vomiting
1240	Weight Gain Assistance	Facilitating gain of body weight
1260	Weight Management	Facilitating maintenance of optimal body weight and percent body fat

NIC

1280	Weight Reduction Assistance	Facilitating loss of weight and/or body fat
3660	Wound Care	Prevention of wound complications and promotion of wound healing
3662	Wound Care: Closed Drainage	Maintenance of a pressure drainage system at the wound site
3680	Wound Irrigation	Flushing of an open wound to cleanse and remove debris and excessive drainage

Index

A

Abuse Cessation, as outcome, 621
  with Violence: Other-Directed, Risk for, 611
Abuse Protection, as outcome, 621
  with Protection, Ineffective, 341
  with Rape-Trauma Syndrome, 345
  with Rape-Trauma Syndrome: Compound Reaction,
    348
  with Rape-Trauma Syndrome: Silent Reaction, 353
Abuse Protection Support, as intervention, 639
  for Post-Trauma Syndrome, Risk for, 584
  for Protection, Ineffective, 341
  for Rape-Trauma Syndrome, 345
  for Rape-Trauma Syndrome: Compound Reaction,
    348, 349
  for Rape-Trauma Syndrome: Silent Reaction, 353
  for Self-Esteem: Situational Low, Risk for, 592
  for Sexual Dysfunction, 395
  for Violence: Other-Directed, Risk for, 611
Abuse Protection Support: Child, as intervention, 639
  for Parenting, Impaired, 325, 326
  for Parenting, Risk for Impaired, 577
  for Protection, Ineffective, 341
  for Rape-Trauma Syndrome, 345
  for Rape-Trauma Syndrome: Compound Reaction,
    348
  for Rape-Trauma Syndrome: Silent Reaction, 353
Abuse Protection Support: Domestic Partner, as
    intervention, 639
  for Protection, Ineffective, 341
  for Rape-Trauma Syndrome, 345
  for Rape-Trauma Syndrome: Compound Reaction,
    348
  for Rape-Trauma Syndrome: Silent Reaction, 353
Abuse Protection Support: Elder, as intervention, 639
  for Protection, Ineffective, 341
  for Rape-Trauma Syndrome, 345
  for Rape-Trauma Syndrome: Compound Reaction,
    348
  for Rape-Trauma Syndrome: Silent Reaction, 353
Abuse Protection Support: Religious, as intervention,
    639
Abuse Recovery: Emotional, as outcome, 621
  with Post-Trauma Syndrome, 332
  with Rape-Trauma Syndrome, 345
  with Rape-Trauma Syndrome: Compound Reaction,
    349
  with Rape-Trauma Syndrome: Silent Reaction, 353
Abuse Recovery: Financial, as outcome, 621
  with Post-Trauma Syndrome, 332
Abuse Recovery: Physical, as outcome, 621
  with Rape-Trauma Syndrome: Compound Reaction,
    349

Abuse Recovery: Sexual, as outcome, 621
  with Post-Trauma Syndrome, 333
  with Rape-Trauma Syndrome, 346
  with Rape-Trauma Syndrome: Compound Reaction,
    350
  with Rape-Trauma Syndrome: Silent Reaction, 354
  with Sexual Dysfunction, 395
  with Sexuality Patterns, Ineffective, 398
Abuse Recovery Status, as outcome, 621
  with Post-Trauma Syndrome, Risk for, 584
  with Self-Esteem: Situational Low, Risk for, 592
Abusive Behavior Self-Restraint, as outcome, 621
  with Violence: Other-Directed, Risk for, 612
Acceptance: Health Status, as outcome, 621
  with Adjustment, Impaired, 57
  with Coping, Defensive, 120
  with Coping, Ineffective, 124
  with Coping, Readiness for Enhanced, 132
  with Death Anxiety, 135
  with Denial, Ineffective, 141
  with Sorrow: Chronic, 420
Acid-Base Management, as intervention, 639
  for Fluid Volume, Deficient, 190
  for Gas Exchange, Impaired, 198, 199
Acid-Base Management: Metabolic Acidosis, as
    intervention, 639
Acid-Base Management: Metabolic Alkalosis, as
    intervention, 640
Acid-Base Management: Respiratory Acidosis, as
    intervention, 640
  for Gas Exchange, Impaired, 201
  for Tissue Perfusion: Cardiopulmonary, Ineffective,
    465
Acid-Base Management: Respiratory Alkalosis, as
    intervention, 640
  for Gas Exchange, Impaired, 201
  for Tissue Perfusion: Cardiopulmonary, Ineffective,
    465
Acid-Base Monitoring, as intervention, 640
  for Tissue Perfusion: Cardiopulmonary, Ineffective,
    463
  for Tissue Perfusion: Renal, Ineffective, 482
Active Listening, as intervention, 640
  for Communication, Impaired Verbal, 98
Activity Intolerance, 53-56
Activity Intolerance, Risk for, 511-513
Activity Therapy, as intervention, 640
  for Activity Intolerance, 53, 54, 55
  for Disuse Syndrome, Risk for, 537
  for Fatigue, 183
  for Lifestyle, Sedentary, 273, 274
Activity Tolerance, as outcome, 621
  with Activity Intolerance, 53
  with Activity Intolerance, Risk for, 511

Activity Tolerance, as outcome *(Continued)*
  with Fatigue, 183
  with Lifestyle, Sedentary, 273
Acupressure, as intervention, 640
Adaptation to Physical Disability, as outcome, 621
  with Adjustment, Impaired, 57
  with Body Image, Disturbed, 67
  with Coping, Defensive, 120
  with Coping, Ineffective, 124
  with Coping, Readiness for Enhanced, 132
  with Grieving, Anticipatory, 203
  with Self-Esteem: Situational Low, 377
  with Unilateral Neglect, 487
Adherence Behavior, as outcome, 621
  with Health-Seeking Behavior (Specify), 228
  with Noncompliance, 289
  with Therapeutic Regimen Management, Effective,
    435
  with Therapeutic Regimen Management, Readiness
    for Enhanced, 450
Adjustment, Impaired, 57-60
Admission Care, as intervention, 640
Aggression Self-Control, as outcome, 621
  with Post-Trauma Syndrome, Risk for, 585
  with Violence: Other-Directed, Risk for, 613
Airway Clearance, Ineffective, 61
Airway Insertion and Stabilization, as intervention, 640
Airway Management, as intervention, 640
  for Airway Clearance, Ineffective, 61
  for Aspiration, Risk for, 514
  for Breathing Pattern, Ineffective, 81, 82, 83
  for Gas Exchange, Impaired, 200, 202
  for Latex Allergy Response, 271
  for Suffocation, Risk for, 603, 604
  for Ventilation, Impaired Spontaneous, 499, 501
Airway Suctioning, as intervention, 640
  for Airway Clearance, Ineffective, 61
  for Breathing Pattern, Ineffective, 82
Allergic Response: Localized, as outcome, 622
  with Latex Allergy Response, 271
  with Latex Allergy Response, Risk for, 567
  with Skin Integrity, Impaired, 401
  with Tissue Integrity, Impaired, 459
Allergic Response: Systemic, as outcome, 622
  with Breathing Pattern, Ineffective, 81
  with Gas Exchange, Impaired, 197
  with Latex Allergy Response, 271
  with Ventilation, Impaired Spontaneous, 499
Allergy Management, as intervention, 640
  for Latex Allergy Response, 271
  for Protection, Ineffective, 343
Ambulation, as outcome, 622
  with Mobility: Physical, Impaired, 280
  with Surgical Recovery, Delayed, 427
  with Walking, Impaired, 507
Ambulation: Wheelchair, as outcome, 622
  with Mobility: Physical, Impaired, 280
  with Mobility: Wheelchair, Impaired, 284
American Nurses Association, standard nursing
    languages recognized by, 3-10
Amnioinfusion, as intervention, 640
Amputation Care, as intervention, 640
Analgesic Administration, as intervention, 640
  for Pain, Acute, 305
Analgesic Administration: Intraspinal, as intervention,
    640
Anaphylaxis Management, as intervention, 641
  for Breathing Pattern, Ineffective, 81
  for Gas Exchange, Impaired, 197
  for Latex Allergy Response, 271
Anesthesia Administration, as intervention, 641

Anger Control Assistance, as intervention, 641
  for Post-Trauma Syndrome, Risk for, 585
  for Self-Mutilation, Risk for, 595
  for Violence: Other-Directed, Risk for, 612, 613, 614
Animal-Assisted Therapy, as intervention, 641
Anticipatory Guidance, as intervention, 641
  for Adjustment, Impaired, 57, 60
  for Anxiety, 64
  for Body Image, Disturbed, 72
  for Caregiver Role Strain, 93
  for Coping, Ineffective, 125, 129
  for Coping, Readiness for Enhanced, 132
  for Parental Role Conflict, 315
  for Role Performance, Ineffective, 364
  for Self-Esteem: Situational Low, 378
  for Therapeutic Regimen Management, Effective,
    435, 439
  for Therapeutic Regimen Management, Readiness
    for Enhanced, 450, 452
  for Unilateral Neglect, 487
Anxiety, 62-64
Anxiety Level, as outcome, 622
  with Anxiety, 62
  with Post-Trauma Syndrome, 333
  with Rape-Trauma Syndrome: Silent Reaction, 354
  with Relocation Stress Syndrome, 358
  with Ventilatory Weaning Response, Dysfunctional,
    503
  with Wandering, 510
Anxiety Reduction, as intervention, 641
  for Anxiety, 62, 63
  for Communication, Impaired Verbal, 99
  for Communication, Readiness for Enhanced, 100
  for Confusion, Chronic, 114
  for Coping, Readiness for Enhanced, 134
  for Death Anxiety, 135
  for Denial, Ineffective, 141, 142
  for Environmental Interpretation Syndrome,
    Impaired, 151
  for Fear, 186
  for Memory, Impaired, 275
  for Post-Trauma Syndrome, 333
  for Rape-Trauma Syndrome: Silent Reaction, 354,
    355
  for Relocation Stress Syndrome, 358
  for Relocation Stress Syndrome, Risk for, 590
  for Thought Processes, Disturbed, 455
  for Ventilatory Weaning Response, Dysfunctional,
    503
  for Wandering, 510
Anxiety Self-Control, as outcome, 622
  with Anxiety, 63
  with Death Anxiety, 135
  with Denial, Ineffective, 141
  with Rape-Trauma Syndrome: Silent Reaction, 355
Appetite, as outcome, 622
  with Failure to Thrive, Adult, 153
  with Nausea, 286
  with Nutrition: Imbalanced, Less than Body
    Requirements, 294
  with Sensory Perception: Gustatory, Disturbed, 384
  with Sensory Perception: Olfactory, Disturbed, 389
Area Restriction, as intervention, 641
Aromatherapy, as intervention, 641
Art Therapy, as intervention, 641
Artificial Airway Management, as intervention, 641
  for Breathing Pattern, Ineffective, 81
  for Ventilation, Impaired Spontaneous, 501
Aspiration, Risk for, 514-515
Aspiration Precautions, as intervention, 641
  for Airway Clearance, Ineffective, 61
  for Aspiration, Risk for, 514, 515

Aspiration Precautions, as intervention *(Continued)*
for Suffocation, Risk for, 602
for Swallowing, Impaired, 433, 434
for Ventilation, Impaired Spontaneous, 499
Aspiration Prevention, as outcome, 622
with Airway Clearance, Ineffective, 61
with Aspiration, Risk for, 514
with Suffocation, Risk for, 602
with Swallowing, Impaired, 433
Assertiveness Training, as intervention, 641
for Communication, Readiness for Enhanced, 100
for Decisional Conflict, 140
Asthma Management, as intervention, 641
for Airway Clearance, Ineffective, 61
for Breathing Pattern, Ineffective, 81
for Gas Exchange, Impaired, 197
for Suffocation, Risk for, 603
Asthma Self-Management, as outcome, 622
with Suffocation, Risk for, 603
Attachment Promotion, as intervention, 641
for Breastfeeding, Interrupted, 80
for Caregiver Role Strain, 96
for Development, Risk for Delayed, 525
for Parent/Infant/Child Attachment, Risk for
Impaired, 572
for Parenting, Impaired, 316, 324
Autogenic Training, as intervention, 641
Autonomic Dysreflexia, 65-66
Autonomic Dysreflexia, Risk for, 516-517
Autotransfusion, as intervention, 641

B

Balance, as outcome, 622
with Falls, Risk for, 540
with Mobility: Physical, Impaired, 281
with Mobility: Wheelchair, Impaired, 284
with Sensory Perception: Kinesthetic, Disturbed, 386
with Transfer Ability, Impaired, 484
with Walking, Impaired, 507
Bathing, as intervention, 642
Bed Rest Care, as intervention, 642
for Mobility: Bed, Impaired, 278
for Skin Integrity, Risk for Impaired, 596
for Surgical Recovery, Delayed, 429
Bedside Laboratory Testing, as intervention, 642
Behavior Management, as intervention, 642
for Violence: Other-Directed, Risk for, 611
Behavior Management: Overactivity/Inattention, as
intervention, 642
for Development, Risk for Delayed, 535
for Thought Processes, Disturbed, 455
Behavior Management: Self-Harm, as intervention, 642
for Personal Identity, Disturbed, 331
for Post-Trauma Syndrome, 336
for Self-Mutilation, 380
for Self-Mutilation, Risk for, 594, 595
for Suicide, Risk for, 606
for Violence: Self-Directed, Risk for, 616, 617
Behavior Management: Sexual, as intervention, 642
for Rape-Trauma Syndrome, 347
for Rape-Trauma Syndrome: Silent Reaction, 354
Behavior Modification, as intervention, 642
for Adjustment, Impaired, 58
for Nutrition: Imbalanced, More than Body
Requirements, 299, 300
for Pain, Chronic, 309
for Sexual Dysfunction, 396
for Therapeutic Regimen Management, Ineffective,
442, 449
Behavior Modification: Social Skills, as intervention, 642
for Coping, Defensive, 123
for Development, Risk for Delayed, 536

Behavior Modification: Social Skills, as intervention
(Continued)
for Social Interaction, Impaired, 413
for Social Isolation, 418
Bibliotherapy, as intervention, 642
Biofeedback, as intervention, 642
Bioterrorism Preparedness, as intervention, 642
for Community Coping, Ineffective, 101
for Community Coping, Readiness for Enhanced, 105
Birthing, as intervention, 642
Bladder Irrigation, as intervention, 642
Bleeding Precautions, as intervention, 642
for Protection, Ineffective, 341
Bleeding Reduction, as intervention, 642
for Cardiac Output, Decreased, 84
for Surgical Recovery, Delayed, 427
Bleeding Reduction: Antepartum Uterus, as
intervention, 642
Bleeding Reduction: Gastrointestinal, as intervention,
642
Bleeding Reduction: Nasal, as intervention, 642
Bleeding Reduction: Postpartum Uterus, as
intervention, 642
Bleeding Reduction: Wound, as intervention, 643
Blood Coagulation, as outcome, 622
with Protection, Ineffective, 341
Blood Glucose Level, as outcome, 622
with Therapeutic Regimen Management,
Ineffective, 440
Blood Loss Severity, as outcome, 622
with Cardiac Output, Decreased, 84
with Surgical Recovery, Delayed, 427
Blood Products Administration, as intervention, 643
Blood Transfusion Reaction, as outcome, 622
Body Image, as outcome, 622
with Body Image, Disturbed, 67
with Self-Concept, Readiness for Enhanced, 374
with Sexuality Patterns, Ineffective, 398
Body Image, Disturbed, 67-72
Body Image Enhancement, as intervention, 643
for Body Image, Disturbed, 67
for Coping, Defensive, 120
for Grieving, Anticipatory, 203
for Self-Concept, Readiness for Enhanced, 374
for Self-Esteem: Situational Low, 377
for Sexuality Patterns, Ineffective, 398
Body Mechanics Performance, as outcome, 622
with Mobility: Bed, Impaired, 277
with Mobility: Physical, Impaired, 281
Body Mechanics Promotion, as intervention, 643
for Falls, Risk for, 540
for Knowledge, Deficient (Specify), 257
for Mobility: Bed, Impaired, 277
for Mobility: Physical, Impaired, 281, 283
for Sensory Perception: Kinesthetic, Disturbed,
386, 387, 388
Body Positioning: Self-Initiated, as outcome, 622
with Mobility: Bed, Impaired, 277
with Sensory Perception: Kinesthetic, Disturbed, 386
with Transfer Ability, Impaired, 484
with Unilateral Neglect, 487
Body Temperature, Risk for Imbalanced, 518
Bone Healing, as outcome, 622
Bottle Feeding, as intervention, 643
for Breastfeeding Interrupted, 79
for Infant Feeding Pattern, Ineffective, 253
Bowel Continence, as outcome, 622
with Bowel Incontinence, 73
with Diarrhea, 144
Bowel Elimination, as outcome, 622
with Bowel Incontinence, 73
with Constipation, 117
with Constipation, Perceived, 119

Bowel Elimination, as outcome *(Continued)*
  with Constipation, Risk for, 524
  with Diarrhea, 144
Bowel Incontinence, 73
Bowel Incontinence Care, as intervention, 643
  for Bowel Incontinence, 73
Bowel Incontinence Care: Encopresis, as intervention,
    643
Bowel Irrigation, as intervention, 643
Bowel Management, as intervention, 643
  for Bowel Incontinence, 73
  for Constipation, 117
  for Constipation, Perceived, 119
  for Diarrhea, 144
  for Self-Care Deficit: Toileting, 372, 373
Bowel Training, as intervention, 643
  for Bowel Incontinence, 73
Breast Examination, as intervention, 643
Breastfeeding, Effective, 74-75
Breastfeeding, Ineffective, 76-78
Breastfeeding Assistance, as intervention, 643
  for Breastfeeding, Effective, 74
  for Breastfeeding, Ineffective, 76, 77, 78
  for Infant Feeding Pattern, Ineffective, 252, 253
  for Knowledge, Deficient (Specify), 257
  for Nutrition: Imbalanced, Less than Body
      Requirements, 294
Breastfeeding Establishment: Infant, as outcome, 623
  with Breastfeeding, Effective, 74
  with Breastfeeding, Ineffective, 76
  with Infant Feeding Pattern, Ineffective, 252
  with Nutrition: Imbalanced, Less than Body
      Requirements, 294
Breastfeeding Establishment: Maternal, as outcome,
    623
  with Breastfeeding, Effective, 74
  with Breastfeeding, Ineffective, 77
Breastfeeding Interrupted, 79-80
Breastfeeding Maintenance, as outcome, 623
  with Breastfeeding, Effective, 75
  with Breastfeeding, Ineffective, 78
  with Breastfeeding, Interrupted, 79
  with Infant Feeding Pattern, Ineffective, 252
Breastfeeding Weaning, as outcome, 623
  with Breastfeeding, Effective, 75
  with Breastfeeding, Ineffective, 78
  with Breastfeeding, Interrupted, 79
Breathing Pattern, Ineffective, 81-83
Bulechek, Gloria, 4

C

Calming Technique, as intervention, 643
  for Anxiety, 62, 63
  for Denial, Ineffective, 142
  for Fear, 186, 187
Capillary Blood Sample, as intervention, 643
Cardiac Care, as intervention, 643
  for Cardiac Output, Decreased, 85
Cardiac Care: Acute, as intervention, 643
  for Cardiac Output, Decreased, 85
  for Tissue Perfusion: Cardiopulmonary, Ineffective,
      462, 463, 464
Cardiac Care: Rehabilitative, as intervention, 643
Cardiac Disease Self-Management, as outcome, 623
  with Therapeutic Regimen Management,
      Ineffective, 441
Cardiac Output, Decreased, 84-90
Cardiac Precautions, as intervention, 644
  for Health-Seeking Behavior (Specify), 234
  for Therapeutic Regimen Management, Ineffective,
      441

Cardiac Pump Effectiveness, as outcome, 623
  with Cardiac Output, Decreased, 85
  with Tissue Perfusion: Cardiopulmonary,
      Ineffective, 462
Care planning, linkage use in, 21-23
Caregiver Adaptation to Patient Institutionalization, as
    outcome, 623
  with Coping, Ineffective, 125
  with Parental Role Conflict, 311
Caregiver Emotional Health, as outcome, 623
  with Caregiver Role Strain, 91
  with Caregiver Role Strain, Risk for, 519
  with Family Coping, Compromised, 156
Caregiver Home Care Readiness, as outcome, 623
  with Caregiver Role Strain, Risk for, 520
  with Parental Role Conflict, 312
Caregiver Lifestyle Disruption, as outcome, 623
  with Caregiver Role Strain, 92
  with Parental Role Conflict, 312
  with Role Performance, Ineffective, 364
Caregiver-Patient Relationship, as outcome, 623
  with Caregiver Role Strain, 92
  with Family Coping, Compromised, 156
  with Family Coping, Disabled, 160
Caregiver Performance: Direct Care, as outcome, 623
  with Caregiver Role Strain, 93
  with Family Coping, Compromised, 157
  with Family Coping, Disabled, 161
  with Noncompliance, 290
Caregiver Performance: Indirect Care, as outcome, 623
  with Caregiver Role Strain, 94
  with Family Coping, Compromised, 157
  with Family Coping, Disabled, 161
  with Noncompliance, 290
Caregiver Physical Health, as outcome, 623
  with Caregiver Role Strain, 94
  with Caregiver Role Strain, Risk for, 521
Caregiver Role Strain, 91-97
Caregiver Role Strain, Risk for, 519-523
Caregiver Stressors, as outcome, 623
  with Caregiver Role Strain, Risk for, 521
Caregiver Support, as intervention, 644
  for Caregiver Role Strain, 91, 92, 95
  for Caregiver Role Strain, Risk for, 519, 520, 521,
      522
  for Family Coping, Compromised, 156, 157, 158
  for Family Coping, Disabled, 160, 161, 162
  for Family Coping, Readiness for Enhanced, 164
  for Noncompliance, 290
  for Parental Role Conflict, 311, 312
Caregiver Well-Being, as outcome, 623
  with Caregiver Role Strain, 95
  with Family Coping, Disabled, 162
  with Family Coping, Readiness for Enhanced, 164
Caregiving Endurance Potential, as outcome, 623
  with Caregiver Role Strain, Risk for, 522
  with Family Coping, Compromised, 158
  with Family Coping, Disabled, 162
Case Management, as intervention, 644
  for Community Coping, Ineffective, 103
Cast Care: Maintenance, as intervention, 644
Cast Care: Wet, as intervention, 644
Cerebral Edema Management, as intervention, 644
  for Intracranial Adaptive Capacity, Decreased, 254,
      255, 256
Cerebral Perfusion Promotion, as intervention, 644
  for Cardiac Output, Decreased, 88
  for Confusion, Acute, 112
  for Confusion, Chronic, 116
  for Environmental Interpretation Syndrome,
      Impaired, 152
  for Intracranial Adaptive Capacity, Decreased, 254,
      255, 256

Cerebral Perfusion Promotion, as intervention
  (*Continued*)
  for Memory, Impaired, 276
  for Thought Processes, Disturbed, 458
  for Tissue Perfusion: Cerebral, Ineffective, 467,
     468, 469
Cesarean Section Care, as intervention, 644
Chemical Restraint, as intervention, 644
Chemotherapy Management, as intervention, 644
Chest Physiotherapy, as intervention, 644
Child Adaptation to Hospitalization, as outcome, 623
  with Coping, Ineffective, 125
  with Relocation Stress Syndrome, 359
Child Development: 1 Month, as outcome, 624
  with Development, Risk for Delayed, 525
  with Growth and Development, Delayed, 209
  with Infant Behavior, Disorganized, 246
  with Infant Behavior: Organized, Readiness for
     Enhanced, 249
  with Infant Behavior, Risk for Disorganized, 555
  with Parenting, Impaired, 316
Child Development: 2 Months, as outcome, 624
  with Development, Risk for Delayed, 526
  with Growth and Development, Delayed, 209
  with Infant Behavior, Disorganized, 246
  with Infant Behavior: Organized, Readiness for
     Enhanced, 249
  with Infant Behavior, Risk for Disorganized, 555
  with Parenting, Impaired, 317
Child Development: 4 Months, as outcome, 624
  with Development, Risk for Delayed, 526
  with Growth and Development, Delayed, 210
  with Infant Behavior: Organized, Readiness for
     Enhanced, 250
  with Infant Behavior, Risk for Disorganized, 556
  with Parenting, Impaired, 318
Child Development: 6 Months, as outcome, 624
  with Development, Risk for Delayed, 527
  with Growth, Risk for Disproportionate, 550
  with Growth and Development, Delayed, 210
  with Parenting, Impaired, 318
Child Development: 12 Months, as outcome, 624
  with Development, Risk for Delayed, 528
  with Growth, Risk for Disproportionate, 550
  with Growth and Development, Delayed, 211
  with Parenting, Impaired, 319
Child Development: 2 Years, as outcome, 624
  with Body Image, Disturbed, 68
  with Development, Risk for Delayed, 529
  with Growth, Risk for Disproportionate, 551
  with Growth and Development, Delayed, 212
  with Parenting, Impaired, 320
Child Development: 3 Years, as outcome, 624
  with Body Image, Disturbed, 68
  with Development, Risk for Delayed, 530
  with Growth, Risk for Disproportionate, 551
  with Growth and Development, Delayed, 213
  with Parenting, Impaired, 321
Child Development: 4 Years, as outcome, 624
  with Body Image, Disturbed, 69
  with Development, Risk for Delayed, 531
  with Growth, Risk for Disproportionate, 551
  with Growth and Development, Delayed, 214
  with Parenting, Impaired, 321
Child Development: 5 Years, as outcome, 624
  with Body Image, Disturbed, 69
  with Development, Risk for Delayed, 532
  with Growth, Risk for Disproportionate, 552
  with Growth and Development, Delayed, 215
  with Parenting, Impaired, 322
Child Development: Adolescence, as outcome, 624
  with Body Image, Disturbed, 71
  with Coping, Defensive, 121

Child Development: Adolescence, as outcome
  (*Continued*)
  with Development, Risk for Delayed, 534
  with Growth, Risk for Disproportionate, 553
  with Growth and Development, Delayed, 217
  with Parenting, Impaired, 323
  with Social Interaction, Impaired, 411
Child Development: Middle Childhood, as outcome, 624
  with Body Image, Disturbed, 70
  with Development, Risk for Delayed, 533
  with Growth, Risk for Disproportionate, 552
  with Growth and Development, Delayed, 216
  with Parenting, Impaired, 322
  with Social Interaction, Impaired, 410
Childbirth Preparation, as intervention, 644
  for Knowledge, Deficient (Specify), 264, 266
Circulation Status, as outcome, 624
  with Cardiac Output, Decreased, 86
  with Perioperative Positioning Injury, Risk for, 579
  with Tissue Perfusion: Cardiopulmonary,
     Ineffective, 463
  with Tissue Perfusion: Cerebral, Ineffective, 467
  with Tissue Perfusion: Gastrointestinal, Ineffective,
     471
  with Tissue Perfusion: Peripheral, Ineffective, 475
  with Tissue Perfusion: Renal, Ineffective, 479
Circulatory Care: Arterial Insufficiency, as
     intervention, 644
  for Cardiac Output, Decreased, 86, 87, 88, 89
  for Infection, Risk for, 561
  for Perioperative Positioning Injury, Risk for, 579
  for Peripheral Neurovascular Dysfunction, Risk for,
     582
  for Tissue Perfusion: Peripheral, Ineffective, 475, 477
Circulatory Care: Mechanical Assist Device, as
     intervention, 644
  for Cardiac Output, Decreased, 86
Circulatory Care: Venous Insufficiency, as
     intervention, 644
  for Cardiac Output, Decreased, 86, 87, 89
  for Perioperative Positioning Injury, Risk for, 579
  for Peripheral Neurovascular Dysfunction, Risk for,
     582
  for Tissue Perfusion: Peripheral, Ineffective, 475, 477
Circulatory Precautions, as intervention, 645
  for Peripheral Neurovascular Dysfunction, Risk for,
     582
Circumcision Care, as intervention, 645
Client Satisfaction: Access to Care Resources, as
     outcome, 624
Client Satisfaction: Caring, as outcome, 624
Client Satisfaction: Communication, as outcome, 624
Client Satisfaction: Continuity of Care, as outcome, 624
Client Satisfaction: Cultural Needs Fulfillment, as
     outcome, 624
Client Satisfaction: Functional Assistance, as outcome,
     624
Client Satisfaction: Physical Care, as outcome, 625
Client Satisfaction: Physical Environment, as outcome,
     625
Client Satisfaction: Protection of Rights, as outcome, 625
Client Satisfaction: Psychological Care, as outcome, 625
Client Satisfaction: Safety, as outcome, 625
Client Satisfaction: Symptom Control, as outcome, 625
Client Satisfaction: Teaching, as outcome, 625
Client Satisfaction: Technical Aspects of Care, as
     outcome, 625
Clinical decision-making, linkage use in teaching, 24-25
Code Management, as intervention, 645
Cognition, as outcome, 625
  with Confusion, Chronic, 113
  with Failure to Thrive, Adult, 153
  with Memory, Impaired, 275

Cognition, as outcome *(Continued)*
   with Thought Processes, Disturbed, 454
   with Tissue Perfusion: Cerebral, Ineffective, 467
Cognitive Orientation, as outcome, 625
   with Confusion, Acute, 111
   with Confusion, Chronic, 113
   with Environmental Interpretation Syndrome,
      Impaired, 151
   with Memory, Impaired, 275
   with Sensory Perception: Auditory, Disturbed, 381
   with Thought Processes, Disturbed, 454
Cognitive Restructuring, as intervention, 645
   for Confusion, Chronic, 115
   for Pain, Chronic, 307
   for Powerlessness, 337
   for Self-Mutilation, 379
   for Thought Processes, Disturbed, 456
Cognitive Stimulation, as intervention, 645
   for Confusion, Acute, 112
   for Confusion, Chronic, 113, 114, 115
   for Disuse Syndrome, Risk for, 539
   for Environmental Interpretation Syndrome,
      Impaired, 151
   for Failure to Thrive, Adult, 153
   for Memory, Impaired, 275
   for Sensory Perception: Auditory, Disturbed, 381
   for Thought Processes, Disturbed, 457
Comfort Level, as outcome, 625
   with Energy Field, Disturbed, 149
   with Nausea, 286
   with Pain, Acute, 303
   with Pain, Chronic, 306
   with Sleep, Readiness for Enhanced, 408
Comfortable Death, as outcome, 625
   for Death Anxiety, 136
Communicable Disease Management, as intervention,
   645
   for Community Coping, Ineffective, 102, 103
   for Community Coping, Readiness for Enhanced,
      106
   for Community Therapeutic Regimen Management,
      Ineffective, 110
   for Infection, Risk for, 557
Communication, as outcome, 625
   with Communication, Impaired Verbal, 98
   with Communication, Readiness for Enhanced,
      100
Communication: Expressive, as outcome, 625
   with Communication, Impaired Verbal, 98
   with Communication, Readiness for Enhanced,
      100
Communication, Impaired Verbal, 98-99
Communication, Readiness for Enhanced, 100
Communication: Receptive, as outcome, 625
   with Communication, Impaired Verbal, 98
   with Communication, Readiness for Enhanced, 100
   with Sensory Perception: Auditory, Disturbed, 381
Communication Enhancement: Hearing Deficit, as
     intervention, 645
   for Communication, Impaired Verbal, 98
   for Communication, Readiness for Enhanced, 100
   for Injury, Risk for, 566
   for Sensory Perception: Auditory, Disturbed, 381,
     382, 383
Communication Enhancement: Speech Deficit, as
     intervention, 645
   for Communication, Impaired Verbal, 98
   for Communication, Readiness for Enhanced, 100
Communication Enhancement: Visual Deficit, as
     intervention, 645
   for Communication, Impaired Verbal, 98
   for Injury, Risk for, 566
   for Sensory Perception: Visual, Disturbed, 393, 394

Community Competence, as outcome, 625
   with Community Coping, Ineffective, 101
   with Community Coping, Readiness for Enhanced,
     105
   with Community Therapeutic Regimen
     Management, Ineffective, 108
Community Coping, Ineffective, 101-104
Community Coping, Readiness for Enhanced, 105-108
Community Disaster Preparedness, as intervention, 645
   for Community Coping, Ineffective, 101
   for Community Coping, Readiness for Enhanced,
     105
Community Disaster Readiness, as outcome, 625
   with Community Coping, Ineffective, 101
   with Community Coping, Readiness for Enhanced,
     105
Community Health Development, as intervention, 645
   for Community Coping, Ineffective, 101, 102
   for Community Therapeutic Regimen Management,
     Ineffective, 108, 109
Community Health Status, as outcome, 625
   with Community Coping, Ineffective, 102
   with Community Therapeutic Regimen
     Management, Ineffective, 109
Community Health Status: Immunity, as outcome, 626
   with Community Coping, Ineffective, 102
   with Community Coping, Readiness for Enhanced,
     106
   with Community Therapeutic Regimen
     Management, Ineffective, 109
Community Risk Control: Chronic Disease, as
     outcome, 626
   with Community Coping, Ineffective, 103
   with Community Therapeutic Regimen
     Management, Ineffective, 110
Community Risk Control: Communicable Disease, as
     outcome, 626
   with Community Coping, Ineffective, 103
   with Community Coping, Readiness for Enhanced,
     106
   with Community Therapeutic Regimen
     Management, Ineffective, 110
   with Infection, Risk for, 557
Community Risk Control: Lead Exposure, as outcome,
     626
   with Community Coping, Ineffective, 103
   with Community Coping, Readiness for Enhanced,
     106
   with Community Therapeutic Regimen
     Management, Ineffective, 110
Community Risk Control: Violence, as outcome, 626
   with Community Coping, Ineffective, 104
Community Therapeutic Regimen Management,
     Ineffective, 108-110
Community Violence Level, as outcome, 626
   with Community Coping, Ineffective, 104
   with Community Coping, Readiness for Enhanced,
     107
   with Protection, Ineffective, 341
Complex Relationship Building, as intervention, 645
   for Communication, Readiness for Enhanced, 100
   for Coping, Defensive, 123
   for Social Interaction, Impaired, 413
   for Social Isolation, 418
Compliance Behavior, as outcome, 626
   with Adjustment, Impaired, 58
   with Noncompliance, 291
   with Therapeutic Regimen Management, Effective,
     436
   with Therapeutic Regimen Management,
     Ineffective, 442
   with Therapeutic Regimen Management, Readiness
     for Enhanced, 450

Concentration, as outcome, 626
  with Anxiety, 63
  with Confusion, Chronic, 114
  with Environmental Interpretation Syndrome,
    Impaired, 151
  with Memory, Impaired, 275
  with Thought Processes, Disturbed, 455
Conflict Mediation, as intervention, 645
Confusion, Acute, 111-112
Confusion, Chronic, 113-116
Constipation, 117-118
Constipation, Perceived, 119
Constipation, Risk for, 524
Constipation/Impaction Management, as intervention,
  645
  for Constipation, 117, 118
  for Constipation, Risk for, 524
Consultation, as intervention, 645
  for Caregiver Role Strain, 94
Contact Lens Care, as intervention, 645
Controlled Substance Checking, as intervention, 646
Coordinated Movement, as outcome, 626
  with Falls, Risk for, 540
  with Mobility: Bed, Impaired, 277
  with Mobility: Physical, Impaired, 281
  with Mobility: Wheelchair, Impaired, 285
  with Peripheral Neurovascular Dysfunction, Risk
    for, 581
  with Sensory Perception: Kinesthetic, Disturbed, 387
  with Transfer Ability, Impaired, 485
  with Walking, Impaired, 508
Coping, as outcome, 626
  with Adjustment, Impaired, 58
  with Anxiety, 64
  with Coping, Defensive, 121
  with Coping, Ineffective, 126
  with Coping, Readiness for Enhanced, 133
  with Grieving, Anticipatory, 203
  with Grieving, Dysfunctional, 206
  with Grieving, Dysfunctional, Risk for, 548
  with Parental Role Conflict, 313
  with Post-Trauma Syndrome, 334
  with Post-Trauma Syndrome, Risk for, 586
  with Rape-Trauma Syndrome, 347
  with Rape-Trauma Syndrome: Compound Reaction,
    351
  with Relocation Stress Syndrome, 360
  with Role Performance, Ineffective, 364
Coping, Defensive, 120-123
Coping, Ineffective, 124-131
Coping, Readiness for Enhanced, 132-134
Coping Enhancement, as intervention, 646
  for Adjustment, Impaired, 57, 58, 60
  for Anxiety, 64
  for Body Image, Disturbed, 72
  for Caregiver Role Strain, 91, 92
  for Caregiver Role Strain, Risk for, 521, 522
  for Coping, Defensive, 120, 121
  for Coping, Ineffective, 124, 125, 126, 128, 129, 130
  for Coping, Readiness for Enhanced, 132, 133, 134
  for Death Anxiety, 135, 138
  for Denial, Ineffective, 141
  for Family Coping, Compromised, 158
  for Family Coping, Disabled, 162, 163
  for Family Processes, Dysfunctional: Alcoholism, 168
  for Family Processes, Interrupted, 172
  for Family Processes, Readiness for Enhanced, 177
  for Family Therapeutic Regimen Management,
    Ineffective, 180, 182
  for Fear, 188
  for Grieving, Anticipatory, 203
  for Grieving, Dysfunctional, 206, 207, 208
  for Grieving, Dysfunctional, Risk for, 548

Coping Enhancement, as intervention (*Continued*)
  for Hopelessness, 242
  for Pain, Chronic, 309
  for Parental Role Conflict, 313, 315
  for Parenting, Impaired, 323
  for Post-Trauma Syndrome, 332, 334
  for Post-Trauma Syndrome, Risk for, 584, 586
  for Rape-Trauma Syndrome, 347
  for Rape-Trauma Syndrome: Compound Reaction,
    349, 351
  for Rape-Trauma Syndrome: Silent Reaction, 353
  for Relocation Stress Syndrome, 359, 360, 362, 363
  for Relocation Stress Syndrome, Risk for, 591
  for Role Performance, Ineffective, 364
  for Self-Esteem: Situational Low, 378
  for Sexual Dysfunction, 395
  for Sexuality Patterns, Ineffective, 398
  for Sleep Pattern, Disturbed, 407
  for Social Isolation, 417
  for Sorrow: Chronic, 420, 422
  for Unilateral Neglect, 487
Cost Containment, as intervention, 646
Cough Enhancement, as intervention, 646
  for Airway Clearance, Ineffective, 61
Counseling, as intervention, 646
  for Adjustment, Impaired, 58
  for Coping, Defensive, 121
  for Coping, Ineffective, 126
  for Denial, Ineffective, 141
  for Hopelessness, 241
  for Parental Role Conflict, 313
  for Post-Trauma Syndrome, 332, 333, 334, 336
  for Post-Trauma Syndrome, Risk for, 586
  for Rape-Trauma Syndrome, 345, 346
  for Rape-Trauma Syndrome: Compound Reaction,
    349
  for Rape-Trauma Syndrome: Silent Reaction, 353
  for Self-Esteem: Situational Low, Risk for, 592
  for Sexual Dysfunction, 395
Crisis Intervention, as intervention, 646
  for Adjustment, Impaired, 58
  for Parental Role Conflict, 313, 314
  for Post-Trauma Syndrome, Risk for, 584, 586
  for Rape-Trauma Syndrome, 347
  for Rape-Trauma Syndrome: Compound Reaction,
    350, 351
Critical Path Development, as intervention, 646
Culture Brokerage, as intervention, 646
Cumulative Index to Nursing and Allied Health
  Literature (CINAHL), 10
Curriculum planning, linkage use in, 25
Cutaneous Stimulation, as intervention, 646

D

Death Anxiety, 135-138
Decision-Making, as outcome, 626
  with Confusion, Chronic, 114
  with Coping, Ineffective, 127
  with Decisional Conflict, 139
  with Thought Processes, Disturbed, 455
Decision-making, linkages in teaching, 24-25
Decision-Making Support, as intervention, 646
  for Adjustment, Impaired, 59
  for Confusion, Chronic, 114, 115
  for Coping, Ineffective, 126, 127
  for Death Anxiety, 137
  for Decisional Conflict, 139, 140
  for Family Coping, Readiness for Enhanced, 167
  for Family Therapeutic Regimen Management,
    Ineffective, 181
  for Health Maintenance, Ineffective, 221, 223
  for Health-Seeking Behavior (Specify), 230

Decision-Making Support, as intervention *(Continued)*
  for Parental Role Conflict, 311
  for Powerlessness, 337, 338, 340
  for Powerlessness, Risk for, 588
  for Rape-Trauma Syndrome: Compound Reaction, 351
  for Therapeutic Regimen Management, Effective, 438, 439
  for Therapeutic Regimen Management, Ineffective, 445
  for Therapeutic Regimen Management, Readiness for Enhanced, 451
  for Thought Processes, Disturbed, 455
Decision support, linkages in, 24
Decisional Conflict (Specify), 139-140
Delegation, as intervention, 646
Delirium Management, as intervention, 646
  for Confusion, Acute, 111
  for Memory, Impaired, 275
Delusion Management, as intervention, 646
  for Confusion, Acute, 111
  for Confusion, Chronic, 114
  for Personal Identity, Disturbed, 330
  for Sensory Perception: Auditory, Disturbed, 382
  for Sensory Perception: Tactile, Disturbed, 391
  for Sensory Perception: Visual, Disturbed, 393
  for Thought Processes, Disturbed, 456
Dementia Management, as intervention, 647
  for Confusion, Chronic, 113, 114
  for Environmental Interpretation Syndrome, Impaired, 151, 152
  for Memory, Impaired, 275, 276
  for Thought Processes, Disturbed, 454, 457
  for Wandering, 510
Dementia Management: Bathing, as intervention, 647
Denial, Ineffective, 141-142
Dentition, Impaired, 143
Deposition/Testimony, as intervention, 647
Depression Level, as outcome, 626
  with Death Anxiety, 137
  with Hopelessness, 239
  with Pain, Chronic, 306
  with Post-Trauma Syndrome, 334
  with Relocation Stress Syndrome, 360
  with Role Performance, Ineffective, 365
  with Self-Esteem: Chronic Low, 375
  with Sorrow: Chronic, 420
Depression Self-Control, as outcome, 626
  with Hopelessness, 239
  with Pain, Chronic, 307
  with Post-Trauma Syndrome, Risk for, 586
  with Powerlessness, 337
  with Sorrow: Chronic, 421
Development, Risk for Delayed, 525-536
Developmental Care, as intervention, 647
  for Development, Risk for Delayed, 535
  for Infant Behavior, Disorganized, 246, 247
  for Infant Behavior: Organized, Readiness for Enhanced, 249, 250
  for Infant Behavior, Risk for Disorganized, 556
  for Sudden Infant Death Syndrome, Risk for, 601
Developmental Enhancement: Adolescent, as intervention, 647
  for Body Image, Disturbed, 71
  for Development, Risk for Delayed, 534, 536
  for Growth and Development, Delayed, 217, 220
  for Health Maintenance, Ineffective, 226
  for Parenting, Impaired, 322, 324
  for Parenting, Readiness for Enhanced, 328, 329
  for Parenting, Risk for Impaired, 576
  for Social Interaction, Impaired, 71

Developmental Enhancement: Child, as intervention, 647
  for Body Image, Disturbed, 68, 69, 70
  for Development, Risk for Delayed, 529, 530, 531, 532, 533, 535, 536
  for Growth and Development, Delayed, 209-216
  for Health Maintenance, Ineffective, 226
  for Parenting, Impaired, 320, 321, 322, 324, 325
  for Parenting, Readiness for Enhanced, 328, 329
  for Parenting, Risk for Impaired, 576
  for Social Interaction, Impaired, 410
Diabetes Self-Management, as outcome, 626
  with Therapeutic Regimen Management, Ineffective, 443
Diagnoses. *See* Nursing diagnoses.
Dialysis Access Maintenance, as intervention, 647
  for Skin Integrity, Impaired, 401
Diarrhea, 144-146
Diarrhea Management, as intervention, 647
  for Diarrhea, 144, 145, 146
Diet Staging, as intervention, 647
Dignified Life Closure, as outcome, 626
  with Death Anxiety, 137
  with Spiritual Distress, 423
Discharge Planning, as intervention, 647
  for Relocation Stress Syndrome, 361
  for Relocation Stress Syndrome, Risk for, 590
Discharge Readiness: Independent Living, as outcome, 626
  with Relocation Stress Syndrome, 361
Discharge Readiness: Supported Living, as outcome, 626
  with Relocation Stress Syndrome, Risk for, 590
Distorted Thought Self-Control, as outcome, 626
  with Confusion, Acute, 111
  with Confusion, Chronic, 114
  with Personal Identity, Disturbed, 330
  with Sensory Perception: Auditory, Disturbed, 382
  with Sensory Perception: Tactile, Disturbed, 391
  with Sensory Perception: Visual, Disturbed, 393
  with Thought Processes, Disturbed, 456
Distraction, as intervention, 647
Disuse Syndrome, Risk for, 537-539
Diversional Activity Deficit, 147-148
Dochterman, Joanne, 4
Documentation, as intervention, 647
Dressing, as intervention, 647
  for Self-Care Deficit: Dressing/Grooming, 369
Dying Care, as intervention, 647
  for Death Anxiety, 135, 136, 137
  for Spiritual Distress, 423
Dysreflexia Management, as intervention, 647
  for Autonomic Dysreflexia, 65
  for Autonomic Dysreflexia, Risk for, 516, 517
Dysrhythmia Management, as intervention, 647
  for Tissue Perfusion: Cardiopulmonary, Ineffective, 462

E

Ear Care, as intervention, 647
Eating Disorders Management, as intervention, 648
  for Nutrition: Imbalanced, Less than Body Requirements, 295, 298
Electroconvulsive Therapy (ECT) Management, as intervention, 648
Electrolyte and Acid/Base Balance, as outcome, 626
  with Diarrhea, 145
  with Fluid Volume, Deficient, 190
  with Fluid Volume, Excess, 193
  with Fluid Volume, Risk for Deficient, 542
  with Fluid Volume, Risk for Imbalanced, 545

Electrolyte and Acid/Base Balance, as outcome
    (*Continued*)
  with Gas Exchange, Impaired, 198
  with Tissue Perfusion: Gastrointestinal, Ineffective,
      471
  with Tissue Perfusion: Renal, Ineffective, 480
Electrolyte Management, as intervention, 648
  for Diarrhea, 145
  for Fluid Volume, Deficient, 190
  for Fluid Volume, Risk for Deficient, 542
  for Fluid Volume, Risk for Imbalanced, 545
  for Gas Exchange, Impaired, 198
  for Nutrition: Imbalanced, Less than Body
      Requirements, 296
  for Tissue Perfusion: Gastrointestinal, Ineffective, 471
  for Tissue Perfusion: Renal, Ineffective, 480, 482
Electrolyte Management: Hypercalcemia, as
    intervention, 648
Electrolyte Management: Hyperkalemia, as
    intervention, 648
Electrolyte Management: Hypermagnesemia, as
    intervention, 648
Electrolyte Management: Hypernatremia, as
    intervention, 648
Electrolyte Management: Hyperphosphatemia, as
    intervention, 648
Electrolyte Management: Hypocalcemia, as
    intervention, 648
Electrolyte Management: Hypokalemia, as
    intervention, 648
Electrolyte Management: Hypomagnesemia, as
    intervention, 648
Electrolyte Management: Hyponatremia, as
    intervention, 648
Electrolyte Management: Hypophosphatemia, as
    intervention, 648
Electrolyte Monitoring, as intervention, 648
  for Nutrition: Imbalanced, Less than Body
      Requirements, 296
Electronic Fetal Monitoring: Antepartum, as
    intervention, 649
  for Protection, Ineffective, 342
Electronic Fetal Monitoring: Intrapartum, as
    intervention, 649
  for Injury, Risk for, 562
  for Protection, Ineffective, 342
Elopement Precautions, as intervention, 649
  for Wandering, 510
Embolus Care: Peripheral, as intervention, 649
  for Cardiac Output, Decreased, 89
Embolus Care: Pulmonary, as intervention, 649
  for Cardiac Output, Decreased, 89
  for Gas Exchange, Impaired, 201
  for Tissue Perfusion: Cardiopulmonary, Ineffective,
      465
Embolus Precautions, as intervention, 649
  for Surgical Recovery, Delayed, 429
Emergency Care, as intervention, 649
  for Latex Allergy Response, 271
  for Ventilation, Impaired Spontaneous, 499
Emergency Cart Checking, as intervention, 649
Emotional Support, as intervention, 649
  for Adjustment, Impaired, 57
  for Anxiety, 64
  for Breastfeeding, Interrupted, 79
  for Caregiver Role Strain, Risk for, 519
  for Coping, Defensive, 120
  for Coping, Ineffective, 124, 125
  for Death Anxiety, 135
  for Denial, Ineffective, 141
  for Family Coping, Compromised, 156
  for Grieving, Anticipatory, 203
  for Powerlessness, 339

Emotional Support, as intervention (*Continued*)
  for Religiosity, Impaired, Risk for, 589
  for Spiritual Distress, 423
Endotracheal Extubation, as intervention, 649
Endurance, as outcome, 626
  with Activity Intolerance, 54
  with Activity Intolerance, Risk for, 511
  with Disuse Syndrome, Risk for, 537
  with Fatigue, 183
  with Lifestyle, Sedentary, 273
  with Surgical Recovery, Delayed, 428
  with Walking, Impaired, 508
Energy Conservation, as outcome, 627
  with Activity Intolerance, 54
  with Activity Intolerance, Risk for, 513
  with Fatigue, 184
Energy Field, Disturbed, 149-150
Energy Management, as intervention, 649
  for Activity Intolerance, 54, 55
  for Activity Intolerance, Risk for, 511, 512, 513
  for Caregiver Role Strain, 94
  for Caregiver Role Strain, Risk for, 521
  for Disuse Syndrome, Risk for, 537, 538
  for Fatigue, 183, 184, 185
  for Sleep Deprivation, 405
  for Surgical Recovery, Delayed, 428
  for Walking, Impaired, 508
Enteral Tube Feeding, as intervention, 649
  for Infant Feeding Pattern, Ineffective, 253
Environmental Interpretation Syndrome, Impaired,
    151-152
Environmental Management, as intervention, 649
  for Activity Intolerance, 54
  for Disuse Syndrome, Risk for, 539
  for Failure to Thrive, Adult, 154
  for Fatigue, 184
  for Infant Behavior, Disorganized, 247
  for Sensory Perception: Olfactory, Disturbed, 389
  for Sensory Perception: Visual, Disturbed, 394
Environmental Management: Attachment Process, as
    intervention, 649
  for Breastfeeding, Interrupted, 80
  for Development, Risk for Delayed, 535
  for Infant Behavior, Risk for Disorganized, 556
  for Parent/Infant/Child Attachment, Risk for
      Impaired, 572
  for Parenting, Impaired, 324
Environmental Management: Comfort, as
    intervention, 649
  for Energy Field, Disturbed, 149
  for Sleep, Readiness for Enhanced, 408
  for Sleep Pattern, Disturbed, 407
Environmental Management: Community, as
    intervention, 649
  for Community Coping, Ineffective, 101, 103, 104
  for Community Coping, Readiness for Enhanced, 106
  for Community Therapeutic Regimen Management,
      Ineffective, 109, 110
  for Protection, Ineffective, 341
Environmental Management: Home Preparation, as
    intervention, 650
Environmental Management: Safety, as intervention, 650
  for Development, Risk for Delayed, 529, 530
  for Environmental Interpretation Syndrome,
      Impaired, 151, 152
  for Falls, Risk for, 541
  for Home Maintenance, Impaired, 238
  for Injury, Risk for, 563, 565, 566
  for Parenting, Impaired, 320, 321, 327
  for Poisoning, Risk for, 583
  for Self-Mutilation, Risk for, 595
  for Sensory Perception: Tactile, Disturbed, 391
  for Thought Processes, Disturbed, 454, 458

Environmental Management: Safety, as intervention
(*Continued*)
for Trauma, Risk for, 608
for Wandering, 510
Environmental Management: Violence Prevention, as
intervention, 650
for Community Coping, Ineffective, 104
for Community Coping, Readiness for Enhanced,
107
for Personal Identity, Disturbed, 331
for Violence: Other-Directed, Risk for, 612, 613
for Violence: Self-Directed, Risk for, 616, 617
Environmental Management: Worker Safety, as
intervention, 650
Environmental Risk Protection, as intervention, 650
for Community Coping, Ineffective, 103
for Community Coping, Readiness for Enhanced, 106
for Community Therapeutic Regimen Management,
Ineffective, 110
for Health-Seeking Behavior (Specify), 235, 236
Examination Assistance, as intervention, 650
Exercise Promotion, as intervention, 650
for Activity Intolerance, Risk for, 511
for Lifestyle, Sedentary, 273
Exercise Promotion: Strength Training, as
intervention, 650
for Activity Intolerance, 53, 54, 55, 56
for Activity Intolerance, Risk for, 511, 512
for Lifestyle, Sedentary, 273
for Mobility: Bed, Impaired, 277, 278, 279
for Mobility: Physical, Impaired, 280, 281, 283
for Mobility: Wheelchair, Impaired, 284, 285
for Peripheral Neurovascular Dysfunction, Risk for,
581
for Sensory Perception: Kinesthetic, Disturbed, 386
for Transfer Ability, Impaired, 484, 485, 486
Exercise Promotion: Stretching, as intervention, 650
Exercise Therapy: Ambulation, as intervention, 650
for Disuse Syndrome, Risk for, 539
for Mobility: Physical, Impaired, 280, 281, 282, 283
for Surgical Recovery, Delayed, 427
for Transfer Ability, Impaired, 485
for Walking, Impaired, 507, 509
Exercise Therapy: Balance, as intervention, 650
for Disuse Syndrome, Risk for, 539
for Falls, Risk for, 540
for Mobility: Physical, Impaired, 281, 282
for Mobility: Wheelchair, Impaired, 284
for Sensory Perception: Kinesthetic, Disturbed,
386, 388
for Transfer Ability, Impaired, 484, 485
for Walking, Impaired, 507
Exercise Therapy: Joint Mobility, as intervention, 650
for Activity Intolerance, 53
for Disuse Syndrome, Risk for, 539
for Mobility: Bed, Impaired, 278
for Mobility: Physical, Impaired, 282
for Peripheral Neurovascular Dysfunction, Risk for,
581
for Surgical Recovery, Delayed, 429
for Transfer Ability, Impaired, 485
for Walking, Impaired, 508
Exercise Therapy: Muscle Control, as intervention, 650
for Activity Intolerance, 53
for Disuse Syndrome, Risk for, 539
for Falls, Risk for, 540
for Mobility: Bed, Impaired, 277, 279
for Mobility: Physical, Impaired, 281, 282, 283
for Mobility: Wheelchair, Impaired, 284
for Peripheral Neurovascular Dysfunction, Risk for,
581
for Sensory Perception: Kinesthetic, Disturbed,
386, 387

Exercise Therapy: Muscle Control, as intervention
(*Continued*)
for Transfer Ability, Impaired, 484, 485
for Unilateral Neglect, 488
for Walking, Impaired, 508
Eye Care, as intervention, 650

F

Failure to Thrive, Adult, 153-155
Fall Prevention, as intervention, 650
for Environmental Interpretation Syndrome,
Impaired, 151
for Falls, Risk for, 540, 541
for Injury, Risk for, 562, 564
for Knowledge, Deficient (Specify), 260
for Transfer Ability, Impaired, 484
for Wandering, 510
Fall Prevention Behavior, as outcome, 627
with Environmental Interpretation Syndrome,
Impaired, 151
with Falls, Risk for, 541
with Wandering, 510
Falls, Risk for, 540-541
Falls Occurrence, as outcome, 627
with Falls, Risk for, 541
with Injury, Risk for, 562
Family Coping, as outcome, 627
with Family Coping, Compromised, 158
with Family Coping, Disabled, 163
with Family Coping, Readiness for Enhanced, 164
with Family Processes, Dysfunctional: Alcoholism,
168
with Family Processes, Interrupted, 172
with Family Processes, Readiness for Enhanced,
177
with Family Therapeutic Regimen Management,
Ineffective, 180
with Grieving, Anticipatory, 204
with Grieving, Dysfunctional, 207
with Grieving, Dysfunctional, Risk for, 548
with Parenting, Impaired, 323
Family Coping, Compromised, 156-159
Family Coping, Disabled, 160-163
Family Coping, Readiness for Enhanced, 164-167
Family Functioning, as outcome, 627
with Family Coping, Readiness for Enhanced, 165
with Family Processes, Dysfunctional: Alcoholism,
168
with Family Processes, Interrupted, 173
with Family Processes, Readiness for Enhanced,
177
with Family Therapeutic Regimen Management,
Ineffective, 180
with Home Maintenance, Impaired, 237
with Parental Role Conflict, 313
with Parenting, Impaired, 324
with Parenting, Readiness for Enhanced, 328
Family Health Status, as outcome, 627
with Family Processes, Readiness for Enhanced, 178
Family Integrity, as outcome, 627
with Family Processes, Readiness for Enhanced,
178
Family Integrity Promotion, as intervention, 650
for Family Processes, Dysfunctional: Alcoholism, 168
for Family Processes, Interrupted, 173, 174
for Family Processes, Readiness for Enhanced, 178,
179
for Family Therapeutic Regimen Management,
Ineffective, 180
for Grieving, Anticipatory, 204
for Grieving, Dysfunctional, 207
for Home Maintenance, Impaired, 237

Family Integrity Promotion, as intervention
    (Continued)
  for Parenting, Impaired, 324
  for Parenting, Readiness for Enhanced, 328
  for Social Interaction, Impaired, 411
  for Social Isolation, 415
Family Integrity Promotion: Childbearing Family, as
    intervention, 651
  for Family Processes, Dysfunctional: Alcoholism, 170
  for Family Processes, Readiness for Enhanced, 177,
    178
  for Home Maintenance, Impaired, 237
  for Parenting, Impaired, 317, 318, 319, 324
  for Parenting, Risk for Impaired, 576, 577
Family Involvement Promotion, as intervention, 651
  for Caregiver Role Strain, Risk for, 520
  for Confusion, Chronic, 114
  for Family Coping, Compromised, 158
  for Family Coping, Readiness for Enhanced, 164
  for Family Processes, Interrupted, 175
  for Family Therapeutic Regimen Management,
    Ineffective, 180, 181
  for Health Maintenance, Ineffective, 226
  for Parental Role Conflict, 312
  for Parenting, Impaired, 327
  for Powerlessness, 337
  for Relocation Stress Syndrome, 361
  for Social Isolation, 419
  for Therapeutic Regimen Management, Effective, 436
Family Mobilization, as intervention, 651
  for Family Coping, Compromised, 158
  for Family Processes, Readiness for Enhanced, 177
  for Family Therapeutic Regimen Management,
    Ineffective, 181
Family Normalization, as outcome, 627
  with Family Coping, Compromised, 159
  with Family Coping, Disabled, 163
  with Family Coping, Readiness for Enhanced, 165
  with Family Processes, Interrupted, 173
  with Family Therapeutic Regimen Management,
    Ineffective, 181
Family Participation in Professional Care, as outcome,
    627
  with Family Therapeutic Regimen Management,
    Ineffective, 181
  with Powerlessness, 337
  with Therapeutic Regimen Management, Effective,
    436
Family Physical Environment, as outcome, 627
  with Home Maintenance, Impaired, 237
Family Planning: Contraception, as intervention, 651
  for Health-Seeking Behavior (Specify), 236
  for Knowledge, Deficient (Specify), 258
Family Planning: Infertility, as intervention, 651
  for Knowledge, Deficient (Specify), 260
Family Planning: Unplanned Pregnancy, as
    intervention, 651
Family Presence Facilitation, as intervention, 651
  for Family Processes, Interrupted, 175
Family Process Maintenance, as intervention, 651
  for Diversional Activity Deficit, 147
  for Family Coping, Compromised, 159
  for Family Processes, Dysfunctional: Alcoholism,
    168, 169
  for Family Processes, Interrupted, 173, 174
  for Family Therapeutic Regimen Management,
    Ineffective, 180
  for Parental Role Conflict, 313, 314
  for Parenting, Impaired, 323, 324
  for Social Interaction, Impaired, 411
Family Processes, Dysfunctional: Alcoholism, 168-171
Family Processes, Interrupted, 172-176
Family Processes, Readiness for Enhanced, 177-179

Family Resiliency, as outcome, 627
  with Family Processes, Dysfunctional: Alcoholism,
    169
  with Family Processes, Interrupted, 174
  with Family Processes, Readiness for Enhanced, 179
  with Family Therapeutic Regimen Management,
    Ineffective, 182
  with Grieving, Dysfunctional, 207
Family Social Climate, as outcome, 627
  with Diversional Activity Deficit, 147
  with Family Processes, Dysfunctional: Alcoholism, 169
  with Family Processes, Interrupted, 174
  with Family Processes, Readiness for Enhanced, 179
  with Grieving, Anticipatory, 204
  with Parental Role Conflict, 314
  with Parenting, Impaired, 324
  with Social Interaction, Impaired, 411
  with Social Isolation, 415
Family Support, as intervention, 651
  for Diversional Activity Deficit, 147
  for Family Coping, Compromised, 159
  for Family Coping, Disabled, 163
  for Family Coping, Readiness for Enhanced, 164, 165
  for Family Processes, Interrupted, 172
  for Grieving, Anticipatory, 204
  for Grieving, Dysfunctional, 207
  for Parenting, Impaired, 323
Family Support During Treatment, as outcome, 627
  with Family Processes, Interrupted, 175
Family Therapeutic Regimen Management,
    Ineffective, 180-182
Family Therapy, as intervention, 651
  for Family Coping, Disabled, 163
  for Family Processes, Dysfunctional: Alcoholism, 169
  for Grieving, Dysfunctional, Risk for, 548
Fatigue, 183-185
Fear, 186-188
Fear Level, as outcome, 627
  with Fear, 186
  with Post-Trauma Syndrome, 334
Fear Level: Child, as outcome, 627
  with Fear, 187
  with Post-Trauma Syndrome, 335
Fear Self-Control, as outcome, 627
  with Death Anxiety, 138
  with Denial, Ineffective, 142
  with Fear, 188
Feeding, as intervention, 651
  for Self-Care Deficit: Feeding, 370
Fertility Preservation, as intervention, 651
  for Knowledge, Deficient (Specify), 260
Fetal Status: Antepartum, as outcome, 628
  with Protection, Ineffective, 342
Fetal Status: Intrapartum, as outcome, 628
  with Injury, Risk for, 562
  with Protection, Ineffective, 342
Fever Treatment, as intervention, 651
  for Hyperthermia, 243
Financial Resource Assistance, as intervention, 651
  for Health Maintenance, Ineffective, 221
  for Post-Trauma Syndrome, 332
  for Powerlessness, 339
Fire-Setting Precautions, as intervention, 651
First Aid, as intervention, 651
Fiscal Resource Management, as intervention, 651
Flatulence Reduction, as intervention, 651
Fluid Balance, as outcome, 628
  with Diarrhea, 145
  with Fluid Balance, Readiness for Enhanced, 189
  with Fluid Volume, Deficient, 191
  with Fluid Volume, Excess, 194
  with Fluid Volume, Risk for Deficient, 543
  with Fluid Volume, Risk for Imbalanced, 546

Fluid Balance, as outcome *(Continued)*
  with Tissue Perfusion: Gastrointestinal, Ineffective, 472
  with Tissue Perfusion: Renal, Ineffective, 481
Fluid Balance, Readiness for Enhanced, 189
Fluid/Electrolyte Management, as intervention, 651
  for Constipation, 117
  for Diarrhea, 145
  for Fluid Volume, Deficient, 190
  for Fluid Volume, Excess, 193, 195, 196
  for Fluid Volume, Risk for Imbalanced, 545
  for Nausea, 286
  for Nutrition: Imbalanced, Less than Body
      Requirements, 296
  for Tissue Perfusion: Gastrointestinal, Ineffective,
      471, 472, 473
  for Tissue Perfusion: Peripheral, Ineffective, 476
  for Tissue Perfusion: Renal, Ineffective, 480, 481,
      482, 483
Fluid Management, as intervention, 652
  for Constipation, 117
  for Diarrhea, 145, 146
  for Fluid Balance, Readiness for Enhanced, 189
  for Fluid Volume, Deficient, 191, 192
  for Fluid Volume, Excess, 193, 194, 196
  for Fluid Volume, Risk for Deficient, 542, 543, 544
  for Fluid Volume, Risk for Imbalanced, 545, 546,
      547
  for Surgical Recovery, Delayed, 427, 428
  for Tissue Perfusion: Gastrointestinal, Ineffective,
      472
  for Tissue Perfusion: Peripheral, Ineffective, 476
  for Tissue Perfusion: Renal, Ineffective, 481
Fluid Monitoring, as intervention, 652
  for Failure to Thrive, Adult, 154
  for Fluid Balance, Readiness for Enhanced, 189
  for Fluid Volume, Deficient, 191, 192
  for Fluid Volume, Excess, 193, 194
  for Fluid Volume, Risk for Deficient, 543, 544
  for Fluid Volume, Risk for Imbalanced, 546, 547
  for Infant Feeding Pattern, Ineffective, 252
  for Nausea, 288
  for Nutrition: Imbalanced, Less than Body
      Requirements, 297
  for Sensory Perception: Gustatory, Disturbed, 384
Fluid Overload Severity, as outcome, 628
  with Fluid Volume, Excess, 195
  with Surgical Recovery, Delayed, 428
  with Tissue Perfusion: Peripheral, Ineffective, 476
  with Tissue Perfusion: Renal, Ineffective, 482
Fluid Resuscitation, as intervention, 652
Fluid Volume, Deficient, 190-192
Fluid Volume, Excess, 193-196
Fluid Volume, Risk for Deficient, 542-544
Fluid Volume, Risk for Imbalanced, 545-547
Foot Care, as intervention, 652
Forgiveness Facilitation, as intervention, 652

G

Gas Exchange, Impaired, 197-202
Gastrointestinal Intubation, as intervention, 652
Genetic Counseling, as intervention, 652
Grief Resolution, as outcome, 628
  with Grieving, Anticipatory, 205
  with Grieving, Dysfunctional, 208
  with Grieving, Dysfunctional, Risk for, 549
  with Self-Esteem: Situational Low, 377
  with Sorrow: Chronic, 421
Grief Work Facilitation, as intervention, 652
  for Grieving, Anticipatory, 203, 204
  for Grieving, Dysfunctional, 206, 207, 208
  for Grieving, Dysfunctional, Risk for, 548, 549

Grief Work Facilitation, as intervention *(Continued)*
  for Self-Esteem: Situational Low, 377
  for Sorrow: Chronic, 421, 422
Grief Work Facilitation: Perinatal Death, as
    intervention, 652
  for Grieving, Anticipatory, 203, 204
  for Grieving, Dysfunctional, 206, 207, 208
  for Grieving, Dysfunctional, Risk for, 548, 549
  for Self-Esteem: Situational Low, 377
  for Sorrow: Chronic, 421
Grieving, Anticipatory, 203-205
Grieving, Dysfunctional, 206-208
Grieving, Dysfunctional, Risk for, 548-549
Growth, as outcome, 628
  with Growth, Risk for Disproportionate, 554
  with Growth and Development, Delayed, 218
Growth, Risk for Disproportionate, 550-554
Growth and Development, Delayed, 209-220
Guilt Work Facilitation, as intervention, 652

H

Hair Care, as intervention, 652
  for Self-Care Deficit: Dressing/Grooming, 369
Hallucination Management, as intervention, 652
  for Confusion, Acute, 111
  for Personal Identity, Disturbed, 330
  for Sensory Perception: Auditory, Disturbed, 382
  for Sensory Perception: Tactile, Disturbed, 391
  for Sensory Perception: Visual, Disturbed, 393
  for Thought Processes, Disturbed, 456
Health Beliefs, as outcome, 628
  with Constipation, Perceived, 119
  with Health-Seeking Behavior (Specify), 228
  with Powerlessness, 338
Health Beliefs: Perceived Ability to Perform, as
    outcome, 628
  with Powerlessness, 338
  with Powerlessness, Risk for, 587
Health Beliefs: Perceived Control, as outcome, 628
  with Powerlessness, 338
  with Powerlessness, Risk for, 587
Health Beliefs: Perceived Resources, as outcome, 628
  with Health Maintenance, Ineffective, 221
  with Powerlessness, 339
Health Beliefs: Perceived Threat, as outcome, 628
  with Denial, Ineffective, 142
Health Care Information Exchange, as intervention, 652
Health Education, as intervention, 652
  for Adjustment, Impaired, 59
  for Community Coping, Ineffective, 103
  for Community Therapeutic Regimen Management,
      Ineffective, 110
  for Constipation, Perceived, 119
  for Denial, Ineffective, 142
  for Family Coping, Readiness for Enhanced, 166
  for Health Maintenance, Ineffective, 221, 222, 224,
      226
  for Health-Seeking Behavior (Specify), 228, 229,
      230, 231, 233, 234, 235
  for Injury, Risk for, 563, 565
  for Knowledge, Deficient (Specify), 261, 265, 266,
      267
  for Knowledge (Specify), Readiness for Enhanced,
      269, 270
  for Noncompliance, 289
  for Poisoning, Risk for, 583
  for Powerlessness, 338
  for Protection, Ineffective, 342
  for Therapeutic Regimen Management, Effective,
      435, 438
  for Therapeutic Regimen Management, Readiness
      for Enhanced, 450, 452

Health Level 7 (HL7), 24
Health Maintenance, Ineffective, 221-227
Health Orientation, as outcome, 628
  with Health-Seeking Behavior (Specify), 228
Health Policy Monitoring, as intervention, 652
  for Community Coping, Readiness for Enhanced, 105
  for Community Therapeutic Regimen Management, Ineffective, 108
Health Promoting Behavior, as outcome, 628
  with Family Coping, Readiness for Enhanced, 166
  with Health Maintenance, Ineffective, 221
  with Health-Seeking Behavior (Specify), 229
  with Protection, Ineffective, 342
Health Screening, as intervention, 652
  for Caregiver Role Strain, Risk for, 521
  for Community Coping, Ineffective, 102
  for Development, Risk for Delayed, 530, 531, 532, 533
  for Growth, Risk for Disproportionate, 521
  for Growth and Development, Delayed, 210-220
  for Health Maintenance, Ineffective, 224, 226
  for Health-Seeking Behavior (Specify), 231, 234
  for Infant Behavior: Organized, Readiness for Enhanced, 250
  for Infection, Risk for, 557
Health Seeking Behavior, as outcome, 628
  with Adjustment, Impaired, 59
  with Family Coping, Readiness for Enhanced, 166
  with Health Maintenance, Ineffective, 221
  with Health-Seeking Behavior (Specify), 230
Health-Seeking Behavior (Specify), 228-236
Health System Guidance, as intervention, 653
  for Caregiver Role Strain, 94
  for Coping, Ineffective, 129
  for Decisional Conflict, 140
  for Family Coping, Compromised, 157
  for Family Coping, Disabled, 161
  for Family Coping, Readiness for Enhanced, 167
  for Family Processes, Readiness for Enhanced, 178
  for Family Therapeutic Regimen Management, Ineffective, 181
  for Health Maintenance, Ineffective, 221, 222, 223
  for Health-Seeking Behavior (Specify), 230
  for Knowledge, Deficient (Specify), 262
  for Knowledge (Specify), Readiness for Enhanced, 270
  for Noncompliance, 290, 291
  for Powerlessness, 339, 340
  for Relocation Stress Syndrome, 361
  for Therapeutic Regimen Management, Effective, 435, 438
  for Therapeutic Regimen Management, Ineffective, 445
  for Therapeutic Regimen Management, Readiness for Enhanced, 451
Hearing Compensation Behavior, as outcome, 628
  with Sensory Perception: Auditory, Disturbed, 382
Heat/Cold Application, as intervention, 653
Heat Exposure Treatment, as intervention, 653
Hemodialysis Access, as outcome, 628
  with Skin Integrity, Impaired, 401
Hemodialysis Therapy, as intervention, 653
  for Therapeutic Regimen Management, Ineffective, 448
  for Tissue Perfusion: Renal, Ineffective, 481, 482
Hemodynamic Regulation, as intervention, 653
  for Cardiac Output, Decreased, 85, 90
  for Gas Exchange, Impaired, 201
  for Tissue Perfusion: Cardiopulmonary, Ineffective, 462, 463, 464, 466
  for Tissue Perfusion: Gastrointestinal, Ineffective, 471

Hemofiltration Therapy, as intervention, 653
  for Therapeutic Regimen Management, Ineffective, 448
  for Tissue Perfusion: Renal, Ineffective, 482
Hemorrhage Control, as intervention, 653
  for Cardiac Output, Decreased, 84
High-Risk Pregnancy Care, as intervention, 653
Home Maintenance, Impaired, 237-238
Home Maintenance Assistance, as intervention, 653
  for Activity Intolerance, 56
  for Failure to Thrive, Adult, 154
  for Home Maintenance, Impaired, 237
Hope, as outcome, 628
  with Death Anxiety, 138
  with Hopelessness, 240
  with Powerlessness, 339
  with Sorrow: Chronic, 421
  with Spiritual Distress, 424
  with Spiritual Distress, Risk for, 599
  with Spiritual Well-Being, Readiness for Enhanced, 425
Hope Instillation, as intervention, 653
  for Death Anxiety, 137, 138
  for Energy Field, Disturbed, 150
  for Failure to Thrive, Adult, 153, 155
  for Hopelessness, 239, 240, 242
  for Powerlessness, 339
  for Relocation Stress Syndrome, 360
  for Role Performance, Ineffective, 365
  for Self-Esteem: Chronic Low, 375
  for Sorrow: Chronic, 420, 421
  for Spiritual Distress, 424
  for Spiritual Distress, Risk for, 599, 600
  for Spiritual Well-Being, Readiness for Enhanced, 425
  for Suicide, Risk for, 607
Hopelessness, 239-242
Hormone Replacement Therapy, as intervention, 653
Humor, as intervention, 653
Hydration, as outcome, 628
  with Constipation, 117
  with Diarrhea, 146
  with Fluid Balance, Readiness for Enhanced, 189
  with Fluid Volume, Deficient, 192
  with Fluid Volume, Risk for Deficient, 544
  with Fluid Volume, Risk for Imbalanced, 547
  with Infant Feeding Pattern, Ineffective, 252
  with Nausea, 286
  with Tissue Perfusion: Gastrointestinal, Ineffective, 473
Hyperactivity Level, as outcome, 628
  with Development, Risk for Delayed, 535
Hyperglycemia Management, as intervention, 653
  for Therapeutic Regimen Management, Ineffective, 440
Hyperthermia, 243-244
Hypervolemia Management, as intervention, 653
  for Fluid Volume, Excess, 194, 195
  for Surgical Recovery, Delayed, 428
  for Tissue Perfusion: Peripheral, Ineffective, 476
Hypnosis, as intervention, 653
Hypoglycemia Management, as intervention, 653
  for Therapeutic Regimen Management, Ineffective, 440
Hypothermia, 245
Hypothermia Treatment, as intervention, 654
  for Hypothermia, 245
Hypovolemia Management, as intervention, 654
  for Fluid Volume, Deficient, 191, 192
  for Fluid Volume, Risk for Deficient, 543, 544
  for Surgical Recovery, Delayed, 427
  for Tissue Perfusion: Gastrointestinal, Ineffective, 471, 473, 474
  for Tissue Perfusion: Renal, Ineffective, 479, 483

I

Identity, as outcome, 628
  with Confusion, Chronic, 115
  with Personal Identity, Disturbed, 330
  with Self-Mutilation, 379
  with Thought Processes, Disturbed, 456
Immobility Consequences: Physiological, as outcome, 628
  with Disuse Syndrome, Risk for, 538
  with Mobility: Bed, Impaired, 278
  with Skin Integrity, Risk for Impaired, 596
  with Surgical Recovery, Delayed, 429
Immobility Consequences: Psycho-Cognitive, as outcome, 629
  with Disuse Syndrome, Risk for, 539
Immune Hypersensitivity Response, as outcome, 629
  with Protection, Ineffective, 343
Immune Status, as outcome, 629
  with Infection, Risk for, 557
  with Protection, Ineffective, 343
Immunization Behavior, as outcome, 629
  with Protection, Ineffective, 344
Immunization/Vaccination Management, as intervention, 654
  for Community Coping, Ineffective, 102, 103
  for Community Coping, Readiness for Enhanced, 106
  for Community Therapeutic Regimen Management, Ineffective, 109
  for Infection, Risk for, 557, 558
  for Protection, Ineffective, 344
Impulse Control Training, as intervention, 654
  for Coping, Ineffective, 128
  for Post-Trauma Syndrome, 335
  for Post-Trauma Syndrome, Risk for, 585
  for Self-Mutilation, 379, 380
  for Self-Mutilation, Risk for, 594
  for Violence: Other-Directed, Risk for, 614
  for Violence: Self-Directed, Risk for, 615
Impulse Self-Control, as outcome, 629
  with Coping, Ineffective, 128
  with Post-Trauma Syndrome, 335
  with Self-Mutilation, 379
  with Self-Mutilation, Risk for, 594
  with Violence: Other-Directed, Risk for, 614
  with Violence: Self-Directed, Risk for, 615
Incident Reporting, as intervention, 654
Incision Site Care, as intervention, 654
  for Infection, Risk for, 560
  for Skin Integrity, Impaired, 403
  for Skin Integrity, Risk for Impaired, 598
  for Surgical Recovery, Delayed, 429, 431, 432
  for Tissue Integrity, Impaired, 461
Infant Behavior, Disorganized, 246-248
Infant Behavior: Organized, Readiness for Enhanced, 249-251
Infant Behavior, Risk for Disorganized, 555-556
Infant Care, as intervention, 654
  for Development, Risk for Delayed, 526, 527, 528
  for Growth, Risk for Disproportionate, 550
  for Growth and Development, Delayed, 209, 210
  for Infant Behavior, Disorganized, 246
  for Infant Behavior: Organized, Readiness for Enhanced, 249, 250
  for Infant Behavior, Risk for Disorganized, 555, 556
  for Infant Feeding Pattern, Ineffective, 252
Infant Feeding Pattern, Ineffective, 252-253
Infection, Risk for, 557-561
Infection Control, as intervention, 654
  for Infection, Risk for, 558, 559, 561
  for Surgical Recovery, Delayed, 429

Infection Control: Intraoperative, as intervention, 654
Infection Protection, as intervention, 654
  for Infection, Risk for, 558, 559
  for Knowledge, Deficient (Specify), 263
  for Protection, Ineffective, 343
  for Sexual Dysfunction, 396
  for Tissue Integrity, Impaired, 461
Infection Severity, as outcome, 629
  with Infection, Risk for, 558
  with Surgical Recovery, Delayed, 429
Infection Severity: Newborn, as outcome, 629
  with Infection, Risk for, 559
Information databases, linkage use in, 23-24
Information Processing, as outcome, 629
  with Communication, Impaired Verbal, 99
  with Confusion, Acute, 112
  with Confusion, Chronic, 115
  with Decisional Conflict, 139
  with Thought Processes, Disturbed, 457
Injury, Risk for, 562-567
Insurance Authorization, as intervention, 654
Intellectual skills, of nursing, 21-28
Intervention. *See* Nursing intervention(s).
Intracranial Adaptive Capacity, Decreased, 254-256
Intracranial Pressure (ICP) Monitoring, as intervention, 654
  for Intracranial Adaptive Capacity, Decreased, 254, 256
  for Tissue Perfusion: Cerebral, Ineffective, 468
Intrapartal Care, as intervention, 654
Intrapartal Care: High-Risk Delivery, as intervention, 654
  for Injury, Risk for, 562
Intravenous (IV) Insertion, as intervention, 654
Intravenous (IV) Therapy, as intervention, 654
  for Cardiac Output, Decreased, 87
  for Fluid Volume, Deficient, 192
  for Fluid Volume, Risk for Deficient, 543
  for Tissue Perfusion: Gastrointestinal, Ineffective, 474
Invasive hemodynamic Monitoring, as intervention, 654

J

Johnson, Marion, 7
Joint Movement: (Specify Joint), as outcome
  with Mobility: Bed, Impaired, 278
  with Mobility: Physical, Impaired, 282
Joint Movement: Ankle, as outcome, 629
  with Walking, Impaired, 508
Joint Movement: Elbow, as outcome, 629
Joint Movement: Fingers, as outcome, 629
Joint Movement: Hip, as outcome, 629
  with Walking, Impaired, 508
Joint Movement: Knee, as outcome, 629
  with Walking, Impaired, 508
Joint Movement: Neck, as outcome, 629
Joint Movement: Passive, as outcome, 629
  with Mobility: Bed, Impaired, 278
Joint Movement: Shoulder, as outcome, 629
Joint Movement: Spine, as outcome, 629
Joint Movement: Wrist, as outcome, 629

K

Kangaroo Care, as intervention, 655
for Parenting, Impaired, 324
Kidney Function, as outcome, 629
  with Fluid Balance, Readiness for Enhanced, 189
  with Fluid Volume, Excess, 196
  with Tissue Perfusion: Renal, Ineffective, 482

Knowledge: Body Mechanics, as outcome, 629
  with Knowledge, Deficient (Specify), 257
Knowledge: Breastfeeding, as outcome, 629
  with Breastfeeding, Interrupted, 80
  with Breastfeeding Ineffective, 78
  with Knowledge, Deficient (Specify), 257
Knowledge: Cardiac Disease Management, as
  outcome, 629
  with Knowledge, Deficient (Specify), 257
Knowledge: Child Physical Safety, as outcome, 630
  with Knowledge, Deficient (Specify), 258
  with Parenting, Readiness for Enhanced, 328
Knowledge: Conception Prevention, as outcome, 630
  with Knowledge, Deficient (Specify), 258
Knowledge, Deficient (Specify), 257-268
Knowledge: Diabetes Management, as outcome, 630
  with Knowledge, Deficient (Specify), 258
Knowledge: Diet, as outcome, 630
  with Knowledge, Deficient (Specify), 259
  with Nutrition, Readiness for Enhanced, 301
  with Therapeutic Regimen Management,
    Ineffective, 443
Knowledge: Disease Process, as outcome, 630
  with Knowledge, Deficient (Specify), 259
Knowledge: Energy Conservation, as outcome, 630
  with Knowledge, Deficient (Specify), 259
Knowledge: Fall Prevention, as outcome, 630
  with Falls, Risk for, 541
  with Knowledge, Deficient (Specify), 260
Knowledge: Fertility Promotion, as outcome, 630
  with Knowledge, Deficient (Specify), 260
Knowledge: Health Behavior, as outcome, 630
  with Constipation, Perceived, 119
  with Health Maintenance, Ineffective, 222
  with Knowledge, Deficient (Specify), 261
  with Knowledge (Specify), Readiness for Enhanced,
    269
Knowledge: Health Promotion, as outcome, 630
  with Health Maintenance, Ineffective, 222
  with Health-Seeking Behavior (Specify), 230
  with Knowledge, Deficient (Specify), 261
  with Knowledge (Specify), Readiness for Enhanced,
    270
Knowledge: Health Resources, as outcome, 630
  with Coping, Ineffective, 129
  with Health Maintenance, Ineffective, 222
  with Health-Seeking Behavior (Specify), 230
  with Knowledge, Deficient (Specify), 262
  with Knowledge (Specify), Readiness for Enhanced,
    270
Knowledge: Illness Care, as outcome, 630
  with Knowledge, Deficient (Specify), 262
Knowledge: Infant Care, as outcome, 630
  with Knowledge, Deficient (Specify), 263
  with Parenting, Readiness for Enhanced, 328
Knowledge: Infection Control, as outcome, 630
  with Knowledge, Deficient (Specify), 263
Knowledge: Labor and Delivery, as outcome, 630
  with Knowledge, Deficient (Specify), 264
Knowledge: Medication, as outcome, 630
  with Knowledge, Deficient (Specify), 264
Knowledge: Ostomy Care, as outcome, 630
  with Knowledge, Deficient (Specify), 264
  with Self-Care Deficit: Toileting, 372
Knowledge: Parenting, as outcome, 630
  with Knowledge, Deficient (Specify), 265
  with Parenting, Readiness for Enhanced, 329
Knowledge: Personal Safety, as outcome, 630
  with Knowledge, Deficient (Specify), 265
Knowledge: Postpartum Maternal Health, as outcome,
  631
  with Knowledge, Deficient (Specify), 266

Knowledge: Preconception Maternal Health, as
  outcome, 631
  with Knowledge, Deficient (Specify), 266
Knowledge: Pregnancy, as outcome, 631
  with Knowledge, Deficient (Specify), 266
Knowledge: Prescribed Activity, as outcome, 631
  with Knowledge, Deficient (Specify), 267
Knowledge: Sexual Functioning, as outcome, 631
  with Knowledge, Deficient (Specify), 267
Knowledge: Substance Use Control, as outcome, 631
  with Knowledge, Deficient (Specify), 267
Knowledge: Treatment Procedure(s), as outcome, 631
  with Knowledge, Deficient (Specify), 268
Knowledge: Treatment Regimen, as outcome, 631
  with Family Therapeutic Regimen Management,
    Ineffective, 182
  with Health Maintenance, Ineffective, 223
  with Knowledge, Deficient (Specify), 268
  with Therapeutic Regimen Management, Effective,
    437
  with Therapeutic Regimen Management,
    Ineffective, 444
  with Therapeutic Regimen Management, Readiness
    for Enhanced, 451
Knowledge (Specify), Readiness for Enhanced, 269-
  270
Knowledge development, nursing, linkage use in, 25-
  26

L

Labor Induction, as intervention, 655
  for Injury, Risk for, 562
Labor Suppression, as intervention, 655
Laboratory Data Interpretation, as intervention, 655
  for Gas Exchange, Impaired, 198
Lactation Counseling, as intervention, 655
  for Breastfeeding, Effective, 74, 75
  for Breastfeeding, Ineffective, 76, 77, 78
  for Breastfeeding, Interrupted, 79, 80
  for Infant Feeding Pattern, Ineffective, 252
  for Knowledge, Deficient (Specify), 257, 266
  for Nutrition: Imbalanced, Less than Body
    Requirements, 294
Lactation Suppression, as intervention, 655
  for Breastfeeding, Effective, 75
  for Breastfeeding, Ineffective, 78
  for Breastfeeding, Interrupted, 79, 80
Laser Precautions, as intervention, 655
Latex Allergy Response, 271-272
Latex Allergy Response, Risk for, 567
Latex Precautions, as intervention, 655
  for Latex Allergy Response, 271, 272
  for Latex Allergy Response, Risk for, 567
  for Skin Integrity, Impaired, 401
Learning Facilitation, as intervention, 655
  for Decisional Conflict, 139
  for Family Coping, Compromised, 157
  for Family Coping, Disabled, 161
  for Family Coping, Readiness for Enhanced, 166
  for Knowledge (Specify), Readiness for Enhanced,
    269, 270
  for Noncompliance, 290
Learning Readiness Enhancement, as intervention,
  655
  for Knowledge (Specify), Readiness for Enhanced,
    269, 270
Leech Therapy, as intervention, 655
Leisure Participation, as outcome, 631
  with Diversional Activity Deficit, 147
  with Social Interaction, Impaired, 412
  with Social Isolation, 415

Lifestyle, Sedentary, 273-274
Likert scale, 9
Limit Setting, as intervention, 655
Linkage(s), 13
    aggregate data basis of, 13-14, 14t
    application of, 21-48
    in care planning, 21-23
    case studies in, 28-48
    in clinical decision-making, 24-25
    in computerized information databases, 23-24
    references on, 26-27
    in research and knowledge development, 25-26
    case studies in application of, 28-48
    study 1 of, 28-30
    study 2 of, 31-34
    study 3 of, 35-37
    study 4 of, 38-42
    study 5 of, 43-48
    concept names and definitions of, sources, 13-14
    definition of, 13
    description of, 13-15
    development of, 15-19
    first edition, 15-17
    second edition, 17-19
    entry point for, 14
    and judgment of practitioner, 13
    references on, 19
Loneliness, Risk for, 568-569
Loneliness Severity, as outcome, 631
    with Loneliness, Risk for, 568
    with Relocation Stress Syndrome, 361
    with Social Isolation, 416
Lower Extremity Monitoring, as intervention, 655
    for Sensory Perception: Tactile, Disturbed, 392

M

Maas, Meridean, 7
Malignant Hyperthermia Precautions, as intervention, 655
    for Hyperthermia, 243
Maternal Status: Intrapartum, as outcome, 631
    with Injury, Risk for, 562
Maternal Status: Postpartum, as outcome, 631
McCloskey, Joanne. See Dochterman, Joanne.
Mechanical Ventilation, as intervention, 655
    for Breathing Pattern, Ineffective, 81, 82
    for Gas Exchange, Impaired, 199
    for Ventilation, Impaired Spontaneous, 499
    for Ventilatory Weaning Response, Dysfunctional, 504, 505
Mechanical Ventilation Response: Adult, as outcome, 631
    with Breathing Pattern, Ineffective, 81
    with Gas Exchange, Impaired, 199
    with Ventilation, Impaired Spontaneous, 499
Mechanical Ventilation Weaning Response: Adult, as outcome, 631
    with Breathing Pattern, Ineffective, 82
    with Ventilatory Weaning Response, Dysfunctional, 504
Mechanical Ventilatory Weaning, as intervention, 655
    for Breathing Pattern, Ineffective, 82
    for Ventilatory Weaning Response, Dysfunctional, 504, 505
Medication Administration, as intervention, 655
    for Skin Integrity, Impaired, 401
Medication Administration: Ear, as intervention, 655
Medication Administration: Enteral, as intervention, 655
Medication Administration: Eye, as intervention, 656
Medication Administration: Inhalation, as intervention, 656
Medication Administration: Interpleural, as intervention, 656
Medication Administration: Intradermal, as intervention, 656
Medication Administration: Intramuscular (IM), as intervention, 656
    for Ventilation, Impaired Spontaneous, 499
Medication Administration: Intraosseous, as intervention, 656
Medication Administration: Intraspinal, as intervention, 656
Medication Administration: Intravenous (IV), as intervention, 656
    for Ventilation, Impaired Spontaneous, 499
Medication Administration: Nasal, as intervention, 656
Medication Administration: Oral, as intervention, 656
Medication Administration: Rectal, as intervention, 656
Medication Administration: Skin, as intervention, 656
Medication Administration: Subcutaneous, as intervention, 656
Medication Administration: Vaginal, as intervention, 656
Medication Administration: Ventricular Reservoir, as intervention, 656
Medication Management, as intervention, 656
    for Nausea, 286, 287
    for Pain, Acute, 303, 304
    for Pain, Chronic, 306, 308
    for Sleep Deprivation, 405
Medication Prescribing, as intervention, 656
Medication Response, as outcome, 631
    with Therapeutic Regimen Management, Ineffective, 445
Meditation Facilitation, as intervention, 656
Memory, as outcome, 631
    with Confusion, Chronic, 115
    with Environmental Interpretation Syndrome, Impaired, 152
    with Memory, Impaired, 276
    with Thought Processes, Disturbed, 457
Memory, Impaired, 275-276
Memory Training, as intervention, 656
    for Communication, Impaired Verbal, 99
    for Confusion, Chronic, 115
    for Environmental Interpretation Syndrome, Impaired, 152
    for Memory, Impaired, 275, 276
    for Thought Processes, Disturbed, 457
Milieu Therapy, as intervention, 656
Mobility, as outcome, 631
    with Disuse Syndrome, Risk for, 539
    with Mobility: Bed, Impaired, 279
    with Mobility: Physical, Impaired, 282
    with Mobility: Wheelchair, Impaired, 285
    with Transfer Ability, Impaired, 485
    with Walking, Impaired, 509
Mobility: Bed, Impaired, 277-279
Mobility: Physical, Impaired, 280-283
Mobility: Wheelchair, Impaired, 284-285
Mood Equilibrium, as outcome, 632
    with Hopelessness, 240
    with Sleep Deprivation, 405
    with Social Isolation, 417
    with Sorrow: Chronic, 422
    with Suicide, Risk for, 605
Mood Management, as intervention, 656
    for Activity Intolerance, 55
    for Fatigue, 185
    for Hopelessness, 239, 240, 241
    for Pain, Chronic, 306, 307
    for Post-Trauma Syndrome, 334
    for Post-Trauma Syndrome, Risk for, 586

Mood Management, as intervention *(Continued)*
  for Powerlessness, 337
  for Relocation Stress Syndrome, 360
  for Role Performance, Ineffective, 365
  for Self-Esteem: Chronic Low, 375
  for Sleep Deprivation, 405
  for Social Isolation, 417
  for Sorrow: Chronic, 420, 421, 422
  for Suicide, Risk for, 605
Motivation, as outcome, 632
  with Adjustment, Impaired, 59
  with Diversional Activity Deficit, 147
  with Noncompliance, 292
Multidisciplinary Care Conference, as intervention, 657
Music Therapy, as intervention, 657
Mutual Goal Setting, as intervention, 657
  for Adjustment, Impaired, 58
  for Decisional Conflict, 139
  for Noncompliance, 291
  for Powerlessness, 338
  for Therapeutic Regimen Management, Effective, 436
  for Therapeutic Regimen Management, Ineffective, 442
  for Therapeutic Regimen Management, Readiness for Enhanced, 450

N

Nail Care, as intervention, 657
NANDA International
  diagnoses developed by, 3. *See also* Nursing diagnoses, NANDA.
  overview of, 4
  publications of, 4
Web address of, 4
Nausea, 286-288
Nausea and Vomiting: Disruptive Effects, as outcome, 632
  with Nausea, 287
Nausea and Vomiting Control, as outcome, 632
  with Nausea, 287
Nausea and Vomiting Severity, as outcome, 632
  with Nausea, 288
  with Surgical Recovery, Delayed, 430
Nausea Management, as intervention, 657
  for Nausea, 286, 287, 288
  for Sensory Perception: Gustatory, Disturbed, 384, 385
  for Surgical Recovery, Delayed, 430
Neglect Cessation, as outcome, 632
Neglect Recovery, as outcome, 632
  with Self-Esteem: Situational Low, Risk for, 592
Neurologic Monitoring, as intervention, 657
  for Autonomic Dysreflexia, Risk for, 516
  for Cardiac Output, Decreased, 88
  for Confusion, Acute, 112
  for Confusion, Chronic, 116
  for Environmental Interpretation Syndrome, Impaired, 152
  for Infant Behavior, Disorganized, 246, 247
  for Intracranial Adaptive Capacity, Decreased, 254, 255
  for Memory, Impaired, 276
  for Sensory Perception: Auditory, Disturbed, 383
  for Sensory Perception: Kinesthetic, Disturbed, 387
  for Sensory Perception: Olfactory, Disturbed, 389
  for Sensory Perception: Visual, Disturbed, 389
  for Thought Processes, Disturbed, 458
  for Tissue Perfusion: Cerebral, Ineffective, 467, 468, 469
  for Tissue Perfusion: Peripheral, Ineffective, 476
Neurological Status, as outcome, 632
  with Autonomic Dysreflexia, 65
  with Infant Behavior, Disorganized, 247

Neurological Status, as outcome *(Continued)*
  with Intracranial Adaptive Capacity, Decreased, 254
  with Memory, Impaired, 276
  with Tissue Perfusion: Cerebral, Ineffective, 468
Neurological Status: Autonomic, as outcome, 632
  with Autonomic Dysreflexia, 65
  with Autonomic Dysreflexia, Risk for, 516
  with Urinary Incontinence: Reflex, 493
Neurological Status: Central Motor Control, as outcome, 632
  with Sensory Perception: Kinesthetic, Disturbed, 387
Neurological Status: Consciousness, as outcome, 632
  with Confusion, Acute, 112
  with Confusion, Chronic, 116
  with Environmental Interpretation Syndrome, Impaired, 152
  with Intracranial Adaptive Capacity, Decreased, 255
  with Thought Processes, Disturbed, 458
  with Tissue Perfusion: Cerebral, Ineffective, 469
Neurological Status: Cranial Sensory/Motor Function, as outcome, 632
  with Sensory Perception: Auditory, Disturbed, 383
  with Sensory Perception: Olfactory, Disturbed, 389
  with Sensory Perception: Visual, Disturbed, 393
Neurological Status: Spinal Sensory/Motor Function, as outcome, 632
  with Perioperative Positioning Injury, Risk for, 579
  with Peripheral Neurovascular Dysfunction, Risk for, 581
  with Sensory Perception: Tactile, Disturbed, 391
Newborn Adaptation, as outcome, 632
  with Infant Behavior: Organized, Readiness for Enhanced, 250
Newborn Care, as intervention, 657
  for Body Temperature, Risk for Imbalanced, 518
  for Development, Risk for Delayed, 525
  for Growth and Development, Delayed, 209
  for Hyperthermia, 243
  for Hypothermia, 245
  for Infant Behavior, Disorganized, 246, 248
  for Infant Behavior: Organized, Readiness for Enhanced, 249, 250
  for Infant Behavior, Risk for Disorganized, 555, 556
  for Parenting, Impaired, 316
  for Thermoregulation, Ineffective, 453
Newborn Monitoring, as intervention, 657
NIC. *See* Nursing Interventions Classification.
NOC. *See* Nursing Outcomes Classification.
Noncompliance, 289-293
Nonnutritive Sucking, as intervention, 657
  for Infant Feeding Pattern, Ineffective, 253
Normalization Promotion, as intervention, 657
  for Family Coping, Compromised, 159
  for Family Coping, Disabled, 163
  for Family Coping, Readiness for Enhanced, 165
  for Family Processes, Interrupted, 173
  for Family Therapeutic Regimen Management, Ineffective, 181
North American Nursing Diagnosis Association. *See* NANDA International.
Nursing diagnoses, NANDA
  actual and potential, 4
  components of, 4
  definition of, 4
  determining, 21-22
  as entry points for linkages, 14, 22
  example of, 5t
  for group of patients, 22
  and intervention selection, 22-23
  nursing interventions linked to, 4-7
  nursing outcomes linked to, 7-10
  and outcome selection, 22

Nursing diagnoses, NANDA *(Continued)*
 references on, 10-11
 term rearrangement in, for alphabetical ordering,
  14-15
Nursing intervention(s)
 components of, 4, 6
 definition(s) of, 4, 639-670
 direct and indirect, 4
 example of, 6t
 interdisciplinary use of, 7
 labels of, 639-670
 and linkage to NANDA diagnoses, 7
 selecting, 22-23
Nursing Interventions Classification (NIC), 3, 4-7
 development of, 4
 publications of, 7
 references on, 10-11
Nursing language. *See* Standardized nursing
  language(s).
Nursing outcome(s)
 components of, 7, 9
 correlated with nursing care, 9
 definition(s) of, 7, 621-638
 example of, 8t-9t
 labels of, 621-638
 linkage of, 9
 selecting, 22
Nursing Outcomes Classification (NOC), 3, 7-10
 development of, 3, 7, 9
 publications of, 9
 references on, 10-11
Nutrition: Imbalanced, Less than Body Requirements,
  294-298
Nutrition: Imbalanced, More than Body
  Requirements, 299-300
Nutrition: Imbalanced, Risk for More than Body
  Requirements, 570-571
Nutrition, Readiness for Enhanced, 301
Nutrition Management, as intervention, 657
 for Caregiver Role Strain, 94
 for Failure to Thrive, Adult, 153
 for Fatigue, 184
 for Fluid Volume, Deficient, 192
 for Growth, Risk for Disproportionate, 552, 553, 554
 for Growth and Development, Delayed, 218
 for Nutrition: Imbalanced, Less than Body
   Requirements, 295, 297
 for Nutrition: Imbalanced, More than Body
   Requirements, 299
 for Nutrition: Imbalanced, Risk for More than Body
   Requirements, 570, 571
 for Nutrition, Readiness for Enhanced, 301
 for Self-Care Deficit: Feeding, 370
 for Sensory Perception: Gustatory, Disturbed, 384,
   385
 for Sensory Perception: Olfactory, Disturbed, 389,
   390
 for Surgical Recovery, Delayed, 432
Nutrition Therapy, as intervention, 657
 for Failure to Thrive, Adult, 153
 for Growth and Development, Delayed, 218
 for Nutrition: Imbalanced, Less than Body
   Requirements, 294
 for Protection, Ineffective, 344
Nutritional Counseling, as intervention, 657
 for Nutrition: Imbalanced, More than Body
   Requirements, 299
 for Nutrition, Readiness for Enhanced, 301
 for Protection, Ineffective, 344
 for Self-Care Deficit: Feeding, 370
Nutritional Monitoring, as intervention, 657
 for Failure to Thrive, Adult, 153, 154
 for Fluid Volume, Deficient, 192

Nutritional Monitoring, as intervention *(Continued)*
 for Fluid Volume, Risk for Deficient, 544
 for Growth, Risk for Disproportionate, 551, 552, 554
 for Growth and Development, Delayed, 209
 for Nausea, 286, 288
 for Nutrition: Imbalanced, Less than Body
   Requirements, 294, 297
 for Nutrition: Imbalanced, More than Body
   Requirements, 299
 for Nutrition: Imbalanced, Risk for More than Body
   Requirements, 570
 for Self-Care Deficit: Feeding, 370
 for Sensory Perception: Gustatory, Disturbed, 384
Nutritional Status, as outcome, 632
 with Failure to Thrive, Adult, 153
 with Nutrition: Imbalanced, Less than Body
   Requirements, 295
 with Nutrition: Imbalanced, More than Body
   Requirements, 299
 with Nutrition, Readiness for Enhanced, 301
 with Protection, Ineffective, 344
 with Self-Care Deficit: Feeding, 370
Nutritional Status: Biochemical Measures, as outcome,
  632
 with Nutrition: Imbalanced, Less than Body
   Requirements, 296
Nutritional Status: Energy, as outcome, 632
 with Fatigue, 184
Nutritional Status: Food and Fluid Intake, as outcome,
  632
 with Failure to Thrive, Adult, 154
 with Fluid Volume, Deficient, 192
 with Fluid Volume, Risk for Deficient, 544
 with Infant Feeding Pattern, Ineffective, 253
 with Nausea, 288
 with Nutrition: Imbalanced, Less than Body
   Requirements, 297
 with Nutrition: Imbalanced, More than Body
   Requirements, 299
 with Nutrition: Imbalanced, Risk for More than
   Body Requirements, 570
 with Self-Care Deficit: Feeding, 370
 with Sensory Perception: Gustatory, Disturbed, 384
 with Sensory Perception: Olfactory, Disturbed, 389
Nutritional Status: Nutrient Intake, as outcome, 632
 with Nutrition: Imbalanced, Less than Body
   Requirements, 297
 with Nutrition: Imbalanced, More than Body
   Requirements, 299
 with Nutrition: Imbalanced, Risk for More than
   Body Requirements, 570
 with Nutrition, Readiness for Enhanced, 301

O

Oral Health Maintenance, as intervention, 657
 for Dentition, Impaired, 143
 for Self-Care Deficit: Bathing/Hygiene, 368
 for Tissue Integrity, Impaired, 460
Oral Health Promotion, as intervention, 657
Oral Health Restoration, as intervention, 657
 for Dentition, Impaired, 143
 for Oral Mucous Membrane, Impaired, 302
Oral Hygiene, as outcome, 632
 with Dentition, Impaired, 143
 with Oral Mucous Membrane, Impaired, 302
Oral Mucous Membrane, Impaired, 302
Order Transcription, as intervention, 658
Organ Procurement, as intervention, 658
Ostomy Care, as intervention, 658
 for Diarrhea, 146
 for Knowledge, Deficient (Specify), 264

Ostomy Care, as intervention (*Continued*)
　　for Self-Care Deficit: Bathing/Hygiene, 367
　　for Self-Care Deficit: Toileting, 372
　　for Tissue Integrity, Impaired, 459
Ostomy Self-Care, as outcome, 633
　with Diarrhea, 146
　with Self-Care Deficit: Bathing/Hygiene, 367
　with Self-Care Deficit: Toileting, 372
　with Tissue Integrity, Impaired, 459
Outcome. *See* Nursing outcome(s).
Outcome-Present State Test (OPT) model, 25
Oxygen Therapy, as intervention, 658
　for Gas Exchange, Impaired, 199
　for Tissue Perfusion: Cardiopulmonary, Ineffective,
　　463
　for Ventilation, Impaired Spontaneous, 499, 500

P

Pain, Acute, 303-305
Pain: Adverse Psychological Response, as outcome,
　633
　with Pain, Chronic, 307
Pain, Chronic, 306-310
Pain: Disruptive Effects, as outcome, 633
　with Pain, Chronic, 309
Pain Control, as outcome, 633
　with Pain, Acute, 304
　with Pain, Chronic, 308
Pain Level, as outcome, 633
　with Energy Field, Disturbed, 149
　with Pain, Acute, 305
　with Pain, Chronic, 310
　with Surgical Recovery, Delayed, 430
Pain Management, as intervention, 658
　for Death Anxiety, 136
　for Energy Field, Disturbed, 149
　for Pain, Acute, 303, 304, 305
　for Pain, Chronic, 306, 307, 308, 310
　for Surgical Recovery, Delayed, 430, 431
Parent Education: Adolescent, as intervention, 658
　for Body Image, Disturbed, 71
　for Development, Risk for Delayed, 534
　for Family Processes, Interrupted, 176
　for Home Maintenance, Impaired, 238
　for Knowledge, Deficient (Specify), 265
　for Parenting, Impaired, 326
　for Parenting, Readiness for Enhanced, 329
　for Parenting, Risk for Impaired, 575
Parent Education: Childrearing Family, as
　　intervention, 658
　for Body Image, Disturbed, 68, 69, 70
　for Caregiver Role Strain, Risk for, 523
　for Family Processes, Interrupted, 176
　for Growth and Development, Delayed, 212, 213,
　　214
　for Home Maintenance, Impaired, 238
　for Knowledge, Deficient (Specify), 265
　for Parenting, Impaired, 322, 326
　for Parenting, Readiness for Enhanced, 329
　for Parenting, Risk for Impaired, 575
Parent Education: Infant, as intervention, 658
　for Caregiver Role Strain, Risk for, 523
　for Development, Risk for Delayed, 526, 528
　for Family Processes, Interrupted, 176
　for Infant Behavior, Risk for Disorganized, 555
　for Knowledge, Deficient (Specify), 263, 265
　for Parent/Infant/Child Attachment, Risk for
　　Impaired, 572, 573
　for Parenting, Impaired, 317, 318, 326
　for Parenting, Readiness for Enhanced, 328, 329
　for Sudden Infant Death Syndrome, Risk for, 601

Parent-Infant Attachment, as outcome, 633
　with Breastfeeding, Interrupted, 80
　with Parent/Infant/Child Attachment, Risk for
　　Impaired, 572
　with Parenting, Impaired, 324
Parent/Infant/Child Attachment, Risk for Impaired,
　572-574
Parental Role Conflict, 311-315
Parenting: Adolescent Physical Safety, as outcome, 633
　with Parenting, Risk for Impaired, 575
Parenting: Early/Middle Childhood Physical Safety, as
　　outcome, 633
　with Parenting, Risk for Impaired, 575
Parenting, Impaired, 316-327
Parenting: Infant/Toddler Physical Safety, as outcome,
　633
　with Parenting, Risk for Impaired, 576
　with Sudden Infant Death Syndrome, Risk for, 601
Parenting: Psychosocial Safety, as outcome, 633
　with Home Maintenance, Impaired, 238
　with Parenting, Impaired, 326
　with Parenting, Readiness for Enhanced, 329
　with Parenting, Risk for Impaired, 577
Parenting, Readiness for Enhanced, 328-329
Parenting, Risk for Impaired, 575-578
Parenting Performance, as outcome, 633
　with Caregiver Role Strain, 96
　with Caregiver Role Strain, Risk for, 523
　with Family Processes, Dysfunctional: Alcoholism,
　　170
　with Family Processes, Interrupted, 176
　with Home Maintenance, Impaired, 237
　with Parent/Infant/Child Attachment, Risk for
　　Impaired, 573
　with Parental Role Conflict, 314
　with Parenting, Impaired, 325
　with Parenting, Readiness for Enhanced, 329
　with Parenting, Risk for Impaired, 576
　with Role Performance, Ineffective, 365
Parenting Promotion, as intervention, 658
　for Caregiver Role Strain, 96
　for Caregiver Role Strain, Risk for, 520, 523
　for Family Processes, Dysfunctional: Alcoholism,
　　170
　for Family Processes, Interrupted, 176
　for Growth and Development, Delayed, 209, 210,
　　211
　for Home Maintenance, Impaired, 237
　for Parent/Infant/Child Attachment, Risk for
　　Impaired, 573, 574
　for Parental Role Conflict, 314, 315
　for Parenting, Impaired, 317-323, 325
　for Parenting, Readiness for Enhanced, 329
　for Parenting, Risk for Impaired, 576, 578
　for Role Performance, Ineffective, 365
Participation in Health Care Decisions, as outcome,
　633
　with Decisional Conflict, 140
　with Family Coping, Readiness for Enhanced, 167
　with Health Maintenance, Ineffective, 223
　with Powerlessness, 340
　with Therapeutic Regimen Management, Effective,
　　438
　with Therapeutic Regimen Management,
　　Ineffective, 445
　with Therapeutic Regimen Management, Readiness
　　for Enhanced, 451
Pass Facilitation, as intervention, 658
Patient Contracting, as intervention, 658
　for Adjustment, Impaired, 58
　for Noncompliance, 291
　for Pain, Chronic, 307

Patient Contracting, as intervention *(Continued)*
  for Therapeutic Regimen Management, Effective,
    436
  for Therapeutic Regimen Management, Ineffective,
    442
Patient Controlled Analgesia (PCA) Assistance, as
    intervention, 658
  for Pain, Acute, 304
  for Pain, Chronic, 310
Patient Rights Protection, as intervention, 658
  for Powerlessness, 340
Peer Review, as intervention, 658
Pelvic Muscle Exercise, as intervention, 658
  for Urinary Incontinence: Stress, 495
Perineal Care, as intervention, 658
  for Bowel Incontinence, 73
  for Urinary Incontinence: Reflex, 493
Perioperative Positioning Injury, Risk for, 579-580
Peripheral Neurovascular Dysfunction, Risk for,
    581-582
Peripheral Sensation Management, as intervention,
    658
  for Peripheral Neurovascular Dysfunction, Risk for,
    581
  for Sensory Perception: Tactile, Disturbed, 391, 392
  for Tissue Perfusion: Peripheral, Ineffective, 476
Peripherally Inserted Central (PIC) Catheter Care, as
    intervention, 659
Peritoneal Dialysis Therapy, as intervention, 659
  for Therapeutic Regimen Management, Ineffective,
    448
  for Tissue Perfusion: Renal, Ineffective, 481, 482
Personal Autonomy, as outcome, 633
  with Decisional Conflict, 140
  with Powerlessness, 340
  with Powerlessness, Risk for, 588
  with Rape-Trauma Syndrome: Compound Reaction,
    351
  with Self-Concept, Readiness for Enhanced, 374
Personal Health Status, as outcome, 633
  with Health Maintenance, Ineffective, 224
  with Health-Seeking Behavior (Specify), 231
  with Relocation Stress Syndrome, Risk for, 590
Personal Identity, Disturbed, 330-331
Personal Safety Behavior, as outcome, 633
  with Injury, Risk for, 563
  with Poisoning, Risk for, 583
  with Trauma, Risk for, 608
Personal Well-Being, as outcome, 633
  with Coping, Readiness for Enhanced, 133
  with Energy Field, Disturbed, 150
  with Health-Seeking Behavior (Specify), 232
  with Religiosity, Readiness for Enhanced, 357
  with Sleep Pattern, Disturbed, 407
  with Social Isolation, 417
  with Spiritual Well-Being, Readiness for Enhanced,
    425
Pessary Management, as intervention, 659
Phlebotomy: Arterial Blood Sample, as intervention,
    659
Phlebotomy: Blood Unit Acquisition, as intervention,
    659
Phlebotomy: Cannulated Vessel, as intervention, 659
Phlebotomy: Venous Blood Sample, as intervention,
    659
Phototherapy: Mood/Sleep Regulation, as
    intervention, 659
Phototherapy: Neonate, as intervention, 659
Physical Aging, as outcome, 633
  with Failure to Thrive, Adult, 154
  with Growth and Development, Delayed, 219
  with Sexual Dysfunction, 396

Physical Fitness, as outcome, 633
  with Activity Intolerance, 55
  with Lifestyle, Sedentary, 274
Physical Injury Severity, as outcome, 633
  with Injury, Risk for, 564
  with Poisoning, Risk for, 583
  with Trauma, Risk for, 608
Physical Maturation: Female, as outcome, 633
  for Growth and Development, Delayed, 220
  for Sexuality Patterns, Ineffective, 399
Physical Maturation: Male, as outcome, 633
  for Growth and Development, Delayed, 220
  for Sexuality Patterns, Ineffective, 399
Physical Restraint, as intervention, 659
Physician Support, as intervention, 659
Play Participation, as outcome, 634
  with Diversional Activity Deficit, 148
  with Social Interaction, Impaired, 412
  with Social Isolation, 418
Pneumatic Tourniquet Precautions, as intervention,
    659
Poisoning, Risk for, 583
Positioning, as intervention, 659
  for Airway Clearance, Ineffective, 61
  for Infant Behavior, Risk for Disorganized, 556
  for Mobility: Bed, Impaired, 278
  for Swallowing, Impaired, 433
Positioning: Intraoperative, as intervention, 659
  for Perioperative Positioning Injury, Risk for, 579, 580
Positioning: Neurologic, as intervention, 659
  for Peripheral Neurovascular Dysfunction, Risk for,
    581
Positioning: Wheelchair, as intervention, 660
  for Mobility: Physical, Impaired, 280
  for Mobility: Wheelchair, Impaired, 284, 285
Post Procedure Recovery Status, as outcome, 634
  with Surgical Recovery, Delayed, 431
Post-Trauma Syndrome, 332-336
Post-Trauma Syndrome, Risk for, 584-586
Postanesthesia Care, as intervention, 660
Postmortem Care, as intervention, 660
Postpartal Care, as intervention, 660
Powerlessness, 337-340
Powerlessness, Risk for, 587-588
Preceptor: Employee, as intervention, 660
Preceptor: Student, as intervention, 660
Preconception Counseling, as intervention, 660
  for Health-Seeking Behavior (Specify), 233
  for Knowledge, Deficient (Specify), 266
Pregnancy Termination Care, as intervention, 660
Premenstrual Syndrome (PMS) Management, as
    intervention, 660
Prenatal Care, as intervention, 660
  for Health-Seeking Behavior (Specify), 233
Prenatal Health Behavior, as outcome, 634
  with Health-Seeking Behavior (Specify), 233
Preoperative Coordination, as intervention, 660
Preparatory Sensory Information, as intervention, 660
  for Knowledge, Deficient (Specify), 268
  for Ventilatory Weaning Response, Dysfunctional,
    503
Presence, as intervention, 660
  for Caregiver Role Strain, 92
  for Death Anxiety, 136
  for Fear, 186, 187
Pressure Management, as intervention, 660
  for Perioperative Positioning Injury, Risk for, 580
  for Skin Integrity, Impaired, 402
  for Skin Integrity, Risk for Impaired, 596, 597
  for Trauma, Risk for, 609
Pressure Ulcer Care, as intervention, 660
  for Skin Integrity, Impaired, 402, 404

Pressure Ulcer Prevention, as intervention, 660
  for Skin Integrity, Risk for Impaired, 597
  for Tissue Integrity, Impaired, 460
Preterm Infant Organization, as outcome, 634
  with Development, Risk for Delayed, 535
  with Infant Behavior, Disorganized, 247
  with Infant Behavior, Risk for Disorganized, 556
  with Sudden Infant Death Syndrome, Risk for, 601
Product Evaluation, as intervention, 660
Program Development, as intervention, 661
  for Community Coping, Ineffective, 103
  for Community Coping, Readiness for Enhanced,
    105, 106
  for Community Therapeutic Regimen Management,
    Ineffective, 108, 110
Progressive Muscle Relaxation, as intervention, 661
Prompted Voiding, as intervention, 661
  for Urinary Incontinence: Functional, 492
Prosthesis Care, as intervention, 661
Protection, Ineffective, 341-344
Pruritus Management, as intervention, 661
  for Skin Integrity, Impaired, 401
Psychomotor Energy, as outcome, 634
  with Activity Intolerance, 55
  with Fatigue, 185
  with Hopelessness, 241
Psychosocial Adjustment: Life Change, as outcome,
    634
  with Adjustment, Impaired, 60
  with Body Image, Disturbed, 72
  with Coping, Ineffective, 129
  with Grieving, Anticipatory, 205
  with Grieving, Dysfunctional, 208
  with Parental Role Conflict, 315
  with Relocation Stress Syndrome, 362
  with Relocation Stress Syndrome, Risk for, 591
  with Role Performance, Ineffective, 366
  with Self-Esteem: Situational Low, 378
  with Sorrow: Chronic, 422

Q

Quality Monitoring, as intervention, 661
Quality of Life, as outcome, 634
  with Hopelessness, 241
  with Relocation Stress Syndrome, 362
  with Self-Esteem: Chronic Low, 375
  with Spiritual Well-Being, Readiness for Enhanced,
    426

R

Radiation Therapy Management, as intervention, 661
Rape-Trauma Syndrome, 345-347
Rape-Trauma Syndrome: Compound Reaction, 348-
    352
Rape-Trauma Syndrome: Silent Reaction, 353-355
Rape-Trauma Treatment, as intervention, 661
  for Post-Trauma Syndrome, 333
  for Rape-Trauma Syndrome, 345, 346, 347
  for Rape-Trauma Syndrome: Compound Reaction,
    349, 351, 352
  for Rape-Trauma Syndrome: Silent Reaction, 353,
    354
Reality Orientation, as intervention, 661
  for Confusion, Acute, 111
  for Confusion, Chronic, 113, 115, 116
  for Environmental Interpretation Syndrome,
    Impaired, 151
  for Memory, Impaired, 275
  for Sensory Perception: Auditory, Disturbed, 381
  for Thought Processes, Disturbed, 454

Recreation Therapy, as intervention, 661
  for Diversional Activity Deficit, 147
  for Social Interaction, Impaired, 412
  for Social Isolation, 415
Rectal Prolapse Management, as intervention, 661
Referral, as intervention, 661
  for Self-Care Deficit: Feeding, 371
Religiosity, Impaired, 356
Religiosity, Impaired, Risk for, 589
Religiosity, Readiness for Enhanced, 357
Religious Addiction Prevention, as intervention, 661
Religious Ritual Enhancement, as intervention, 661
  for Death Anxiety, 138
  for Religiosity, Readiness for Enhanced, 357
Relocation Stress Reduction, as intervention, 661
  for Relocation Stress Syndrome, 358, 360, 361, 362,
    363
  for Relocation Stress Syndrome, Risk for, 590, 591
Relocation Stress Syndrome, 358-363
Relocation Stress Syndrome, Risk for, 590-591
Reminiscence Therapy, as intervention, 661
Reproductive Technology Management, as
    intervention, 661
  for Knowledge, Deficient (Specify), 260
Research, nursing, linkage use in, 25-26
Research Data Collection, as intervention, 661
Resiliency Promotion, as intervention, 662
  for Coping, Readiness for Enhanced, 133
  for Family Processes, Dysfunctional: Alcoholism,
    169
  for Family Processes, Interrupted, 174
  for Family Processes, Readiness for Enhanced, 179
  for Family Therapeutic Regimen Management,
    Ineffective, 182
  for Grieving, Dysfunctional, 207
  for Hopelessness, 239
Respiratory Monitoring, as intervention, 662
  for Airway Clearance, Ineffective, 61
  for Aspiration, Risk for, 514
  for Breathing Pattern, Ineffective, 83
  for Gas Exchange, Impaired, 200, 202
  for Latex Allergy Response, 271
  for Suffocation, Risk for, 602, 604
  for Tissue Perfusion: Cardiopulmonary, Ineffective,
    463
  for Ventilation, Impaired Spontaneous, 500, 501, 502
  for Ventilatory Weaning Response, Dysfunctional,
    505, 506
Respiratory Status: Airway Patency, as outcome, 634
  with Airway Clearance, Ineffective, 61
  with Breathing Pattern, Ineffective, 82
Respiratory Status: Gas Exchange, as outcome, 634
  with Gas Exchange, Impaired, 199
  with Tissue Perfusion: Cardiopulmonary,
    Ineffective, 463
  with Ventilation, Impaired Spontaneous, 500
  with Ventilatory Weaning Response, Dysfunctional,
    505
Respiratory Status: Ventilation, as outcome, 634
  with Airway Clearance, Ineffective, 61
  with Aspiration, Risk for, 514
  with Breathing Pattern, Ineffective, 83
  with Gas Exchange, Impaired, 200
  with Suffocation, Risk for, 604
  with Ventilation, Impaired Spontaneous, 501
  with Ventilatory Weaning Response, Dysfunctional,
    505
Respite Care, as intervention, 662
  for Caregiver Role Strain, 91, 92, 95
  for Caregiver Role Strain, Risk for, 519, 521
  for Family Coping, Compromised, 156, 158
  for Family Coping, Disabled, 162
  for Family Coping, Readiness for Enhanced, 164

Rest, as outcome, 634
  with Sleep, Readiness for Enhanced, 408
  with Sleep Deprivation, 405
Resuscitation, as intervention, 662
Resuscitation: Fetus, as intervention, 662
Resuscitation: Neonate, as intervention, 662
Risk Control, as outcome, 634
  with Injury, Risk for, 565
  with Therapeutic Regimen Management, Effective,
    438
  with Therapeutic Regimen Management, Readiness
    for Enhanced, 452
Risk Control: Alcohol Use, as outcome, 634
  with Coping, Ineffective, 130
  with Health-Seeking Behavior (Specify), 234
Risk Control: Cancer, as outcome, 634
  with Health-Seeking Behavior (Specify), 234
Risk Control: Cardiovascular Health, as outcome, 634
  with Health-Seeking Behavior (Specify), 234
Risk Control: Drug Use, as outcome, 634
  with Coping, Ineffective, 130
  with Health-Seeking Behavior (Specify), 235
Risk Control: Hearing Impairment, as outcome, 634
  with Health-Seeking Behavior (Specify), 235
Risk Control: Sexually Transmitted Disease (STD), as
    outcome, 634
  with Health-Seeking Behavior (Specify), 235
  with Infection, Risk for, 559
  with Sexual Dysfunction, 396
Risk Control: Tobacco Use, as outcome, 634
  with Health-Seeking Behavior (Specify), 236
Risk Control: Unintended Pregnancy, as outcome, 635
  with Health-Seeking Behavior (Specify), 236
Risk Control: Visual Impairment, as outcome, 635
  with Health-Seeking Behavior (Specify), 236
Risk Detection, as outcome, 635
  with Health Maintenance, Ineffective, 224
Risk Identification, as intervention, 662
  for Body Image, Disturbed, 70, 71
  for Development, Risk for Delayed, 529, 530, 531,
    532, 533, 534
  for Failure to Thrive, Adult, 154
  for Falls, Risk for, 541
  for Growth and Development, Delayed, 217, 219
  for Health Maintenance, Ineffective, 224
  for Health-Seeking Behavior (Specify), 232, 235, 236
  for Infant Behavior, Risk for Disorganized, 555, 556
  for Injury, Risk for, 565
  for Knowledge, Deficient (Specify), 263
  for Protection, Ineffective, 343, 344
  for Sexual Dysfunction, 396
  for Therapeutic Regimen Management, Effective,
    438
  for Therapeutic Regimen Management, Readiness
    for Enhanced, 452
Risk Identification: Childbearing Family, as
    intervention, 662
  for Health Maintenance, Ineffective, 224
  for Home Maintenance, Impaired, 238
  for Parenting, Impaired, 326
Risk Identification: Genetic, as intervention, 662
Role Enhancement, as intervention, 662
  for Caregiver Role Strain, 92, 93, 96, 97
  for Coping, Ineffective, 131
  for Coping, Readiness for Enhanced, 134
  for Family Processes, Dysfunctional: Alcoholism,
    170
  for Grieving, Dysfunctional, 208
  for Home Maintenance, Impaired, 238
  for Parent/Infant/Child Attachment, Risk for
    Impaired, 574
  for Parental Role Conflict, 312, 315
  for Parenting, Impaired, 326

Risk Identification: Childbearing Family *(Continued)*
  for Parenting, Risk for Impaired, 578
  for Role Performance, Ineffective, 364, 365
  for Sexuality Patterns, Ineffective, 399
Role Performance, as outcome, 635
  with Caregiver Role Strain, 97
  with Coping, Ineffective, 131
  with Coping, Readiness for Enhanced, 134
  with Family Processes, Dysfunctional: Alcoholism,
    170
  with Grieving, Dysfunctional, 208
  with Home Maintenance, Impaired, 238
  with Parent/Infant/Child Attachment, Risk for
    Impaired, 574
  with Parental Role Conflict, 315
  with Parenting, Impaired, 326
  with Parenting, Risk for Impaired, 578
  with Role Performance, Ineffective, 366
  with Sexuality Patterns, Ineffective, 399
Role Performance, Ineffective, 364-366

S

Safe Home Environment, as outcome, 635
  with Environmental Interpretation Syndrome,
    Impaired, 152
  with Home Maintenance, Impaired, 238
  with Injury, Risk for, 565
  with Parenting, Impaired, 327
  with Poisoning, Risk for, 583
  with Wandering, 510
Seclusion, as intervention, 662
Security Enhancement, as intervention, 662
  for Denial, Ineffective, 142
  for Fear, 187, 188
  for Post-Trauma Syndrome, 334
  for Relocation Stress Syndrome, 359
Sedation Management, as intervention, 662
  for Pain, Acute, 305
Seizure Control, as outcome, 635
  with Intracranial Adaptive Capacity, Decreased, 255
Seizure Management, as intervention, 662
  for Intracranial Adaptive Capacity, Decreased, 255
Seizure Precautions, as intervention, 662
  for Intracranial Adaptive Capacity, Decreased, 255
Self-Awareness Enhancement, as intervention, 663
  for Coping, Defensive, 120
  for Coping, Readiness for Enhanced, 133
  for Denial, Ineffective, 142
  for Energy Field, Disturbed, 150
  for Grieving, Dysfunctional, 208
  for Health-Seeking Behavior (Specify), 228, 232
  for Personal Identity, Disturbed, 330
  for Powerlessness, Risk for, 587
  for Self-Concept, Readiness for Enhanced, 374
  for Self-Mutilation, 379
  for Sexual Dysfunction, 397
  for Social Isolation, 417
  for Spiritual Well-Being, Readiness for Enhanced,
    425
  for Thought Processes, Disturbed, 456
Self-Care: Activities of Daily Living (ADL), as
    outcome, 635
  with Activity Intolerance, 56
  with Failure to Thrive, Adult, 155
  with Self-Care Deficit: Bathing/Hygiene, 367
  with Self-Care Deficit: Dressing/Grooming, 369
  with Self-Care Deficit: Feeding, 370
  with Self-Care Deficit: Toileting, 373
  with Surgical Recovery, Delayed, 431
Self-Care: Bathing, as outcome, 635
  with Self-Care Deficit: Bathing/Hygiene, 367

Self-Care: Dressing, as outcome, 635
  with Self-Care Deficit: Dressing/Grooming, 369
Self-Care: Eating, as outcome, 635
  with Nutrition: Imbalanced, Less than Body
    Requirements, 298
  with Self-Care Deficit: Feeding, 371
Self-Care: Hygiene, as outcome, 635
  with Self-Care Deficit: Bathing/Hygiene, 368
  with Self-Care Deficit: Dressing/Grooming, 369
  with Self-Care Deficit: Toileting, 373
Self-Care: Instrumental Activities of Daily Living
    (IADL), as outcome, 635
  with Activity Intolerance, 56
Self-Care: Non-Parenteral Medication, as outcome, 635
  with Therapeutic Regimen Management,
    Ineffective, 446
Self-Care: Oral Hygiene, as outcome, 635
  with Dentition, Impaired, 143
  with Self-Care Deficit: Bathing/Hygiene, 368
Self-Care: Parenteral Medication, as outcome, 635
  with Therapeutic Regimen Management,
    Ineffective, 447
Self-Care: Toileting, as outcome, 635
  with Constipation, Risk for, 524
  with Self-Care Deficit: Toileting, 373
  with Urinary Incontinence: Functional, 492
Self-Care Assistance, as intervention, 663
  for Activity Intolerance, 56
  for Failure to Thrive, Adult, 155
  for Health Maintenance, Ineffective, 225
  for Mobility: Bed, Impaired, 277
  for Surgical Recovery, Delayed, 431
  for Therapeutic Regimen Management, Ineffective,
    446
  for Unilateral Neglect, 487, 488
Self-Care Assistance: Bathing/Hygiene, as
    intervention, 663
  for Self-Care Deficit: Bathing/Hygiene, 367, 368
  for Self-Care Deficit: Toileting, 373
Self-Care Assistance: Dressing/Grooming, as
    intervention, 663
  for Self-Care Deficit: Dressing/Grooming, 369
Self-Care Assistance: Feeding, as intervention, 663
  for Nutrition: Imbalanced, Less than Body
    Requirements, 298
  for Self-Care Deficit: Feeding, 370, 371
Self-Care Assistance: Instrumental Activities of Daily
    Living (IADL), as intervention, 663
  for Activity Intolerance, 56
  for Health Maintenance, Ineffective, 225
Self-Care Assistance: Toileting, as intervention, 663
  for Constipation, Risk for, 524
  for Self-Care Deficit: Toileting, 373
  for Urinary Incontinence: Functional, 492
  for Urinary Incontinence: Urge, 497
Self-Care Assistance: Transfer, as intervention, 663
  for Mobility: Physical, Impaired, 283
  for Mobility: Wheelchair, Impaired, 285
  for Transfer Ability, Impaired, 486
Self-Care Deficit: Bathing/Hygiene, 367-368
Self-Care Deficit: Dressing/Grooming, 369
Self-Care Deficit: Feeding, 370-371
Self-Care Deficit: Toileting, 372-373
Self-Care Status, as outcome, 635
  with Health Maintenance, Ineffective, 225
Self-Concept, Readiness for Enhanced, 374
Self-Direction of Care, as outcome, 636
  with Health Maintenance, Ineffective, 225
Self-Esteem, as outcome, 636
  with Body Image, Disturbed, 72
  with Coping, Defensive, 122
  with Rape-Trauma Syndrome: Compound Reaction,
    352

Self-Esteem, as outcome *(Continued)*
  with Self-Concept, Readiness for Enhanced, 374
  with Self-Esteem: Chronic Low, 376
  with Self-Esteem: Situational Low, 378
  with Self-Esteem: Situational Low, Risk for, 593
  with Sexuality Patterns, Ineffective, 400
Self-Esteem: Chronic Low, 375-376
Self-Esteem: Situational Low, 377-378
Self-Esteem: Situational Low, Risk for, 592-593
Self-Esteem Enhancement, as intervention, 663
  for Body Image, Disturbed, 67, 71, 72
  for Coping, Defensive, 121, 122
  for Coping, Ineffective, 124
  for Personal Identity, Disturbed, 330
  for Powerlessness, 337, 338
  for Powerlessness, Risk for, 587, 588
  for Rape-Trauma Syndrome: Compound Reaction,
    352
  for Self-Concept, Readiness for Enhanced, 374
  for Self-Esteem: Chronic Low, 375, 376
  for Self-Esteem: Situational Low, 377, 378
  for Self-Esteem: Situational Low, Risk for, 592, 593
  for Sexuality Patterns, Ineffective, 398, 400
  for Social Interaction, Impaired, 411
  for Spiritual Well-Being, Readiness for Enhanced, 425
  for Thought Processes, Disturbed, 456
Self-Hypnosis Facilitation, as intervention, 663
Self-Modification Assistance, as intervention, 663
  for Adjustment, Impaired, 59
  for Denial, Ineffective, 142
  for Family Coping, Readiness for Enhanced, 166
  for Health Maintenance, Ineffective, 221
  for Health-Seeking Behavior (Specify), 228, 229
  for Hopelessness, 239
  for Noncompliance, 289, 292
  for Protection, Ineffective, 342
  for Therapeutic Regimen Management, Effective,
    438, 439
  for Therapeutic Regimen Management, Ineffective,
    442, 447
  for Therapeutic Regimen Management, Readiness
    for Enhanced, 450, 452
Self-Mutilation, 379-380
Self-Mutilation, Risk for, 594-595
Self-Mutilation Restraint, as outcome, 636
  with Personal Identity, Disturbed, 331
  with Post-Trauma Syndrome, 336
  with Self-Mutilation, 380
  with Self-Mutilation, Risk for, 595
  with Violence: Self-Directed, Risk for, 616
Self-Responsibility Facilitation, as intervention, 663
  for Adjustment, Impaired, 59
  for Coping, Defensive, 121
  for Denial, Ineffective, 142
  for Diversional Activity Deficit, 147
  for Family Processes, Dysfunctional: Alcoholism,
    170
  for Growth and Development, Delayed, 217
  for Health Maintenance, Ineffective, 221, 225, 227
  for Health-Seeking Behavior (Specify), 236
  for Noncompliance, 289, 292, 293
  for Pain, Chronic, 308
  for Powerlessness, 338, 340
  for Powerlessness, Risk for, 587
  for Therapeutic Regimen Management, Ineffective,
    449
Sensory Function: Cutaneous, as outcome, 636
  with Autonomic Dysreflexia, 66
  with Sensory Perception: Tactile, Disturbed, 392
  with Tissue Perfusion: Peripheral, Ineffective, 476
Sensory Function: Hearing, as outcome, 636
  with Sensory Perception: Auditory, Disturbed, 383

Sensory Function: Proprioception, as outcome, 636
  with Sensory Perception: Kinesthetic, Disturbed, 388
Sensory Function: Taste and Smell, as outcome, 636
  with Sensory Perception: Gustatory, Disturbed, 385
  with Sensory Perception: Olfactory, Disturbed, 390
Sensory Function: Vision, as outcome, 636
  with Sensory Perception: Visual, Disturbed, 394
Sensory Function Status, as outcome, 636
  with Injury, Risk for, 566
Sensory Perception: Auditory, Disturbed, 381-383
Sensory Perception: Gustatory, Disturbed, 384-385
Sensory Perception: Kinesthetic, Disturbed, 386-388
Sensory Perception: Olfactory, Disturbed, 389-390
Sensory Perception: Tactile, Disturbed, 391-392
Sensory Perception: Visual, Disturbed, 393-394
Sexual Counseling, as intervention, 663
  for Rape-Trauma Syndrome, 347
  for Rape-Trauma Syndrome: Compound Reaction, 352
  for Rape-Trauma Syndrome: Silent Reaction, 354, 355
  for Sexual Dysfunction, 395, 396, 397
  for Sexuality Patterns, Ineffective, 398, 400
Sexual Dysfunction, 395-397
Sexual Functioning, as outcome, 636
  with Rape-Trauma Syndrome, 347
  with Rape-Trauma Syndrome: Compound Reaction, 352
  with Rape-Trauma Syndrome: Silent Reaction, 355
  with Sexual Dysfunction, 397
Sexual Identity, as outcome, 636
  with Sexual Dysfunction, 397
  with Sexuality Patterns, Ineffective, 400
Sexuality Patterns, Ineffective, 398-400
Shift Report, as intervention, 663
Shock Management: Cardiac, as intervention, 663
  for Cardiac Output, Decreased, 85, 88
  for Tissue Perfusion: Cardiopulmonary, Ineffective, 462, 464
Shock Management: Vasogenic, as intervention, 663
Shock Management: Volume, as intervention, 663
  for Cardiac Output, Decreased, 84
Shock Prevention, as intervention, 664
Sibling Support, as intervention, 664
Simple Guided Imagery, as intervention, 664
Simple Massage, as intervention, 664
Simple Relaxation Therapy, as intervention, 664
Skeletal Function, as outcome, 636
  with Mobility: Physical, Impaired, 283
Skin Care: Donor Site, as intervention, 664
Skin Care: Graft Site, as intervention, 664
Skin Care: Topical Treatments, as intervention, 664
  for Tissue Integrity, Impaired, 459
Skin Integrity, Impaired, 401-404
Skin Integrity, Risk for Impaired, 596-598
Skin Surveillance, as intervention, 664
  for Autonomic Dysreflexia, 66
  for Bowel Incontinence, 73
  for Latex Allergy Response, 272
  for Latex Allergy Response, Risk for, 567
  for Skin Integrity, Impaired, 402
  for Skin Integrity, Risk for Impaired, 597
  for Tissue Integrity, Impaired, 459
  for Tissue Perfusion: Peripheral, Ineffective, 477
  for Trauma, Risk for, 609
  for Urinary Incontinence: Total, 496
Sleep, as outcome, 636
  with Infant Behavior, Disorganized, 248
  with Infant Behavior: Organized, Readiness for Enhanced, 251
  with Sleep, Readiness for Enhanced, 409
  with Sleep Deprivation, 406
  with Sleep Pattern, Disturbed, 407

Sleep, Readiness for Enhanced, 408-409
Sleep Deprivation, 405-406
Sleep Enhancement, as intervention, 664
  for Infant Behavior, Disorganized, 248
  for Infant Behavior: Organized, Readiness for Enhanced, 251
  for Sleep, Readiness for Enhanced, 408, 409
  for Sleep Deprivation, 405, 406
  for Sleep Pattern, Disturbed, 407
Sleep Pattern, Disturbed, 407
Smoking Cessation Assistance, as intervention, 664
  for Health-Seeking Behavior (Specify), 236
Social Interaction, Impaired, 410-414
Social Interaction Skills, as outcome, 636
  with Coping, Defensive, 123
  with Development, Risk for Delayed, 536
  with Social Interaction, Impaired, 413
  with Social Isolation, 418
Social Involvement, as outcome, 636
  with Diversional Activity Deficit, 148
  with Loneliness, Risk for, 569
  with Social Interaction, Impaired, 414
  with Social Isolation, 419
Social Isolation, 415-419
Social Support, as outcome, 636
  with Health Maintenance, Ineffective, 226
  with Parenting, Impaired, 327
  with Social Isolation, 419
Socialization Enhancement, as intervention, 664
  for Communication, Readiness for Enhanced, 100
  for Diversional Activity Deficit, 148
  for Family Processes, Readiness for Enhanced, 179
  for Loneliness, Risk for, 568, 569
  for Relocation Stress Syndrome, 361
  for Social Interaction, Impaired, 411, 412, 414
  for Social Isolation, 416, 418, 419
Sorrow: Chronic, 420-422
Specimen Management, as intervention, 664
Spiritual Distress, 423-424
Spiritual Distress, Risk for, 599-600
Spiritual Growth Facilitation, as intervention, 664
  for Energy Field, Disturbed, 150
  for Hopelessness, 240
  for Religiosity, Impaired, 356
  for Religiosity, Readiness for Enhanced, 357
  for Spiritual Distress, 424
  for Spiritual Distress, Risk for, 599, 600
  for Spiritual Well-Being, Readiness for Enhanced, 425, 426
Spiritual Health, as outcome, 636
  with Death Anxiety, 138
  with Energy Field, Disturbed, 150
  with Religiosity, Impaired, 356
  with Religiosity, Impaired, Risk for, 589
  with Religiosity, Readiness for Enhanced, 357
  with Spiritual Distress, 424
  with Spiritual Distress, Risk for, 599
  with Spiritual Well-Being, Readiness for Enhanced, 426
Spiritual Support, as intervention, 664
  for Death Anxiety, 137, 138
  for Failure to Thrive, Adult, 155
  for Loneliness, Risk for, 568
  for Religiosity, Impaired, 356
  for Religiosity, Impaired, Risk for, 589
  for Religiosity, Readiness for Enhanced, 357
  for Relocation Stress Syndrome, 361
  for Sorrow: Chronic, 421
  for Spiritual Distress, 423, 424
  for Spiritual Distress, Risk for, 599, 600
  for Spiritual Well-Being, Readiness for Enhanced, 425, 426
  for Suicide, Risk for, 607

Spiritual Well-Being, Readiness for Enhanced, 425-426
Splinting, as intervention, 664
Sports Injury Prevention: Youth, as intervention, 664
Staff Development, as intervention, 664
Staff Supervision, as intervention, 664
Standardized nursing language(s) (SNL), 3-10
   linkages between, 3
   purposes of, 3
   references on, 10-11
   taxonomic structures of, sources for, 15
Stress Level, as outcome, 636
   with Coping, Readiness for Enhanced, 134
   with Relocation Stress Syndrome, 363
Student Health Status, as outcome, 636
   with Health Maintenance, Ineffective, 226
Subarachnoid Hemorrhage Precautions, as
   intervention, 665
Substance Addiction Consequences, as outcome, 637
   with Family Processes, Dysfunctional: Alcoholism,
   171
Substance Use Prevention, as intervention, 665
   for Coping, Ineffective, 130
   for Family Processes, Dysfunctional: Alcoholism, 171
   for Health-Seeking Behavior (Specify), 234, 235
   for Knowledge, Deficient (Specify), 267
Substance Use Treatment, as intervention, 665
   for Family Processes, Dysfunctional: Alcoholism,
   168, 169, 170, 171
Substance Use Treatment: Alcohol Withdrawal, as
   intervention, 665
Substance Use Treatment: Drug Withdrawal, as
   intervention, 665
Substance Use Treatment: Overdose, as intervention,
   665
Sudden Infant Death Syndrome, Risk for, 601
Suffering Severity, as outcome, 637
   with Spiritual Distress, Risk for, 600
Suffocation, Risk for, 602-604
Suicide, Risk for, 605-607
Suicide Prevention, as intervention
   for Post-Trauma Syndrome, 334, 665
   for Suicide, Risk for, 606, 607
   for Violence: Self-Directed, Risk for, 617
Suicide Self-Restraint, as outcome, 637
   with Suicide, Risk for, 606
   with Violence: Self-Directed, Risk for, 617
Supply Management, as intervention, 665
Support Group, as intervention, 665
   for Health Maintenance, Ineffective, 226
   for Parenting, Impaired, 327
Support System Enhancement, as intervention, 665
   for Coping, Readiness for Enhanced, 132, 133
   for Health Maintenance, Ineffective, 221, 226
   for Parenting, Impaired, 327
   for Post-Trauma Syndrome, 332, 333
   for Social Isolation, 416, 419
Surgical Assistance, as intervention, 665
Surgical Precautions, as intervention, 665
Surgical Preparation, as intervention, 665
Surgical Recovery, Delayed, 427-432
Surveillance, as intervention, 665
   for Intracranial Adaptive Capacity, Decreased, 255
Surveillance: Community, as intervention, 665
   for Community Coping, Ineffective, 104
   for Community Coping, Readiness for Enhanced, 107
   for Infection, Risk for, 557
Surveillance: Late Pregnancy, as intervention, 665
Surveillance: Remote Electronic, as intervention, 666
Surveillance: Safety, as intervention, 666
   for Environmental Interpretation Syndrome,
    Impaired, 152
   for Injury, Risk for, 562, 564, 565

Surveillance: Safety, as intervention (*Continued*)
   for Parenting, Impaired, 327
   for Poisoning, Risk for, 583
   for Wandering, 510
Sustenance Support, as intervention, 666
Suturing, as intervention, 666
Swallowing, Impaired, 433-434
Swallowing Status, as outcome, 637
   with Aspiration, Risk for, 515
   with Infant Feeding Pattern, Ineffective, 253
   with Self-Care Deficit: Feeding, 371
   with Swallowing, Impaired, 433
Swallowing Status: Esophageal Phase, as outcome, 637
   with Swallowing, Impaired, 433
Swallowing Status: Oral Phase, as outcome, 637
   with Swallowing, Impaired, 433
Swallowing Status: Pharyngeal Phase, as outcome, 637
   with Swallowing, Impaired, 434
Swallowing Therapy, as intervention, 666
   for Aspiration, Risk for, 514, 515
   for Self-Care Deficit: Feeding, 371
   for Swallowing, Impaired, 433, 434
Symptom Control, as outcome, 637
   with Constipation, 118
   with Denial, Ineffective, 142
   with Therapeutic Regimen Management, Effective,
    439
   with Therapeutic Regimen Management,
    Ineffective, 447
Symptom Severity, as outcome, 637
   with Autonomic Dysreflexia, Risk for, 516
   with Diarrhea, 146
   with Sleep Deprivation, 406
Symptom Severity: Perimenopause, as outcome, 637
Symptom Severity: Premenstrual Syndrome (PMS), as
   outcome, 637
Systematized Nomenclature of Medicine (SNOMED),
   10, 24
Systemic Toxin Clearance: Dialysis, as outcome, 637
   with Therapeutic Regimen Management,
    Ineffective, 448

T

Taxonomy of Nursing Practice, 4, 10, 15
Teaching: Disease Process, as intervention, 666
   for Coping, Readiness for Enhanced, 132
   for Denial, Ineffective, 142
   for Family Therapeutic Regimen Management,
    Ineffective, 182
   for Health Maintenance, Ineffective, 227
   for Knowledge, Deficient (Specify), 257, 258, 259,
    268
   for Noncompliance, 293
   for Therapeutic Regimen Management, Ineffective,
    441, 443, 447, 449
Teaching: Foot Care, as intervention, 666
Teaching: Group, as intervention, 666
Teaching: Individual, as intervention, 666
   for Caregiver Role Strain, 95
   for Constipation, Perceived, 119
   for Health Maintenance, Ineffective, 222
   for Health-Seeking Behavior (Specify), 230
   for Knowledge, Deficient (Specify), 260, 261, 262, 264
   for Noncompliance, 293
   for Nutrition, Readiness for Enhanced, 301
   for Self-Care Deficit: Toileting, 372
   for Therapeutic Regimen Management, Ineffective,
    445
   for Therapeutic Regimen Management, Readiness
    for Enhanced, 451

Teaching: Infant Nutrition, as intervention, 666
  for Development, Risk for Delayed, 527
  for Growth, Risk for Disproportionate, 550
  for Knowledge, Deficient (Specify), 259
  for Parenting, Readiness for Enhanced, 328
Teaching: Infant Safety, as intervention, 666
  for Development, Risk for Delayed, 526
  for Falls, Risk for, 541
  for Knowledge, Deficient (Specify), 258, 265
  for Parenting, Readiness for Enhanced, 328
  for Parenting, Risk for Impaired, 576
  for Sudden Infant Death Syndrome, Risk for, 601
Teaching: Infant Stimulation, as intervention, 666
  for Growth and Development, Delayed, 209
Teaching: Preoperative, as intervention, 666
  for Knowledge, Deficient (Specify), 268
Teaching: Prescribed Activity/Exercise, as intervention,
    666
  for Knowledge, Deficient (Specify), 257, 259, 266, 267
  for Lifestyle, Sedentary, 274
  for Therapeutic Regimen Management, Ineffective,
    441
Teaching: Prescribed Diet, as intervention, 666
  for Knowledge, Deficient (Specify), 258, 259
  for Nutrition, Readiness for Enhanced, 301
  for Therapeutic Regimen Management, Ineffective,
    441, 443
Teaching: Prescribed Medication, as intervention, 666
  for Knowledge, Deficient (Specify), 258, 264
  for Therapeutic Regimen Management, Ineffective,
    441, 443, 445, 446, 447
Teaching: Procedure/Treatment, as intervention, 667
  for Family Therapeutic Regimen Management,
    Ineffective, 182
  for Health Maintenance, Ineffective, 223
  for Knowledge, Deficient (Specify), 262, 268
  for Therapeutic Regimen Management, Effective,
    437
  for Therapeutic Regimen Management, Ineffective,
    444
Teaching: Psychomotor Skill, as intervention, 667
  for Knowledge, Deficient (Specify), 268
  for Therapeutic Regimen Management, Ineffective,
    447
Teaching: Safe Sex, as intervention, 667
  for Health-Seeking Behavior (Specify), 235
  for Infection, Risk for, 559
  for Knowledge, Deficient (Specify), 258, 263, 267
  for Sexual Dysfunction, 396
  for Sexuality Patterns, Ineffective, 399
Teaching: Sexuality, as intervention, 667
  for Infection, Risk for, 559
  for Knowledge, Deficient (Specify), 267
  for Sexuality Patterns, Ineffective, 399
Teaching: Toddler Nutrition, as intervention, 667
  for Growth, Risk for Disproportionate, 551
  for Knowledge, Deficient (Specify), 259
Teaching: Toddler Safety, as intervention, 667
  for Falls, Risk for, 541
  for Knowledge, Deficient (Specify), 258, 265
  for Parenting, Readiness for Enhanced, 328
  for Parenting, Risk for Impaired, 576
Teaching: Toilet Training, as intervention, 667
Technology Management, as intervention, 667
Telephone Consultation, as intervention, 667
Telephone Follow-up, as intervention, 667
Temperature Regulation, as intervention, 667
  for Body Temperature, Risk for Imbalanced, 518
  for Hyperthermia, 243, 244
  for Hypothermia, 245
  for Infant Behavior, Disorganized, 248
  for Thermoregulation, Ineffective, 453

Temperature Regulation: Intraoperative, as
    intervention, 667
  for Body Temperature, Risk for Imbalanced, 518
  for Hypothermia, 245
  for Thermoregulation, Ineffective, 453
Temporary Placement Management, as intervention,
    667
The Journal of Nursing Language and Classification, 4
Therapeutic Play, as intervention, 667
  for Diversional Activity Deficit, 148
  for Social Interaction, Impaired, 412
  for Social Isolation, 418
Therapeutic Regimen Management, Effective, 435-439
Therapeutic Regimen Management, Ineffective,
    440-448
Therapeutic Regimen Management, Readiness for
    Enhanced, 450-452
Therapeutic Touch, as intervention, 667
  for Energy Field, Disturbed, 149, 150
Therapy Group, as intervention, 668
Thermoregulation, as outcome, 637
  with Body Temperature, Risk for Imbalanced, 518
  with Hyperthermia, 243
  with Hypothermia, 245
  with Thermoregulation, Ineffective, 453
Thermoregulation, Ineffective, 453
Thermoregulation: Newborn, as outcome
  with Body Temperature, Risk for Imbalanced, 518
  with Hyperthermia, 243
  with Hypothermia, 245
  with Infant Behavior, Disorganized, 248
  with Thermoregulation, Ineffective, 453
Thought Processes, Disturbed, 454-458
Tissue Integrity, Impaired, 459-461
Tissue Integrity: Skin and Mucous Membranes, as
    outcome, 637
  with Bowel Incontinence, 73
  with Latex Allergy Response, 272
  with Latex Allergy Response, Risk for, 567
  with Oral Mucous Membrane, Impaired, 302
  with Skin Integrity, Impaired, 402
  with Skin Integrity, Risk for Impaired, 597
  with Tissue Integrity, Impaired, 460
  with Tissue Perfusion: Peripheral, Ineffective, 477
  with Trauma, Risk for, 609
  with Urinary Incontinence: Reflex, 493
  with Urinary Incontinence: Total, 496
Tissue Perfusion: Abdominal Organs, as outcome, 637
  with Cardiac Output, Decreased, 87
  with Tissue Perfusion: Gastrointestinal, Ineffective,
    474
  with Tissue Perfusion: Renal, Ineffective, 483
Tissue Perfusion: Cardiac, as outcome, 637
  with Cardiac Output, Decreased, 88
  with Tissue Perfusion: Cardiopulmonary,
    Ineffective, 464
Tissue Perfusion: Cardiopulmonary, Ineffective, 462-
    466
Tissue Perfusion: Cerebral, as outcome, 637
  with Cardiac Output, Decreased, 88
  with Intracranial Adaptive Capacity, Decreased, 256
  with Tissue Perfusion: Cerebral, Ineffective, 470
Tissue Perfusion: Cerebral, Ineffective, 467-470
Tissue Perfusion: Gastrointestinal, Ineffective,
    471-474
Tissue Perfusion: Peripheral, as outcome, 637
  with Cardiac Output, Decreased, 89
  with Perioperative Positioning Injury, Risk for, 580
  with Peripheral Neurovascular Dysfunction, Risk
    for, 582
  with Tissue Perfusion: Peripheral, Ineffective, 478
Tissue Perfusion: Peripheral, Ineffective, 475-478

Tissue Perfusion: Pulmonary, as outcome, 638
  with Cardiac Output, Decreased, 89
  with Gas Exchange, Impaired, 201
  with Tissue Perfusion: Cardiopulmonary,
    Ineffective, 465
Tissue Perfusion: Renal, Ineffective, 479-483
Total Parenteral Nutrition (TPN), as intervention, 668
Touch, as intervention, 668
Traction/Immobilization Care, as intervention, 668
Transcutaneous Electrical Nerve Stimulation (TENS),
  as intervention, 668
Transfer Ability, Impaired, 484-486
Transfer Performance, as outcome, 638
  with Mobility: Physical, Impaired, 283
  with Mobility: Wheelchair, Impaired, 285
  with Transfer Ability, Impaired, 486
Transport, as intervention, 668
Trauma, Risk for, 608-609
Trauma Therapy: Child, as intervention, 668
  for Post-Trauma Syndrome, 335
  for Rape-Trauma Syndrome, 345, 346
  for Relocation Stress Syndrome, 359
Treatment Behavior: Illness or Injury, as outcome, 638
  with Health Maintenance, Ineffective, 227
  with Noncompliance, 293
  with Therapeutic Regimen Management, Effective,
    439
  with Therapeutic Regimen Management,
    Ineffective, 449
  with Therapeutic Regimen Management, Readiness
    for Enhanced, 452
Triage: Disaster, as intervention, 668
Triage: Emergency Center, as intervention, 668
Triage: Telephone, as intervention, 668
Truth Telling, as intervention, 668
Tube Care, as intervention, 668
Tube Care: Chest, as intervention, 668
Tube Care: Gastrointestinal, as intervention, 668
Tube Care: Umbilical Line, as intervention, 668
Tube Care: Urinary, as intervention, 668
Tube Care: Ventriculostomy/Lumbar Drain, as
  intervention, 668

U

Ultrasonography: Limited Obstetric, as intervention, 668
  for Protection, Ineffective, 342
Unified Medical Language System (UMLS), 10
Unilateral Neglect, 487-488
Unilateral Neglect Management, as intervention, 669
  for Unilateral Neglect, 487, 488
University of Iowa, College of Nursing, 7, 9
Urinary Bladder Training, as intervention, 669
  for Urinary Elimination, Impaired, 489
  for Urinary Incontinence: Reflex, 493, 494
  for Urinary Incontinence: Urge, Risk for, 610
Urinary Catheterization, as intervention, 669
  for Urinary Retention, 498
Urinary Catheterization: Intermittent, as intervention,
  669
  for Urinary Incontinence: Reflex, 493, 494
Urinary Continence, as outcome, 638
  with Urinary Elimination, Impaired, 489
  with Urinary Incontinence: Functional, 492
  with Urinary Incontinence: Reflex, 494
  with Urinary Incontinence: Stress, 495
  with Urinary Incontinence: Total, 496
  with Urinary Incontinence: Urge, Risk for, 610
  with Urinary Retention, 498
Urinary Elimination, as outcome, 638
  with Urinary Elimination, Impaired, 490
  with Urinary Elimination, Readiness for Enhanced,
    491

Urinary Elimination, as outcome (Continued)
  with Urinary Incontinence: Functional, 492
  with Urinary Incontinence: Reflex, 494
  with Urinary Incontinence: Stress, 495
  with Urinary Incontinence: Total, 496
  with Urinary Incontinence: Urge, Risk for, 610
  with Urinary Retention, 498
Urinary Elimination, Impaired, 489-490
Urinary Elimination, Readiness for Enhanced, 491
Urinary Elimination Management, as intervention, 669
  for Fluid Balance, Readiness for Enhanced, 189
  for Fluid Volume, Excess, 196
  for Urinary Elimination, Impaired, 489, 490
  for Urinary Elimination, Readiness for Enhanced,
    491
  for Urinary Incontinence: Functional, 492
  for Urinary Incontinence: Reflex, 494
  for Urinary Incontinence: Stress, 495
  for Urinary Incontinence: Total, 496
  for Urinary Incontinence: Urge, 497
  for Urinary Incontinence: Urge, Risk for, 610
  for Urinary Retention, 498
Urinary Habit Training, as intervention, 669
  for Urinary Incontinence: Functional, 492
  for Urinary Incontinence: Urge, 497
  for Urinary Incontinence: Urge, Risk for, 610
Urinary Incontinence: Functional, 492
Urinary Incontinence: Reflex, 493-494
Urinary Incontinence: Stress, 495
Urinary Incontinence: Total, 496
Urinary Incontinence: Urge, 497
Urinary Incontinence: Urge, Risk for, 610
Urinary Incontinence Care, as intervention, 669
  for Urinary Incontinence: Reflex, 493
  for Urinary Incontinence: Stress, 495
  for Urinary Incontinence: Total, 496
  for Urinary Incontinence: Urge, 497
Urinary Incontinence Care: Enuresis, as intervention,
  669
Urinary Retention, 498
Urinary Retention Care, as intervention, 669
for Urinary Retention, 498

V

Values Clarification, as intervention, 669
  for Adjustment, Impaired, 59
  for Constipation, Perceived, 119
  for Health-Seeking Behavior (Specify), 228, 230,
    232
  for Hopelessness, 241
  for Powerlessness, 338
  for Religiosity, Impaired, 356
  for Relocation Stress Syndrome, 362
  for Self-Esteem: Chronic Low, 375
  for Spiritual Well-Being, Readiness for Enhanced,
    426
Vehicle Safety Promotion, as intervention, 669
Venous Access Device (VAD) Maintenance, as
  intervention, 669
Ventilation, Impaired Spontaneous, 499-502
Ventilation Assistance, as intervention, 669
  for Airway Clearance, Ineffective, 61
  for Breathing Pattern, Ineffective, 83
  for Gas Exchange, Impaired, 199, 200
  for Ventilation, Impaired Spontaneous, 500, 501
  for Ventilatory Weaning Response, Dysfunctional,
    504, 505
Ventilatory Weaning Response, Dysfunctional, 503-507
Violence: Other-Directed, Risk for, 611-614
Violence: Self-Directed, Risk for, 615-617
Vision Compensation Behavior, as outcome, 638
  with Sensory Perception: Visual, Disturbed, 394

Visitation Facilitation, as intervention, 669
   for Loneliness, Risk for, 568
Vital Signs, as outcome, 638
   with Autonomic Dysreflexia, 66
   with Autonomic Dysreflexia, Risk for, 517
   with Breathing Pattern, Ineffective, 83
   with Cardiac Output, Decreased, 90
   with Gas Exchange, Impaired, 202
   with Hyperthermia, 244
   with Hypothermia, 245
   with Tissue Perfusion: Cardiopulmonary,
      Ineffective, 466
   with Ventilation, Impaired Spontaneous, 502
   for Ventilatory Weaning Response, Dysfunctional,
      506
Vital Signs Monitoring, as intervention, 669
   for Autonomic Dysreflexia, 65
   for Autonomic Dysreflexia, Risk for, 516, 517
   for Body Temperature, Risk for Imbalanced, 518
   for Breathing Pattern, Ineffective, 83
   for Cardiac Output, Decreased, 90
   for Gas Exchange, Impaired, 202
   for Hyperthermia, 244
   for Hypothermia, 245
   for Surgical Recovery, Delayed, 431
   for Tissue Perfusion: Cardiopulmonary, Ineffective,
      466
   for Ventilation, Impaired Spontaneous, 502
   for Ventilatory Weaning Response, Dysfunctional,
      506
Vomiting Management, as intervention, 669
   for Aspiration, Risk for, 514
   for Nausea, 287, 288
   for Surgical Recovery, Delayed, 430

W

Walking, Impaired, 507-509
Wandering, 510
Weight: Body Mass, as outcome, 638
   with Nutrition: Imbalanced, Less than Body
      Requirements, 298

Weight Control, as outcome, 638
   with Nutrition: Imbalanced, More than Body
      Requirements, 300
   with Nutrition: Imbalanced, Risk for More than
      Body Requirements, 571
Weight Gain Assistance, as intervention, 669
   for Nutrition: Imbalanced, Less than Body
      Requirements, 295, 298
Weight Management, as intervention, 669
   for Growth, Risk for Disproportionate, 552, 553,
      554
   for Nutrition: Imbalanced, Risk for More than Body
      Requirements, 571
Weight Reduction Assistance, as intervention, 670
   for Nutrition: Imbalanced, More than Body
      Requirements, 299, 300
Will to Live, as outcome, 638
   with Failure to Thrive, Adult, 155
   with Hopelessness, 242
   with Suicide, Risk for, 607
Wound Care, as intervention, 670
   for Infection, Risk for, 560, 561
   for Self-Mutilation, 380
   for Skin Integrity, Impaired, 403, 404
   for Skin Integrity, Risk for Impaired, 598
   for Surgical Recovery, Delayed, 432
   for Tissue Integrity, Impaired, 460, 461
Wound Care: Closed Drainage, as intervention, 670
Wound Healing: Primary Intention, as outcome, 638
   with Infection, Risk for, 560
   with Skin Integrity, Impaired, 403
   with Skin Integrity, Risk for Impaired, 598
   with Surgical Recovery, Delayed, 432
   with Tissue Integrity, Impaired, 461
Wound Healing: Secondary Intention, as outcome, 638
   with Infection, Risk for, 561
   with Skin Integrity, Impaired, 404
   with Tissue Integrity, Impaired, 461
Wound Irrigation, as intervention, 670